THE
TRADITIONAL
HEALER'S
HANDBOOK

Also by Hakim G.M. Chishti

The Book of Sufi Healing
Encyclopedia of Natural Medicine
Handbook of Common Herbal Remedies

THE TRADITIONAL HEALER'S HANDBOOK

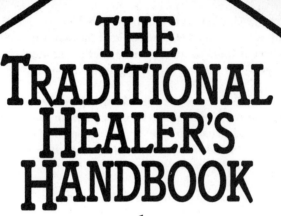

*A
Classic Guide to
the Medicine of
Avicenna*

Hakim G. M. Chishti, N.D.

Healing Arts Press
Rochester, Vermont

Healing Arts Press
One Park Street
Rochester, Vermont 05767
www.InnerTraditions.com

*Note to the reader: This book is intended as an informational guide. The
remedies, approaches, and techniques described herein are meant to supplement, and not to be a substitute for, professional medical care or treatment.
They should not be used to treat a serious ailment without prior consultation
with a qualified healthcare professional.*

Library of Congress Cataloging-in-Publication Data
Chishti, G. M. (Ghulam Moinuddin), 1943–
    The traditional healer's handbook : a classic guide to the
medicine of Avicenna / G. M. Chishti.
        p. cm.
    Rev. ed. of: The traditional healer, c1988.
    Includes bibliographical references and index.
    ISBN 978-0-89281-438-1
    1. Avicenna, 980–1037. 2. Medicine, Arabic. [1. History of
Medicine, Medieval. 2. Medicine, Arabic. 3. Medicine, Herbal.
4. Plants, Medicinal.] I. Chishti,G. M. (Ghulam Moinuddin),
1943– Traditional healer. II. Title.
    [DNLM: WZ 80.5.A8 C54t]
R143.L49 1991
610—dc20   91–20888
                                                 CIP

Printed and bound in the United States

10   9   8   7

Healing Arts Press is a division of Inner Traditions International

To my wife, Iman, *light upon light*

Acknowledgments

There were so many people who assisted me over the course of the past ten years of preparation of this book.

The following persons, listed simply in the order that I can recall them, each made vital contributions to my work: Syed Safdar Ali Shah Chishti, Abu Anees Muhammad Barkat Ali, Pir Syed Daud Iqbali, Hakim Muhammad Abdullah Uzbecki, Hajji Nimayatullah Shahrani, Shaikh Saleh Parwanta, Prof. Dr. Rawan Farhadi, Nasratullah Laheeb, Hassan Kamiab, Hon. Theodore Eliot, Dr. Jon Summers, Parvin, Younus, Zarghuna, Lahli, Muhammad Jan, The American Society at Kabul, Martha Sowerwine, Harmony Noble, Cindy Lynn Cohen, Enayat Shahrani, Dr. Robert Bauman, Dr. Robert Martin, Fred Hills, Peggy Tsukahira, Andrew Weil, M.D., Dr. Ludwig Adamec, Prof. Dr. Annmarie Schimmel, Stephen Moore, M.D., Kathleen Grandison, M.D., Mustafa Omar, M.D., Arjumand Radhwana, M.D., Louis and Nancy Dupree, Dr. Richard M. Eaton, Hakim Mohammad Said, Hakim Abdul Wahid, Dr. Muhammad Qasim, Leslie Colket, Kendra Crossen, Zufar Hussain Khan, Al Zuckerman, Yunous Maharaj, Ahmed Ali Chisti, Khwaja Hamid Ahmad, Abul Kazam Azad Oriental Research Institute, Larry and Nasrin Beck, Ann Thomson, Prof. Bo Utas, Dr. Sheldon Deal, John Heuvelman, Dr. Humbert Santillo, Samuel and Lucy Massa, Dr. Dionysious Skaliotis, Fazl Ahmad Sherfy, Lance Whitney, Angela Werneke, and many others I may not have named but whose help is nonetheless deeply felt and appreciated.

My special thanks are due to my publisher, Mr. Ehud C. Sperling, President of Healing Arts Press, who (with the members of his staff) exhibited a surpassing patience in allowing me the extended time to write and revise the manuscript, and who has dedicated himself to the artistic production of my books.

Finally, my special love and gratitude to the members of my family, who provided the environment of support and encouragement for me to write.

May Allah the Almighty Reward you with His choicest blessings, as many of such things as there are! Amin!

Contents

Notice

The information offered in this book is intended for practical application by physicians and members of other recognized healing professions. It may also have value to those engaged in research and education in the fields of natural medicine, herbology, and other related topics.

Persons who believe they are suffering from serious illness should consult a physician of their choice for diagnosis and treatment. In discussing the use of certain herbs and other procedures, I am not diagnosing or prescribing for any specific ailment, but only presenting the information for educational and scientific interest, without the author's or publisher's endorsement.

I cannot stress enough the necessity of using any information in this book only in cooperation with competent medical advice and guidance.

Illness itself is one of those forms of experience
by which man arrives at the knowledge of God.
As He says, "Sicknesses themselves are My servants,
and are attached to My chosen friends."

—*al-Ghazzali*

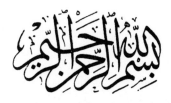

Praise be to Allah, Who is Kind and Merciful, and praise be to His Prophet Muhammad (peace and blessing be upon him) and his sinless followers.

I have written this book due to the interest an ever-growing number of people are showing in various forms of natural healing and because I wish to share the results of my study in one of the great healing traditions of history.

The Traditional Healer is based upon the system of botanical medicine and dietetics developed by the Persian physician Hakim Ibn Sina, known in the West as Avicenna. His *Canon of Medicine* is the most famous book in medical history and has maintained its authority for more than a thousand years of teaching and practice. While his conception of the physical, emotional, and spiritual aspects of health is vast in scope, he once condensed his system into a single statement: "Food is the best medicine."

The Traditional Healer is my own humble effort to contribute to a sensible development of the "new" medicine that is rapidly emerging in the West, a medicine that is shifting from treatment of disease to maintenance of health. It is my sincere hope that as Avicenna's classic texts are now available to a wide audience in the West for the first time, a second millennium of students and practitioners will discover an immense reward in the special and extraordinary genius of Hakim Avicenna, the Prince of Physicians.

Many people may be unaware that herbal medicine served as the primary mode of medical practice in the United States until almost 1935. A review of the then-current physician's drug handbooks shows that physicians routinely used ginger, garlic, valerian, lobelia, and hundreds of other herbs as the primary therapeutic agents. Of course, this practice did change as chemical medicine burst on the scene with penicillin. Yet, prior to 1935—for perhaps two thousand years prior to that date—*all* physicians accepted and adhered to the humoral basis of both human and herbal constitution.

The theory of humors—semivaporous substances that maintain the proper temperament of the organs—are the heart of the medicine of Hippocrates, Galen, and Avicenna, of Chinese and Ayurvedic medicine, and of virtually all other traditional systems. Yet this tremendous consensus among prominent medical authorities for two millennia is ignored. Instead, yielding to the underpinnings of orthodox medicine, even most herbalists today are interested in determining what the "active principles" of drugs are, which is to say, what herb will work as an antibacterial instead of penicillin.

In this book are presented the principles and essential features of practice of the system of healing known as Tibb. This Arabic word literally means "medicine and healing of the physical, mental, and spiritual realms." In practice throughout the world, it is most often called Unani Tibb. *Unan* means "of the Greeks"—in recognition of its origin with Hippocrates.

Ever since 1976, when the World Health Organization formally adopted its policy of promoting traditional remedies, Unani medicine has enjoyed a worldwide upsurge of interest. Unani is most prominent in India and the subcontinent, where 28,382 Unani practitioners are registered, and many more practice along hereditary lines. In India there are 100 fully staffed Unani hospitals, 867 Unani dispensaries, 18 colleges (including 2 offering postgraduate training), a Central Research Institute, 7 Regional Research Institutes, 11 Clinical Research Units, and 17 other related Institutes. At present 19 diseases (arthritis, asthma, liver disorders, etc.) and 46 Unani formulae are being clinically evaluated at these research facilities.

Perhaps most importantly, a program of drug standardization for single and compound Unani herbs of proven efficacy has resulted in published standards for 50 single and 208 compound Unani herbal drugs.

Unani Tibb medicine offers a unified basis of practice and research in all areas of the world. With its 1,000-year-old tradition of literature, Unani traditional healing is vibrant and vigorous today and is being practiced, taught, and researched in twenty-five countries including Afghanistan, Bangladesh, Canada, China, Denmark, Ethiopia, Republic of Germany, Finland, Japan, Netherlands, Norway, Pakistan, Poland, Korea, Saudi Arabia, Sri Lanka, Sweden, Switzerland, Thailand, Turkey, the United Kingdom, and the United States.

The first World Conference on Unani Medicine, jointly sponsored by the World Health Organization, the Government of India's Ministry of Health, and the Central Council for Research in Unani Medicine, was held in New Delhi in February 1987. It attracted 228 noted Unani physicians, scholars, and researchers from the world over.

In 1980 an Institute of Unani Medicine (see Appendix IV for address) was founded to promote its teaching and practice in the United States.

My experience with this tradition of healing began as an innocent encounter in the smoky mists of the old bazaar, deep in the heart of Kabul, Afghanistan. In 1975 I had received a United States government Fulbright Grant to conduct research for an extended period in Afghanistan, a small country generally unknown in the West (even though current events have since thrust it into the forefront of the world's gaze). So in July 1975 my wife and I departed in a high pitch of excitement for an adventurous stay in Afghanistan.

Our plane touched down at the small airport in the autumn dawn, and I felt that overwhelming suddenness of change when arriving in the East, as though we were descending upon an ancient age, something quite like descriptions of life in the Bible. After being whisked through customs formalities and driving through the streets as the slivers of dawn probed from around adobe corners, I sat in silence trying to absorb the sheer force of the absoluteness of the change— men riding donkeys, wearing large baggy pants and turbans, the amber-hued streetlights, the stern and intent gaze of the people.

It took a few days to become acclimated to this entirely "other" way of life. There were so many things to learn and discover, every ten steps brought me to objects of strange shapes and unknown functions, cloths of new and vibrant colors, bazaars fragrant with intriguing odors. Each day we arose with the rest of the populace, before dawn at the call to prayer, and set forth in new directions, tasting, touching, all of our senses being revivified, like children learning life from the start.

And we quickly realized that despite the outwardly fierce demeanor of the Afghans, they turned out to be the friendliest, kindest and most hospitable people on earth.

There was another major adjustment, not simply a matter of intellect, and that was the food we were eating. It was always delicious, healthful, and filling, but since no artificial fertilizers, chemicals, or pesticides were used there, we had to become acclimated to a different microlife in the food we ate. The first signal for me was a rush of loose bowels, and my wife seemed to be developing a serious cough with the early fall temperatures dipping to freezing in the nearly seven-thousand-foot altitude.

We both knew that we would have to seek some kind of medical treatment, as I was without my own stocks of herbal remedies owing to the weight limitations on our flight over. We had to make a decision either to go to the U.S. Embassy's dispensary or find a local healer (a course viewed with unlimited skepticism by our American friends). But by this time, from my study of Persian, I was able to communicate with the local people, and decided to ask an Afghan friend to recommend someone local.

"There is a healer in the old bazaar," he told me, "who saved my life twice when I was a child. He's quite old now, in his nineties, I think, but even so, he's considered the best doctor in the country." My friend told me everyone called him Hakim Sherif, which means Exalted Healer, and gave us instructions how to get to his shop on the central square of Jodi Maiwand just off the entrance to the old bazaar.

We traced our way through the twisting, narrow alleyways, asked some persistent questions, finally located the weatherbeaten wooden door, and entered. Inside the darkened shop, I first saw perhaps twenty men, women, and children lined up on both sides of a slightly raised, pillowed platform upon which an elegant, aged man with a glowing fist-long white beard sat surrounded by several assistants. The walls of the wooden structure were lined floor to ceiling with bottles of odd shapes and of amber, green, and roseate hues. From the center of the room a woodstove cast a snug warmth over us all. Looking up, I noticed there were also a dozen birds in cages—pigeons, white doves, thrushes, nightingales. It was many months before I learned that these feathered creatures had nothing to do with the decor, but rather were used by the Hakim to sensitize his fingertips for pulse diagnosis.

We had both been in the room less than a minute and were transfixed by the scene, so much so that we failed to realize that all the people had stopped what they were doing to stare at these foreigners who must have accidentally stumbled into the Afghans' own medical clinic. I approached the healer, and we exchanged the customary extended greetings. His assistant then told me to sit down at his feet, which I did. I was wondering how I could describe my symptoms of loose bowels without seeming rude or ridiculous in front of all those people (Afghan customs of manners would forbid referring directly to bodily functions in public). To my surprise, Hakim Sherif asked me no questions at all about my ailment. Instead, he took my left hand and pressed the tips of his fingers to my wrist and felt the blood passing through the vessels for perhaps ten seconds. I assumed he had made a superficial examination and had concluded that my pulse was more or less normal. I again braced myself to answer the expected question about my ailment. But he asked nothing and instead reached to the shelf behind him for a small, round can with a mirrored cap and gave it to me. He told me to eat about a thumbnail portion dissolved in hot tea three times a day. Then he nodded and indicated I was to go. Next it was my wife's turn. By now all of the people had gathered about us, enclosing us in a cocoon of bright, astonished faces.

My wife sat down as I had done, and the healer once again asked no questions but felt her pulse at the wrist and on the tips of her fingers. The whole process took less than twenty seconds; this time, though, he called to one of his assistants, who produced a paper funnel of pills, which he gave to her. Then the Hakim and everyone else sat blankly looking at us, waiting for us to leave. I asked how much the treatment would cost, but he just shook his head slightly, indicating that I need not pay. Knowing the small income of the people of Afghanistan, I reached into my pocket and was prepared to argue the point, until the assistant (who I later learned was his son) told me it would be the highest form of insult to the elder Hakim to press the matter.

And so we left, as I had no idea what else we could say to or ask of the man— and apparently nothing else was required for healing our ailments. Both my wife and I, honestly, were leery of eating the substances we had been given until we had even a vague notion of what they were. So we returned home and called my friend over for tea to relate our experience.

When he arrived, he seemed pleased but quite surprised that we had actually gone to the Hakim. "What did he give you?" our friend asked. I showed him the small can and opened it, asking him what it was. "Oh, we all use this," he answered. "It's called *badyan*, some kind of herbs ground up and mixed with ginger and honey."

"Fine, but what's it for?" I asked.

"For loose bowels," he said. "It balances your digestive system, which is what causes the problem with your bowels."

I said nothing further but immediately held out a palmful of the small dark pills the Hakim had given my wife. Our friend likewise knew this was a remedy for cough, but did not know its specific name or what it was composed of— only that it worked.

My initial excitement at having made contact with a healer was increased over the next few days, first of all because the remedies had worked: my stomach settled and my wife's cough disappeared. But even more, because although I had considerable training in Western medicine, this ability of the Hakim seemed practically magical to me—that he could accurately pinpoint a diagnosis and prescribe an effective remedy without either of us giving him so much as a clue to our illness. This was an order of knowledge that seemed to be on an altogether new plane of medical insight.

Over the next few months I managed to become a student of Hakim Hajji Muhammad Sherif and began to discover the basis of this phenomenal system of healing. In addition, I began searching the archives and located many articles and books on the subject of this traditional medicine, called Tibb.

One of the problems of utilizing this system, I soon discovered, was that the Hakims evaluate all of the disease conditions, or what they would call imbalances, by pulse diagnosis. And while I was gaining some understanding of this science, I was by no means proficient enough to rely upon it. Moreover, I knew that if this system was to reach a larger public, I would somehow have to discover the underlying theories that would allow anyone to practice it without spending five or ten years learning pulse diagnosis.

For the whole year Hakim Sherif was adamant in insisting that no book existed to explain these imbalances. But finally, as I was nearing the end of my stay, he revealed that there was *one* book, called *Mizan-ul-tibb* (The Standard of Medicine), where I might find what I needed. But, he added ruefully, it was the rarest of books, and he hadn't even heard of anyone having a copy since the time when his own grandfather was alive.

Undeterred, I went to every bookstall in Kabul and put out a bounty on this book. More months passed, and as I made my regular rounds to check with the shopkeepers, the sad nods of their heads made my search take on a note of grimness and destitution.

One day in late June, I was doing my usual wandering and discovering in the

Shor Bazaar and turned down an alleyway that I had never before encountered. Along the right side was a series of shops housing makers of musical instruments, which were being carved out of the trunks of mulberry trees. I was interested in this process and sat down to chat briefly with one of the craftsmen. During our talk, I asked if he knew any Hakims in the area, and he jerked his head back over the direction of his right shoulder, saying, "Three shops down." I politely took my leave and proceeded to the shop of yet another Hakim.

What transpired during the next four hours is a very long and involved story, but in sum, it turned out that this Hakim did have the book I sought, and after five more days of haggling I had purchased a copy of *Mizan-ul-tibb* for a veritable small fortune.

Over the next year, working with experts in Persian linguistics and the leading professor of pharmacology at Kabul University, I translated *Mizan-ul-tibb* into English. At the same time, I translated a smaller volume called *Rahat-ul-atfal* (The Well-Being of Children). These two volumes, then, form the basis of *The Traditional Healer*.

It would be remiss of me to fail to acknowledge here the great contribution to Tibb made by Dr. O. Cameron Gruner, a British medical doctor who translated into English the first volume of Avicenna's *Canon*. Although Dr. Gruner passed away several years ago, his work was a very great inspiration to me and others, and I feel certain he would be pleased that Tibb is enjoying a resurgence due to his dedicated labor.

Now that I have had almost ten years of experience with this traditional medicine, both in theory and clinical practice, I believe its significance is more apparent to me, and more important to make available to the public, than when I first encountered it in Kabul. It is also of utmost significance, in my opinion, that the Unani Tibb system of traditional medicine include as part of its consideration of treatment the physical, emotional, and spiritual aspects of human life—thus making it a truly unified, holistic medicine.

In this book, all of the information related to the theoretical side of Tibb is presented. I discuss all aspects of the various natural, vital, and psychic functions; the main factors causing health and disease; considerations of life space and homesite selection; the methods of grading foods according to their metabolic values; climatic and atmospheric effects upon health; extensive recipes for constructing diet along humoral lines; urinalysis; pulse diagnosis; fevers; and many other topics, as well as intensive case histories from my own clinical practice of Unani Tibb medicine.

Also, working from clinical experience, I have refined the system of the humors into a process of evaluation, which is explained in simple terms so that anyone can utilize the information in this book without need of further reference materials.

In addition, I include in this volume some specific information on the rules for selecting herbs and define the considerations to keep in view when selecting particular herbs. Such information will, I hope, prove of great interest to practicing herbalists, because so far as I am aware, the basic principles of herbal compounding have never before been presented in the English language.

The remainder of the book consists of the Formulary, which presents recommendations for more than four hundred conditions, presented by body part affected.

I must point out that I am not claiming that Tibb is "better" than Western hospital medicine. I would suggest, however, that the Tibb approach is the element missing from medical practice in the West today, for it supplies all the knowledge of dietetics, prevention, and gentle, noninvasive responses to simple ailments, which allopathic physicians usually treat with agents that are much too powerful.

In transposing the Tibb system from its roots of practice in the Near East and India, I had to deal with two important considerations. First, I have made some amendments to the herbs utilized in Tibb when practiced by fully trained Hakims, or Tibb physicians. Hellbore and belladonna, for example, are used in Tibb formulas by practicing Hakims. Yet they are deleted from the formulas in this book because of the expertise required for the safe use of such potent herbs. This book informs the reader how to correct simple imbalances and also provides considerable information on preventive therapeutics and dietetics. In the Tibb traditional medicine, as with other medical modalities that treat pathology and morbid conditions, each patient is considered unique, and a trained, qualified Tibb physician must personally prescribe treatment for a disease after careful evaluation of that particular case. Still, there is a wide area of self-responsibility that can be assumed by each individual in order to perform all actions necessary to avoid falling ill.

Another matter relating to selection of herbs is that some herbs used in Tibb in India or Afghanistan are not available in the United States (they may be in Europe). As an example, emblemic myrobalen is used in several formulas in the original formulary of *Mizan-ul-tibb*. This herb has great tonic and restorative powers, but it is, for all practical purposes, unavailable in the West. Therefore, in consultation with other Hakims, I arrived at equivalent substitutions using readily available ingredients, according to the imbalance being treated. Nonetheless, out of almost two hundred herbal substances mentioned in *Mizan-ul-tibb*, perhaps 90 percent are available in the West, and some are even imported to India from the United States.

The use of effective drugs for treatment of pain presented another difficulty, because in the West all substances that are effective enough to treat severe pain are restricted to a very few practitioners of one system of medicine, namely, medical doctors. In the usual setting of Tibb practice, one would use opium or one or more forms of cannabis for pain. But these substances are also not permitted to herbal practitioners here (and, even if obtained, may be of uncertain purity, thus posing even greater risks to patients). I have worked out what I consider to be adequate substitutes in the formulas that follow. For many formulas used to palliate pain, I use combinations of saffron, valerian root, asafoetida, and other herbs with anesthetic properties, though they are admittedly milder in effect than morphine or similar chemical drugs.

The second consideration in converting the Tibb system for use in the West concerns the dietary life-styles of Western people. In the East almost no one eats to excess, and it is rare to see an obese person. Despite the propaganda of the media, people in all agriculturally based societies are usually very well nourished and healthy. In fact, their "simple" fare of whole grains, rice, yogurt, and vegetables and fruits in season is as healthy a diet as one could recommend.

In the West, by contrast, eating is caught up in the complex notions of consumerism and becomes a type of contest, a search for ever more stupefying and sumptuous dishes. There is no question that most persons who suffer from disease have exercised very poor dietary habits over long periods.

Therefore, I have devised a special detoxification program that allows a period of eliminating the buildup of toxins and superfluous matters. *The Traditional Healer* is a complete and self-contained volume, and one can discover herein, I believe, recommendations and formulas capable of producing remarkable results within a very reasonable time.

The medicine practiced in Western hospitals has come under attack, and each day the attitude of the public toward the physicians and their techniques seems to become more embittered. The reason for this sad degeneration of respect between patient and physician is because many physicians have lost sight of the basic processes the body uses to heal itself. And it is this knowledge that was most deeply understood by the Tibb physicians. They were trying not to "kill" germs or bombard a disease, but rather to harmonize, to assist, to encourage, and even to love each person, each patient, and guide him or her back to the condition of human happiness and wellness.

Thus *The Traditional Healer* is humbly offered with the hope that it may prove to be a unifying element for those who seek to synthesize all of the various natural health systems.

H.M.C.
Dar-ul-Iman
Oxford, New York
7 Rabi-ul-Awwal
1412 A.H.
September 16, 1991

I
The Practice of
Traditional Healing

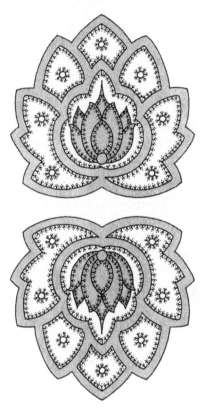

1
The Origins and Development of Unani Tibb

When viewed from the perspective of medical history, Unani Tibb refers to that system of medicine which developed in the late tenth and early eleventh century by the effort of the famous physician Hakim Ibn Sina, called Avicenna in the West.

In order to understand the origin of the theories as well as the present practice of this system, it is necessary to reflect on precisely how "medicine" originated and how it has evolved up to the present time.

Scholars are in general agreement that the origins of medicine are lost in the mists of time. Anthropologists have discovered references to codified medical practice as far back as 10,000 B.C. Treatment by herbs is one of the oldest forms of therapy, with reference to applying herbs found in the Chinese text *Pen tsao* (3000 B.C.). The Egyptian medical papyrus discovered by Georg Moritz Ebers dates from 1550 B.C. and reveals startlingly learned treatises on a wide variety of complex medical treatments.

It is probably fair to assume that ever since the first pain or discomfort was felt by humans, efforts have been made to alleviate human suffering. Religious scholars relate that Adam's first son was inspired with the medicinal powers of herbs and was a healer. The Sufis claim that Hazrat Solomon was the first to record the healing properties of plants, when a succession of hundreds of flowers and plants miraculously appeared before him while he prayed and told him of their healing properties.

Modern scholarship traces the origins of medicine as an art back to ancient Greece, where two distinct schools of medicine flourished. In the older school at Cnidus, emphasis was placed upon subjective symptoms and little attention was paid to the objective evaluation of signs. This school considered an illness affecting one organ to be particular to that organ, and treated it separately. But the diagnosis—based exclusively on symptomatology—was far from accurate and led to great confusion and dissatisfaction with medicine.

Partly as an answer to the disagreement with this school at Cnidus, a band of renegade physicians fled to the nearby island of Cos and established a rival school, which was to become famous as the home of Hippocrates, who is called the Father of Medicine. Hippocrates was the first to set forth the principles of

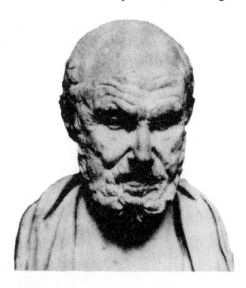

Hippocrates—The medical renegade who came to be called the Father of Medicine.

the humoral theory. He viewed the human body as a complete, integrated whole (as opposed to a collection of parts), and his system of treatments was of a general nature, rather than a specific treatment against one set of symptoms.

Furthermore, Hippocrates eliminated the elements of magic and superstition that had crept into medicine, and laid stress on the careful observation of the mental and physical condition of the patient, as well as on the effects of the surrounding environment. Hippocrates also first introduced the practice of taking case histories of patients, so that a clear record of progress could be followed. He said that the purpose of medicine was to assist nature's recuperative power to throw off disease. In other words, he relied on the body's own self-healing mechanisms rather than introducing external agents.

Perhaps the most important theory developed by Hippocrates was that of *physis*, meaning "the organism in its unity." Hippocrates postulated that life entails a reciprocal relationship between the organism and its environment. In this constant interaction, he saw the origins of disease. Hippocrates held that the organism grows at the expense of the environment, taking from it what is necessary to sustain life and rejecting what is unnecessary. From Hippocrates' viewpoint, disease was the occurrence of severe difficulty in this digestion, or *pepsis*, of the environment by the organism. His term for indigestion—*dyspepsia*—is still used today.

Hippocrates followed the doctrine of his predecessors that the essence of matter was to be found in the four primary elements, fire, water, air, and earth.

He also subscribed to the Pythagorean theory of the four humors. He described the interrelationship of these elements and humors (see diagram) as follows:

> The body of man has in itself blood, phlegm, yellow bile, and black bile; these make up the nature of his body, and through these he feels pain or enjoys health. Now he enjoys the most perfect health when these elements are duly proportioned to one another in respect to compounding, power, and bulk, and when they are prefectly mingled. Pain is felt when one of these elements is in defect or excess, or is isolated in the body without being compounded with all the others.

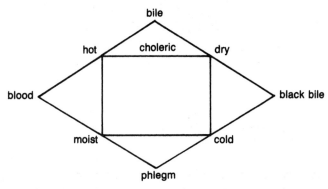

Relation Between Humors and Elements

According to humoral theory, then, pneumonia, for example, is caused by abnormal phlegm arising in the head; when phlegm is admixed with the blood, fever and chills result.

The changing of the seasons of the year were felt to cause major shifts in the proportion of the humors, and in this is found the explanation for seasonal diseases such as colds and flus. Moreover, daily habits of work and sleep, exercise, emotions, geographical changes, and climate all bear an effect upon the humors and thus are considered in determining the cause of disease, that is, which humor is out of balance. For example, the blood humor predominates in spring, yellow bile in summer, black bile in autumn, and phlegm in winter.

The full explanation of the system of humors, along with the diseases associated with imbalances, is covered in Chapters 2 and 3. For now it is important simply to acknowledge that these concepts originated with Hippocrates, who wrote them down and codified them into a science. In sum, Hippocrates introduced a very high standard of ethics, observation, and idealism into medicine, and brought it from the arcane doldrums of superstition into an era of enlightenment and reason. Unfortunately, after his death, his theories became tradition and dogma, and his own contributions were almost destroyed.

The Roman conquest resulted in the stagnation of medicine for more than a thousand years. The Romans were hostile to all Greek thought, and the average Roman citizen considered medicine a lowly occupation, preferring to invoke the gods for a cure rather than rely on medical treatment.

Following this abysmal period of ignorance and hostility to scholarship and medicine, a fresh impetus was breathed into medicine by another brilliant Greek, Galen. Born in 130 A.D., six hundred years after Hippocrates, Galen was a resident of Peragmum in northwest Asia Minor, a culturally distinguished city with a renowned medical college. He was first educated in the sciences, philosophy, and logic at the insistence of his father, who decided, when Galen was seventeen, that the youth would concentrate on a medical curriculum. Thus, Galen was sent to Alexandria for a period of nine years to complete his medical education.

With a vast reach of mind, Galen collected and synthesized not only all of Hippocrates' work, but all medical knowledge that had evolved during the intervening six centuries. According to Galen, there is a force called *pneuma* that pervades or inhabits each living organism. In this *pneuma* Galen saw a "creative force of being," which activated or stimulated all of the faculties of growth, development, and nutrition. Galen was also the first to introduce the idea that the quality of plants (including food plants) was affected by the quality of the soil in which they were grown.

The *pneuma* or vital air identified by Galen was a creative force itself, carried on the breath, originating in the action of the lungs and dispersed throughout the body according to needs of the body. Both Hippocrates and Galen accepted the concept of the humors, which were said to arise at the site of the liver and to be conveyed throughout the body along subtle networks. Galen advanced this idea by suggesting that each food also had its characteristic humor, and thus arose an elaborate system of dietetics.

After Galen, another period of inertia followed for almost nine hundred years while Europe strained to see out from the abyss of the Dark Ages. These veils of darkness were pierced by the appearance of a man who is rightfully called the most famous individual physician in the history of humanity. Hakim Abu Ali al-Husayn Abd Allah Ibn Sina, known in the West as Avicenna, was born in 980 A.D. near Bokhara, in what then was part of Afghanistan. Though that was the center of learning of the age, Avicenna had exhausted all of the most learned teachers while he was still in his teens. His father was a religious man who entertained many learned guests, and the young savant gathered up their discourses with zeal. By the age of ten he had become a *hafiz*—one who has committed the entire Qur'an to memory.

When Avicenna was twenty-one his father died, and this event, coupled with the political turmoil of the era, forced Avicenna into a period of wandering. Ultimately, he found refuge and support from the Bujid prince Shams-ad-Dawlah at Hamadan in Persia. Even such royal patronage was insufficient to shield

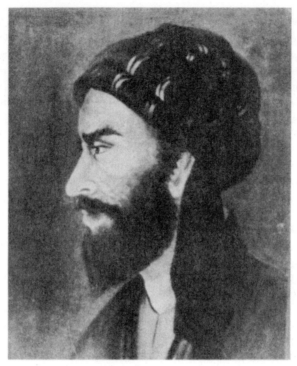

Avicenna, The Prince of Physicians

Avicenna from the epidemic of political intrigues, and he was even imprisoned on one occasion.

But his intellect and physical stamina were so great that Avicenna managed to conduct his work as a physician and scholar despite such dislocations and hardships. Writing with his memory as his primary resource, he composed an astonishing 276 books, most of them in several volumes, covering virtually every subject of human thought and endeavor—medicine, natural history, physics, chemistry, mathematics, music, economics, and moral and religious questions. Two of his medical books have earned undisputed and unparalleled fame. The first, *Kitab al-shifa'* (The Book of Healing), was a monumental work that is generally conceded to be the largest ever produced by one person. In it Avicenna developed his theories of medicine and its relevant allied sciences by expounding the doctrines of logic, natural sciences, psychology, geometry, astronomy, arithmetic, music, and metaphysics. For Avicenna, the evaluation of a "disease" was incomplete until and unless all components of a person's life had been included in the diagnosis.

Like Hippocrates and Galen, Avicenna considered that God was a "necessary existent," and he wrote many books on the nature of Divinity, including the famous *Kitab al-insaf* (Book of Impartial Judgment), in which, at the age of twenty-one, he posed and answered 28,000 questions on the nature of Divinity. Although some Islamic jurists feel that Avicenna misunderstood certain mystic doctrines, and consider some of his religious writings blasphemous, no one disputes his eminence and status as a physician. His fame rests chiefly on his second book, *al-Qanun fi al-Tibb* (The Canon of Medicine), which the *Encyclopaedia Brittanica* calls "the single most famous book in the history of medicine, in East or West." Composed in five long volumes totalling one million words, the *Canon* drew together all of the medical knowledge that existed in the world up to his time, which he refined and codified into the science of medicine. Both *The Book of Healing* and *The Canon of Medicine* were translated widely, first into Latin, then into virtually every other language of the civilized world.*

The *Canon* and other of Avicenna's works became the basis of thought in most of the medieval schools of thought, especially that of the Franciscans. The *Canon* of Avicenna is the medical authority for all therapeutics, and its influence upon the development of all medicine cannot be overestimated. It has maintained its authority through ten centuries of medical teaching and practice, and even today remains the handbook for all practitioners of Tibb medicine. Edward Spicer, an anthropologist at the University of Arizona, has even identified "folk remedies" used by rural Afro-Americans as originating with the *Canon*. Hakim Ibn Sina enjoys a place of honor unequalled by any other individual physician and is often referred to as the Prince of Physicians.

Using the work of Avicenna as their basis and inspiration, Muslim civilizations made several very important contributions to medicine: the founding of medical chemistry in the form of botany, the organization of pharmacy, and the founding of hospitals. Avicenna himself provided much of the basis for later development of fundamental chemical processes such as filtration, distillation, sublimation, and calcination. He invented the procedure of distillation of floral oils and was the first to distill essence of rose.

From the tremendous impetus of advancement of medicine supplied by Avicenna, the Arabs took the huddled masses of sick and established them in sleek and elegant hospitals. Their hospitals were immense structures with courtyards and had features such as lecture halls, libraries, mosques and chapels (they treated people of all religious beliefs), charity wards, kitchens, and dispensaries. All patients were attended by qualified male and female nurses. The mood at the magnificent Mansur Hospital in Cairo is reflected in the following account of the amenities arranged for the benefit of all patients:

---

*English translations of the *Canon* remain incomplete. A treatise on the first volume of the *Canon* was written by O. Cameron Gruner, a British medical doctor who was introduced to the medical teachings of Avicenna and who translated the first volume from Latin and wrote an extensive commentary on the book.

Day and night, fifty reciters intoned the Qur'an aloud. At nightfall, musicians played soft melodies to induce drowsiness in the patients. Professional storytellers entertained the sick with their tales. When the patients left the hospital, they were given enough money so that they would not have to resume work immediately.

By the time of the early eighteenth century, the Tibb system was the basis of virtually all medicine in the civilized world, having been translated and formed as the basis of the work of such men as Father Sebastian Kneipp (1821–1897) and Samuel Hahnemann (1755–1843), the founder of homeopathy, who is reputed to have known Arabic and read Avicenna's works.

In the mid-1800s, there occured a cross-pollinization of medicine between Europe and the United States. Individuals such as William Kellog learned these systems of natural therapeutics, mainly from the European clergy, and spread them among the general population.

All of the modalities of natural therapeutics thrived in Europe and the United States until the beginning of the twentieth century, when chemical medicine began to predominate. This evolution of disease concepts and treatments is important enough to warrant a few words of reflection.

The historical concept of "disease" has changed from the time of the ancient Greeks to modern times. The pre-Hippocratic physicians based their practice only on the study of the diseased individual. But because the variety of signs in disease is so great, it was quickly realized that some system of classification was necessary. Thus the Cnidian physicians introduced nosographical classification. This system required that all symptoms be listed in numerical order and then be evaluated to see which of the symptoms occurred with greatest regularity and frequency. These regularly occurring symptoms received arbitrary names as "diseases," mainly a reflection to the symptoms they represented (e.g., *bursitis*, meaning "inflammation of the bursa," which reveals nothing about the cause). All medicine, from the time of the Cnidians until the beginning of the nineteenth century, was based upon this symptom-complex form of classification.

The dawn of the nineteenth century witnessed the construction of a new class of fictional diseases, based upon the French, British, and Viennese schools of anatomy and clinical studies. The symptomatology of the past was discarded in favor of the series of signs that occurred with regularity in combination and were considered to represent a set of symptoms corresponding to a *specific lesion* or a disturbance in the function of an organ. Thus, the adherents of these anatomical-clinical schools succeeded in switching the *basic concept of disease* from symptom complexes to lesion-anatomical syndromes.

During the third quarter of the nineteenth century (1860–1890), the basic conceptions of disease were again altered by the advent of the bacteriological school, which introduced what was primarily called the etiological (meaning bacteriological) origin of disease. In the past, physicians believed that disease

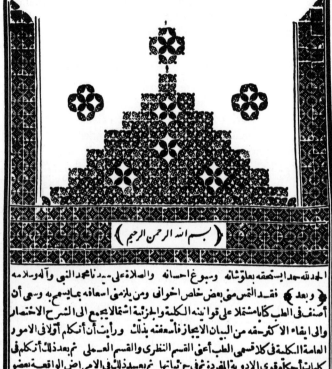

{ بسم الله الرحمن الرحيم }

الحمد لله حمدا يستحقه بعلو شانه وسبوغ احسانه والصلاة على سيد ناامحمد النبي وآله وسلامه
{ وبعد } فقد التمس مني بعض خاص اخواني ومن يلزمني اسعافه بما يسوء هم وسعي أن
أصنف في الطب كتابا مشتملا على قوانينه الكلية والجزئية اشتمالا يجمع الى الشرح الاختصار
والى ايفاء الاكثر حقه من البيان الايجاز فأسعفته بذلك ورأيت أن أتكلم أولا في الامور
العامة الكلية في كلا قسمي الطب أعني القسم النظري والقسم العملي ثم بعد ذلك أن أتكلم في
كليات أحكام قوى الأدوية المفردة ثم في جزئياتها ثم بعد ذلك في الامراض الواقعة بعضو
عضو فأبتدئ أولا بتشريع ذلك العضو ومنفعته وأما تشريح الأعضاء المفردة البسيطة
فيكون قد سبق مني ذكره في الكتاب الاول الكلي وكذلك منافعها ثم اذا فرغت من تشريع
ذلك العضو ابتدأت في أكثر المواضع بالدلالة على كيفية حفظ صحته ثم دللت بالقول المطلق
على كليات أمراضه وأسبابها وطرق الاستدلالات عليها وطرق معالجاتها بالقول الكلي أيضا
فاذا فرغت من هذه الامور الكلية اقبلت على الامراض الجزئية ودللت أولا في أكثرها أيضا
على الحكم الكلي في حدها وأسبابه ودلائله ثم تخلصت الى الأحكام الجزئية ثم أعطيت القانون
الكلي في المعالجة ثم نزلت الى المعالجات الجزئية بدواء دواء بسيط أو مركب وما كان سلف
ذكره من الأدوية المفردة ومنفعته في الامراض في كتاب الأدوية المفردة في الجداول
والاصباغ التي أرى استعمالها هانه كتقف أيها المعلم عليه اذا وصلت اليه ما أكرر الاقلال منه
وما كان من الأدوية المركبة أن ما الاحرى به ان يكون في الاقراباذين الذي أرى ان احمله أخرت
ذكر منافعه وكيفية خلطه اليه ورأيت ان أفرغ عن هذا الكتاب الى الكتاب أيضا في الامور
الجزئية مختص بذكر الامراض التي اذا وقعت تختص بعضو بعينه ونورد هنالك أيضا الكلام
في الزينة وان أسلك في هذا الكتاب أيضا مسلكي في الكتاب الجزئي الذي قبله فاذا تم بتوفيق

*Frontispiece of the Arabic edition of Avicenna's <u>Al-Qanun fi'l at-Tibb</u>
(The Canon of Medicine).*

symptoms revealed some organic malfunction. But with the bateriological school, this idea was abandoned in favor of the notion that there was a "special cause"—usually a microbe or virus—responsible for the symptom.

Physicians of traditional medicine and others who advocate a return to the symptomatology-based mode of disease argue that there can be no such thing as a "single" cause of disease, be it a germ or some other factor. The concept of a single cause or mode of classification is rejected as an illogical fiction because common sense and reason compel one to admit that every morbid condition is the result of not one but many factors, almost always occurring in combination.

The Tibb system follows the traditional mode of evaluation of symptom groups and disregards the idea of germs or viruses as the *primary cause* of disease. The key concept-word in Tibb is *temperament (mizaj)*. This word expresses the various reactional tendencies of the individual, which is an important consideration for physicians from a clinical point of view, especially those endeavoring to defend microbial theories of medicine. For example, it is well known that most physicians attribute the occurrence of influenza to one or more viruses. However, if a particular virus *caused* a particular flu (or cold or any other disease), then one would assume that everyone coming into contact with that causative virus would fall ill. Obviously, such is not the case. Even though many children in one school may get the same flu symptoms, not *every* child falls ill. Physicians use this notion of temperament to "explain" that some people are "disposed" to get the disease. (The term used is "predisposing factor.") Indeed, this being the case, one wonders how anyone has accepted the microbial theories of disease, since to explain viral theory, *some* intemperament is clearly accepted as the initial cause of disease.

In fact, if the viral/bacterial theories were accurate (or complete) then one would assume that no nurse or physician on earth would survive, as such people are constantly exposed to every conceivable form of virulent microbe, yet seldom fall ill. Even though many children for the first several years of life suffer dozens of colds, flus, and infections, the mother virtually never "catches" any of them.

Why do none of these people who are exposed and overexposed to diseases claimed to be caused by serious viruses never fall ill? The answer that Tibb has—and upon which its entire system is built—is the notion of the temperament, or humor. While admitting the existence of microbes, the Tibb system claims that it is the *original imbalance of temperament* that provides an altered biotic environment in which these viruses and bacteria can thrive. And the causes of the initial imbalance of temperament are often to be found in more subtle elements of life, such as rest and activity patterns, work stresses, and interpersonal relations (anger, for example, can dispel moisture in the humor regulating the heart). Treatments of bacterial populations present in disease conditions may kill off all bacteria and provide a temporary "cure," but without restoring the humor to its proper balance, the disease will recur (as happens, for example, with recurring vaginal infections, upper respiratory problems, flus). Today, the knowledge of temperament constitutes for the clinician, from the point of view of physiology as well as of psychology and therapeutics, a notion of primary importance.

The prescriptions used in the Unani Tibb system are classed according to the degree of their temperaments and are administered to restore the temperament to its original equilibrium. These drugs are predominantly of vegetable origin, and their benefit is judged by the effect produced by the whole medical treatment upon the whole person—on the physical, mental, and moral planes of being.

The practitioner of Unani Tibb is known as a *hakim* (masculine) or *hakima* (feminine), an Arabic/Persian word that means both "physician" and "wise." As the Muslim populations begin to interact with Western societies by education and immigration, the concepts of Tibb are gradually being introduced into the mainstream medical thought. A conference was held in 1979 at the University of Arizona Medical School, and international symposia are being held annually in Saudi Arabia, Kuwait, Egypt, India, and Pakistan.

With the foregoing as a background on the origins of traditional healing and some of its important concepts, let us now turn to a full explanation of Tibb's basic principles for evaluating the human being in states of wellness and disease.

2
The Doctrine of the Naturals

The Tibb system is divided into two parts, theory and practice. There are three parts to the theory of Tibb: (1) the theory of naturals, which establishes the standards of the human body, from which disease states are deduced by the deviation from these norms; (2) the theory of causes, which identifies and explains the reasons for the deviations from the norms so that they may be corrected; and (3) the theory of signs, which presents the main diagnostic features for identifying the specific deviation that is causing the imbalance (disease).

There are seven components of the naturals: (1) elements, (2) temperaments, (3) humors, (4) organs, (5) forces, (6) actions, and (7) spirits. By understanding each of these components of the naturals, we can begin to appreciate the viewpoint through which Tibb evaluates human health and wellness.

The Four Elements

The four elements are earth and water (heavy), and fire and air (light). In terms of qualities, the heavy elements are strong, negative, passive, and female. The light elements are weak, positive, active, heavenly, and male.

Earth is an element usually situated at the center of our existence. In its nature it is at rest, and because of its inherent weight, all other elements gravitate toward it, however far away they may be. It is said to be cold and dry in nature, and it appears so to sight and touch, so long as it is not changed by any other elements. It is by means of the earth element that the parts of our bodies are fixed and held in place; thus the outward form of the body is due to the earth element.

Water is a simple substance whose position in nature is exterior to the sphere of the earth and interior to that of air. Water is cold and moist in temperament, although only slightly so. Water is easily dispersed and assumes any shape without permanency. In the construction of "things," the addition of water allows the possibility of their being shaped and molded and spread out. Shapes can readily be made from it, and just as easily dispersed. Moisture dispels dryness, the latter being overruled by the former. Moisture protects dryness from crumbling (as moist earth, or mud), and likewise, dryness prevents moisture from dispersing. Thus the two elements of earth and water are interacting and interdependent. Water is, of course, absolutely essential to life.

Air is positioned in nature above both water and earth, but beneath fire. The temperament of air is hot and moist, and its purpose in nature is to make things finer, lighter, and more delicate and thus more able to ascend into higher spheres. Air is also the agent by which breath moves in and out of the body and causes or makes possible the involuntary movements of the body.

Fire is also a simple substance, situated higher than the other three elements. Fire is hot and dry in temperament, and its role in nature is to rarefy, refine, and intermingle things. Fire has the power to penetrate and can ride through the element of air. It has the capacity to overcome the coldness of the two cold elements, earth and water, and so creates and maintains harmony among the elements.

Each of the elements has a corresponding humor or essence in the body:

Blood humor relates to air.
Phlegm humor relates to water.
Yellow bile humor relates to fire.
Black bile humor relates to earth.

Table 1 summarizes attributes of the elements as they relate to aspects of human physiology:

TABLE 1
ATTRIBUTES OF THE ELEMENTS

	Earth	Water
Tendency	spreading	drooping
Bodily system	skeleton	muscles
Excretion	feces	urine
Sense	touch	taste
Bodily function	form	nutrition
Mentality	torpid	phlegmatic
Mental state	obstinancy, fearfulness	submission, affection

	Air	Fire
Tendency	to and fro	rising
Bodily system	circulation	liver
Excretion	saliva	sweat, tears
Sense	hearing	smell
Bodily function	respiration	digestion, voluntary bodily movements
Mentality	cheerful	emotional
Mental state	humor	weeping, anger

The terms *earth, water, air,* and *fire* do not mean literally clods of dirt, buckets of water, and so forth. The four elements are sometimes referred to as "primary matter," which, when admixed, gives rise to the various forms such as mountains and rivers. Likewise, the burning fire that we see is not the element fire, which is really the potentiality of fire within the substance. For example, green wood has the *element* of fire within, but this may or may not be brought forth as flames, depending on whether it is ever ignited. All of the elements bear this relation between *capacity within* and *reality of form.*

Thus all of the concrete objects of this world—from the most immense mountain to the minutest form of submicroscopic life—are related by the four elements. And through these same four primary elements, all earthly objects are related to (and influenced by) the planets and stars of the zodiac (which also have primary qualities within them).

The movement of these four elements is continually taking place, so that change is a continuous process within the human body. This change can be either cyclical or progressive. The cycle of intake and elimination of food is an example of cyclical change, whereas the growth of a cancerous tumor is an example of a progressive change. In the Tibb system, the monitoring and observation of these changes becomes an important mode of evaluating precisely what is happening within each part of the body. Therefore, a method of classifying these changes has arisen, called temperament.

The Temperaments

There are nine kinds of temperaments: eight are called nonequable and one is called equable. *Equable* means "balanced" or "existing in a state of balance." Of the eight nonequable, four are single: hot, cold, wet, and dry; and four are compound: hot and dry, hot and wet, cold and dry, and cold and wet.

The temperament is that quality which exists by the mutual interaction of the four primary qualities residing within the elements. In other words, blood is characteristically hot and moist. Now, some conditions may arise—such as prolonged sleep or exposure to cold—by which the basic quality of heat may be dissipated, which would allow moisture to build up. Such an event would result in various signs occurring within the body or its organs or parts. Thus, the physician, seeing the evidences of excess heat and other signs, would characterize the imbalance as a cold intemperament of the blood, and he would devise a treatment to correct this primary, single intemperament.

There is a constant interaction among the elements, a rising and falling of influence, and seldom, if ever, do they actually maintain a strictly balanced point. It is well known that while the so-called normal temperature of the body is 98.6 degrees Fahrenheit, the *actual* temperature of the body fluctuates throughout the course of a day by several degrees. If you were to record your own body temperature at intervals, you would discover that it is lower in the morning and higher at or just after noon.

Each part of the body has been evaluated and assigned its own characteristic temperament, ranging through degrees of heat, cold, wetness, and dryness. Table 2 summarizes these temperaments.

TABLE 2

DEGREES OF INHERENT TEMPERAMENT

Heat (1 = Hottest)

1. Breath	6. Spleen
2. Blood	7. Kidneys
3. Liver	8. Walls of arteries
4. Flesh	9. Walls of veins
5. Muscles	10. Skin of palms and soles

Coldness (1 = Coldest)

1. Phlegm humor	7. Membranes
2. Hair	8. Nerves
3. Bones	9. Spinal cord
4. Cartilage	10. Brain
5. Ligaments	11. Fat
6. Tendons	12. Oil of the body
	13. Skin

Moisture (1 = Moistest)

1. Phlegm humor	7. Breasts and testicles
2. Blood	8. Lungs
3. Oil	9. Liver
4. Fat	10. Spleen
5. Brain	11. Kidneys
6. Spinal cord	12. Muscles
	13. Skin

Dryness (1 = Driest)

1. Hair	7. Arteries
2. Bone	8. Veins
3. Cartilage	9. Motor nerves
4. Ligaments	10. Heart
5. Tendons	11. Sensory nerves
6. Serous membranes	12. Skin

Likewise, the seasons and other factors have characteristic temperaments, as related in Table 3.

TABLE 3
COMPOUND TEMPERAMENTS

	Hot & Wet	Hot & Dry	Cold & Dry	Cold & Wet
Season	spring	summer	autumn	winter
Age	childhood	youth	maturity	old age
Region	east	south	west	north
Element	air	fire	earth	water
Humor	blood	yellow bile	black bile	phlegm
Personality	sanguine	choleric	melancholic	phlegmatic

Let us now consider how these temperaments interact to affect health. In the Tibb system, the first diagnostic feature we look for is an *intemperament* of a particular organ or system. There are four main intemperaments:

1. Hot intemperament: hotter than it should be, not moister or drier
2. Cold intemperament: colder than it should be, not moister or drier
3. Dry intemperament: drier than it should be, not hotter or colder
4. Moist intemperament: moister than it should be, not hotter or colder

These four intemperaments are never static, for they are constantly changing and interacting. For example, if a temperament becomes hotter than it should be (hot intemperament), it quickly drives off moisture, which will also lead to a dry intemperament, resulting in a compound intemperament. Thus, there are four compound intemperaments, which occur when the initial simple intemperament persists to the point of affecting a second quality of the innate balance. These four compound intemperaments are: hotter and moister than it should be; hotter and drier; colder and moister; and colder and drier. (Obviously, an intemperament cannot be hotter and colder or drier and more moist.)

In addition, an intemperament is classified as being either qualitative or material. It is qualitative if it does not affect an organ directly (as with a fever), material if the intemperament invades a part of the body and causes change (e.g., invades the colon by excess mucus due to intemperament of the phlegm humor).

Thus there are a total of sixteen intemperaments, or modes of classifying intemperaments. An intemperament is measured by the observable signs occurring in the body or a bodily part. The signs of the four intemperaments are presented in full in Chapter 6. The temperaments are held in place, or kept balanced, by the existence of four humors.

The Theory of Humors in Medicine

The idea of humors originated with Hippocrates, who observed upon examining blood that the red portion of fresh blood is the blood humor, the white material mixed with blood is the phlegm, the yellow-colored froth on top is the yellow bile, and the heavy part that settles down is the black bile (*sauda*). This theory was further refined by Galen, to the extent that he held that all diseases were the result of irregular or improper distribution of the four humors.

Avicenna agreed that these four components are the primary humors, but he added that the intracellular and extracellular fluids in the tissues are secondary humors. According to Avicenna, the four primary humors are derived from the digestion of food and are utilized as nutrient components for the growth and repair of the organs and to yield energy for work. The humors have a normal state as well as abnormal varieties. The worst abnormal humor is black bile, which is believed to be responsible for cancerous growth. It is a toxin.

The origin and action the four humors or essences (Arabic: *akhlat*) and their ultimate fate in the digestive process are presented in the accompanying illustration.

A humor exists in a kinetic state, at all times adjusting and interspersing with the body fluids, tissues, and parts.

All four of these humors arise at the site of the liver, in quantity or predominance according to the nature of the foods eaten and the degree of completeness of their digestion. The blood humor comes into being first and is formed of the choicest parts of nutrients. Second, the phlegm humor arises and accompanies the second-level digestion nutrients. The yellow bile is composed of the third stage of digestion nutrients, which are the coarser and less refined parts, and the black bile is composed of the least digestible and usable parts of nutrients. Each of the four humors has its own characteristic temperament, in accord with the system it regulates. Thus, the blood humor is moist and warm (like blood itself), phlegm humor is cold and moist, yellow bile humor dry and cold, and black bile warm and dry. One humor predominates in each individual.

During the early stages of the Renaissance, the humoral concept of disease was attacked violently and discarded by many. But later, new factors came to light that reawakened interest in humoral medicine. Landsteiner and Garrod began scientific inquiry into humoral theory in 1901, and since then the scientific community has devoted a watchful eye on humoral developments. One of the limitations of this research and attention has been the tendency to consider humor and body fluid as one and the same. While humors share some aspects of nature with body fluids, they are not identical. Urine, for example, is a body fluid but not a humor. The humor associated with the blood and called "sanguine" is not identical with blood drawn by venesection. Nor is the phlegm of the phlegm humor the same as mucus or lymph or phlegm, although it shares some characteristics with them. Dr. Cameron Gruner, a medical doctor who performed exhaustive research into humors, called them "quasi-material." I call them "semigaseous vapors."

The Origin and Fate of the Four Bodily Humors

Mouth takes in food and drink
First digestion
*
To Stomach
Usable parts are acted upon by digestive fluids.
(Unusable parts go to large intestine
and are emitted as excrement.)
*
To Small Intestine
Becomes chyme by mixing with digestive juices
and fluids of meal.
(Travels through mesenteric veins, portal vein.)
*
To Liver
Second digestion
BLOOD HUMOR ARISES
(Hot & Moist)
Superior nutrients are taken in via bloodstream
to heart and dispersed to cells
via general bloodstream.
Third digestion
*
Less choice parts become
*

PHLEGM HUMOR
(Cold & Moist)
Normal digestion converts into mucus,
saliva, and gastric and intestinal mucus.
Abnormal digestion causes excess mucus,
classified as sweet, sour, thick, thin, etc.
*

Remaining nutrients become
BILIOUS HUMOR
(Hot & Dry)
*

Normal bile is formed in liver, affects blood,
and acts in small intestine.
Abnormal humor causes destructive changes in bile.
*
Sediments of precipitates of digestive nutrients become
ATRABILIOUS HUMOR
(Cold & Dry)

Normal humor affects spleen and blood, and mixes with phlegm humor.

Fourth digestion

Abnormal humor is passed out as ash or admixes with blood humor and other humors, producing morbid conditions.

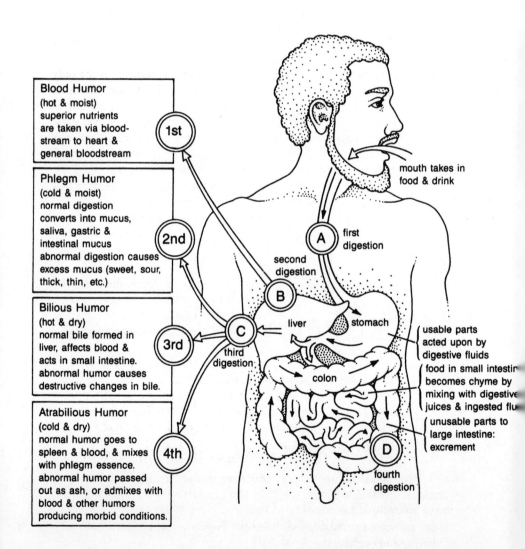

The Process of the Four Humors of the Body

The invention of the microscope has taken us away from the source and origin of the problems associated with disease. For example, most physicians would attribute an infection to one or more bacteria and will produce actual living specimens of those bacteria which they say caused such and such an infection. From the Unani Tibb point of view, the deviation from the normal state of the humor provided a suitable environment for the bacteria to grow to larger than normal populations. While admitting the existence of the bacteria, the Tibb scientist must look deeper to the cause of the imbalance in the humor and its characteristic temperaments. Thus, the mode of current medical practice that "attacks" the red- and white-cell-forming organs does not take into account the fact that blood itself is living and not simply a conglomerate of chemical components.

Thus in Tibb, the dictum "Health is a harmony of the humors" is the only valid point of view if one desires to cure the cause of the disease. Chemical destruction of the abnormal growth of microscopic life may result in a temporary decline or total eradication of the population of microorganisms, but if the imbalance of the humor is not corrected, the disease will recur or will arise in another place in the body. More important, the dramatic effects of the chemical drugs themselves on the humors result in new imbalances, as evidenced by the many so-called side effects of drugs. These concepts will be made clearer when the sections on the causes of disease are read in Chapter 3.

There are several more points to discuss in relation to the naturals: the four main organs, the three forces of activization, and the three spiritual forces.

The Four Organs

There are four organs of primary importance in Tibb: the brain, the heart, the liver, and the testicles or ovaries. Other organs are servants to these main organs. By this is meant that the brain is served by the nerves, the heart by the arteries, the liver by veins, the testicles by spermatic vessels, and the ovaries by the fallopian tubes.

The heart is the source or starting point of the vital power or innate heat of the body. The brain is the seat of the mental faculties, sensation, and movement. The liver is the seat of the nutritive or vegetative faculties. The generative organs (testes, ovaries) give the masculine and feminine form and temperament, and form the generative elements for propagation of the race.

The Three Faculties of the Body

We must distinguish between faculty and function. Faculties originate functions. A faculty is a power, a potentiality. The ultimate faculty is the soul, while the ultimate function is life.

There are three natural faculties: the vital (*haywaniat*), the natural (*taby'yat*), and the psychic (*nafsaniat*).

There are two types of vital forces: the active and the acted upon. An active vital force would be one that causes the heart and arteries to dilate. The acted-upon vital forces are those that underlie anger, contempt, competition for victory, leadership, or fame, and other emotions. Thus, the emotional/psychological aspects of health and disease are considered holistically, as part of the entire person. For example, severe anger is believed to be the result of an excess of moisture in the heart humor, and its correction is accomplished with diet.

There are also two types of natural forces: those that serve other functions and those that are served by others. The natural forces that are served by other forces are three kinds: the generative, the growth-promoting, and the nutritive. The servant natural forces are four: the attractive, the retentive, the digestive, and the propulsive. These various forces interact intimately each with the other. The four servant forces serve the nutritive forces (by attracting, retaining, digesting, and propelling), and the nutritive force serves the growth-promoting force. The first two forces serve the generative force.

The psychic forces perform three functions: (1) to mediate behavior, (2) to cause voluntary movement, and (3) to create sensation. Within these functions are found the various events that serve imagination, create thinking, and underlie memory.

Now, the seat of each of these three forces has a point of origin: the natural forces arise in the liver; the vital forces arise in the heart; and the psychic forces arise in the brain. Over each of these natural forces is a corresponding spirit faculty, which serves as the nexus or interconnecting link with the nonmanifest realms. That is, according to Avicenna, all life is dependent upon the divine permission (*idhn*) for life to begin and continue. The divine permission or cosmic force travels in through the indrawn breath and first alights in the heart, where it is dispersed by the arteries throughout the whole body and activates both the natural forces and psychic forces.

The correction of subtle emotional and spiritual imbalances, while of concern to the Hakim, is often treated by spiritual remedies and practices. My work titled *The Book of Sufi Healing* (Rochester, VT: Inner Traditions, 1991) elaborates the spiritual side of Tibb healing.

Thus, according to the Tibb system, all of the physical, emotional, and spiritual mechanisms of life are included in the evaluation of a person's health. I mentioned before that according to Tibb, the human being possesses a soul (*ruh*), which is independent of and superior to all of the physiological functions of the body—including all mental functions, such as thought processes, memory, and the emotions. Once a human life ends, the activization of the three faculties ends, all physical functions cease, and we observe what is called death.

The science of maintaining the human body in a state of balance, harmony, and vigor is the purpose of Tibb—the treatment of the physical, mental, and spiritual forces of human life. With the foregoing as a necessary explanation of the basic theories of the human being and its parts, we may now turn to the signs that occur to measure health and disease.

3
The Tibb Profile: Six Factors

There are three states of the body: health, disease, and the neutral state between the two, when one is not truly healthy but the signs of disease are not fully manifest.

The neutral state is of three forms: (1) health and disease exist in the same body in different parts (an example would be a blind person, who is healthy apart from the disease of the eyes); (2) neither health nor disease exists to a perfect degree, as with the old and convalescing; (3) the body alternates between healthy and diseased states, as in persons with a hot temperament, who are generally well in the winter and ill in the summer. People with a cold temperament are generally ill in winter and well in summer: those with wet or dry temperament are generally ill in childhood and gain health in maturity and old age.

What we call organic diseases arise when the functions associated with the vital, natural, and psychic forces of the body become "obstructed," or unbalanced, owing to a deviation in the humor away from its characteristic temperament. An example would be an excess of heat affecting the blood humor, altering it to a condition of excess dryness. There are other causes of disease, which need to be treated, although they are generally not the result of disturbance of a humor from metabolic causes. Examples of "disease" conditions of this type are improperly shaped organs (basket head), narrow or expanded ducts, irregular tissue within or without organs (rough uterine-wall tissue), excessive organ size (enlarged heart), displaced organs (transposed liver), small organs (stomach), and conditions arising from occasional causes (poisonous animals and insects). There are other diseases caused by what Tibb calls a break in continuity, or accidents, such as fractures, burns, wounds, and the like.

The treatment of diseases of malformed organs and accidents requires the specialized help of a well-trained physician. Tibb has no herbal treatment for an inverted valve in the bladder, for example, although if this condition were known, the general diet and regimen of the person could be adjusted, until or unless correction by surgical methods was attempted. The treatment of severe injuries and wounds belongs to the realm of Western emergency medicine, which possesses the training, procedures, and technical knowledge to deal with them. In fact, emergency medicine is one of the most legitimate and impressive achievements of orthodox medicine.

The Tibb Profile

Six primary factors are examined in relation to health and disease: (1) the air of one's environment, (2) food and beverages, (3) movement and rest, (4) sleep and wakefulness, (5) eating and evacuation, and (6) emotions. These six factors must be properly apportioned in quantity, quality, time, and sequence in order for there to be health. If these six factors are disturbed in any of the six elements, disease arises and is maintained. With the exception of congenital defects and accidents, it is the changes in the humors caused by these six factors which most often lead to disease.

Before considering each of these factors in turn, we should note that there are some innate characteristics that affect a person's health, or at least are signs by which we can search for the underlying cause of imbalance. These factors are age, complexion, hair color, and eye color.

First we should understand that there are four main stages (or ages) of life: youth, adulthood, maturity, and old age. The years of youth commence with infancy and continue as long as the body is growing, generally up to about thirty years of age. The years of adulthood are those in which growth has ceased but has not yet started to decline. This period usually lasts to about thirty-five years of age. The years of maturity are marked by some decrease in the body and generally end at about sixty years of age. The years of old age are marked by total decline in strength and last from age sixty until death. The temperaments associated with each of these stages are as follows:

Youth: hot and humid
Adulthood: hot and dry
Maturity: cold and dry
Old age: Principal organs are cold and dry; moistures collected in the body are cold and moist.

There are different types of moisture within the body, and it is the drying out of these moistures that ultimately brings on death. There are four types of moisture: moisture of the small vessels; moisture in the small spaces of the body; moisture of the different parts of the organs; and the moisture that holds the body together.

Now, when evaluating a person's health, one must consider first the temperament of the person's age, then the temperament of the particular organ(s) affected. For example, the choice of food and herbs to treat an elderly person with a fever would be quite different from that selected for an infant with a fever, owing to the vastly different innate temperament of each. This is why it is so puzzling to find herbals that, under a heading such as "fever," arbitrarily list many herbs to treat a fever, without any reference to the age or any other factors of the individual.

The complexion also reveals the condition of a person's balance or lack of it. A skin color between white and red—rose—indicates a balanced temperament. Black, yellow, and red colors indicate the dominance of one of the humors: yellow, yellow bile humor; black, black bile humor; red, blood humor; and white and fair, phlegm humor.

The pigmentations of the skin particular to various parts of the world are the result of long exposure to some external environmental factor. The white complexion of the Slavs comes from the cold temperatures of their countries; the black coloration of the Sudanese is from the heat of the desert. Other colors are signs of imbalance, such as yellowish skin due to grief and reddish coloration from shyness.

The effect of skin color on health can be quite significant. For example, persons whose ancestry is in the African deserts cannot "adjust" within a few generations to great climatic changes. The original very hot environment is what the temperament is accustomed to. When the person moves to a very cold environment, the vital force cannot generate enough heat, and, according to Tibb, the person may suffer greatly from sadness, depression, and melancholy.

The color of hair also results from internal conditions. Black hair is from intense heat; red hair is from deficient heat and combustion; blond hair is from a heat level below that caused by red hair; and white hair results from extreme weakness of innate heat and decomposition of putrified phlegm.

The evaluation of eye color also provides information of the metabolic efficiency of a person. There are four basic eye colors: black, blue, gray, and brown. Black eye coloration is from lessening of the spirit faculty (that which activates metabolic functions) of the eyes, lack of moisture in the lens of the eye, and increase in albumin. Blue eyes are caused by the opposites of those producing black eyes. Gray and brown eyes are the result of combining of the black and blue factors. Green eyes are the result of blue pigmentation being admixed with yellowed phlegm deposits.

Table 4 summarizes the various physical faculties of the human being, arranged according to the predominating temperaments and humors.

The Six Factors

Ambient Air

The air of one's environment plays a vital role in the maintenance of health in the human being, and too often this factor is neglected or ignored entirely. Many if not most people live and work in areas that are covered over with in-

TABLE 4

SIGNS OF TEMPERAMENTS AND HUMORS

EVIDENCE	Blood	Phlegm	Yellow Bile	Black Bile
Aspect: General physique	Good	Effeminate; bones slender, joints well covered	Lean, joints large	Emaciated
Color	Flushed	Pale and weak	Yellow tinge in skin and eyes	Dusky; whole body seems dark and hairy
Feel of the skin	Firm	Soft and cool		Flesh hard
State of the skin	Reddens on rubbing Boils			Skin rough, liable to dark eruptions and ulcers
Hair	Full	Absent on chest	Hairy	Hairy
Surface veins		Constricted	Thick and hard	
Vegetative Faculties				
Mouth	Tendency to canker sores	Abundant sticky saliva	Bitter taste	
Tongue	Red		Rough and dry	
Nostrils			Rough and dry	
Pulse		Soft, tends to be slow and infrequent	Rapid	
Urine		White		Dark-colored or black dense
Sensitive Faculties				

Special senses: taste	Unusual sweetness in mouth; senses dull		Bitter taste	Sense of burning at mouth of stomach.
Appetite for food			Poor	Depraved; faulty cravings
Appetite for fluid	Absent unless salt is taken, especially in old people		Thirsty	
Muscular Tone	Weariness not accounted for by exercise	Flaccidity of limbs		
Dreams	Sees red things, blood coming out of the body, swimming in blood, and the like	Sees waters, rivers, snow, rain, cold, thunder	Sees fires, yellow flags, objects not yellow that appear yellow, a conflagration, hot bath, hot sun, etc.	Fear of darkness, of torture; terrifying black things
Movements (gestures)	Yawning, stretching			
Rational faculties: Signs	Reaction time slow; always drowsy	Sleepiness, laziness, tiredness, lassitude	Dull	Sense of anxiety wakefulness
Abnormal Phenomena	Nausea Sense of weight in back of eyes and temples Blood flows out readily from nose, anus, gums	Nausea	Yellow and green bile and acidity Gooseflesh Weak digestion and acid eruptions Severe diarrhea	Splenic disorders often occur, also ulcers

dustrial pollutants, automobile exhaust, and other noxious substances. Not only can these types of pollutants adversely affect health, but also contamination from swamps and sewers and the vapors of lakes create disease.

Let us look at the components of healthy air. By *air* I mean that which is drawn in as breath, including all the bacterial and other life that may reside within it. The substance of air is good when it is not contaminated by extraneous matters, such as those listed above. Moreover, the air should be open to the sky, meaning not shut in by high mountains or confined in caves, high walls, or closed houses. Healthy air should be clear to the sight, which usually testifies to its purity. This is accomplished by winds blowing over the area, a process that continually cleanses the air.

Closely related to the quality of air is the influence of the changes in the atmosphere that accompany seasonal and geographic variations. For example, a hot atmosphere (found in temperate and desert regions) disperses the natural force of the breath and has a relaxing effect. Too great a degree of heat results in a breakdown of the components of the blood and causes diseases of the yellow bile humor. It also causes sweating, diminishes the output of urine, impairs the digestion, and induces constant thirst.

A cold atmosphere has a constricting effect, strengthens digestion, and increases the urine. It also causes the humors to lose their fluid characteristics, so that they are much more slowly broken down into their derivative components and are eliminated with difficulty. People sweat less in a cold atmosphere, and thus the elimination of toxins with perspiration is less. Cold also causes constipation because the anal muscles remain constricted, causing the feces to remain in the rectum longer than normal, so that the watery components are reabsorbed and passed into the urine.

A moist atmosphere softens the skin and generally causes the body to be moist. A dry atmosphere dries the skin and causes it to be rough and lackluster.

A foggy atmosphere causes depression, and disturbs and confuses the humors.

The effects of these basic atmospheric qualities may be present when one lives in a region in which one of these atmospheric conditions predominates. But persons who live in areas exhibiting great seasonal changes are exposed to all of these atmospheres to a greater or lesser degree.

The seasons produce great changes in the body, and many diseases are primarily known by the season in which they occur. Spring is a healthy season, providing a temperament perfectly suited to the temperament of both blood and breath. It is in the spring that the humors—somewhat dormant over winter—begin to stir and disperse themselves more fully throughout the system, which often brings back the signs of chronic disease. People who overeat in the winter and exercise little are prone to springtime diseases.

The diseases often common in spring include nosebleeds, inflammations, carbuncles, anginas, abcesses, aggravation of varicose veins, coughs, bronchitis, pneumonia, influenza, and measles. People in whom the phlegm humor predominates will show a tendency to apoplexy, paralysis, and arthritis. These effects are multiplied if the person undergoes extreme emotional conflicts or adds excess hot spices to the food, for this enhances the effects of the atmosphere on the person. The most effective means to avoid spring diseases, or lessen their severity, are purgatives, fasting or dietary restrictions, increasing fluids, and eliminating intoxicating liquors of all types.

In the summertime the ground temperature is highest and the humors are dispersed, which impairs the faculties and natural functions. The blood and the blood humor are diminished in quantity (summer blood is said to be "thin"). Toward the end of summer, the black bile (atrabilious) humor increases. Older persons feel stronger in summer.

In summer diseases run their course in a shorter period of time, because the warm air helps to disperse and mature disease-producing matter. But persons already weakened by a disease will find it worse in the summer, and may even lose strength and die. The wetter the summer, the more prolonged the disease. Ulcers, for example, will be harder to heal, and may spread and deepen. Diarrhea and loose bowels are common in summer, owing to the general flow of excess humors from the upper body into the lower body. This also explains why people traveling from winter climates to very warm climates (such as Mexico) experience diarrhea (even though it is usually blamed on contaminated food or water). The diseases generally associated with the hot season are fevers (especially continuing ones), emaciation, pains in the ears, eye problems, and furunculosis. For those living where there are southerly winds, deaths are highest in the summer months. Northerly winds are more favorable to health.

Autumn produces many changes in the body, and much disease, for these reasons: (1) the temperature differences between daytime and nighttime are great; (2) the humors are spoiled by eating much fruit, by bad diet, and by accumulation of unresolved excesses within the interior of the body; (3) the general vigor of the body is impaired because of the effects of the preceding hot months. The disorders associated with autumn are fevers, enlargement of the spleen, scanty urine, impetigo, scabies, canker, pustules, angina, pulmonary afflictions, mental disease, diarrhea, sciatica, back and hip pain, and worms.

It must be remembered that all of these conditions which we call disease are the result of the dispersal of the normal quantity and quality of the four humors. In the summertime, because of the heat, the amount of phlegm humor (and phlegm) increases. As the autumn cold comes on increasingly, the body cannot resolve those quantities of mucus rapidly enough. Fever arises as a special heat to rapidly process the excess phlegm into a thinner substance, which is then eliminated as perspiration and/or urine. Moreover, many people do not properly adjust their diet according to these seasonal changes, and thus there is most often an increase in the black bile humor and ashlike toxic by-products of digestion. With impaired and lessened sweating and other elimination, the accumulation of humors produces diseases, according to the inherent strengths and weaknesses of the individual's body. Generally, the autumn season will produce fewer diseases if it is very damp and rainy, because the moisture assists the expulsion of excess phlegm by softening it and making it more liquid. If this does not occur, the excess phlegm becomes hardened and may remain in the body over the winter season.

Wintertime is better for digestion because people eat less. Also, the innate heat of the body is congealed within and fostered because the body responds to lower temperatures by increasing the internal heat. The disorders of winter are primarily associated with the phlegm. The blood humor is very plentiful in winter, and illnesses derived from blood humor imbalance are rarer.

Inflammations of the nose and sinuses are common in winter, and, to a lesser extent, people experience pleurisy, hoarseness, and sore throat. Even rarer are pains in the chest and sides, chronic headache, mental problems, and epileptic seizures. All of these conditions are caused by an increase in the volume of the humors and by their being condensed and confined rather than dispersed. The elderly have the hardest time in the winter, while middle-aged persons enjoy winter the most.

Many other factors connected with wind and atmospheric pressures influence general health. For example, it is said to be especially bad if a dry spring follows a dry winter, because the trees and foliage decay and produce poor feed for the animals, resulting in poor health for the people who eat them. The Chinese have gone so far as to elaborate a system of evaluating the effects of massive disturbances in the atmosphere caused by such phenomena as hurricanes, earthquakes, and tornadoes.

The influence of the atmosphere and seasonal changes has direct and profound effects on the foods growing in the soil and receiving nourishment from the rain. The growth patterns of fungi in various kinds of soil depends on the degree of cold and wetness. An observant and knowledgeable physician ought to be aware of these events of nature and be prepared to include them in evaluation of the patient.

Moreover, there are other factors that indirectly contribute to the quality of the air and atmosphere, such as the types of trees, mines and mineral deposits, cemeteries, dead animals, putrid water, clay soil, and muddy swamps.

A general statement to remember with regard to the effects of the atmosphere and air upon health is that the most harm is done by air that contracts the heart and makes full breathing difficult.

Another factor to be included in environment is the place of residence. While there are many possibilities for selecting where one will live, the following factors should be taken into account: the quality and quantity of the soil; whether the land and house are exposed or sheltered; growth of vegetation and woodlands; water supply (Is it covered or exposed to air? Does it flow down to you, or is it drawn up?); prevailing winds; proximity to ocean, mountains, etc.; mineral content of soil; what types of illnesses are common; construction of house (roomy, good ventilation, wide chimneys, doors and windows facing east and north); amount of light; general temperatures; and humidity. All of these factors have a bearing on health, and one should try and find a place to live where these are as positive as possible, considering the age, sex, and temperament of those who intend to live there.

Movement and Rest

The effect of movement on the body depends on the quantity of exercise, the degree of intensity, the degree of rest taken afterward, and the amount of movement caused to the humors as a result of the exercise. Every kind of exercise will increase the innate heat. Repose always has a cooling effect, thus retaining the humors and interfering with the elimination of waste matters. Sexual intercourse always cools the body, although the net effect may be increase of heat due to physical exertion.

Sleep and Wakefulness

Sleep causes much the same effects as repose. It strengthens all natural functions; makes the breath unclear, restrains strong evacuation, aids digestion, helps expel matter that has lost its vitality, induces sweating, and usually disperses the innate heat. The waking state has the opposite of all of these effects. Excessive sleep draws the innate heat within the body, causing the exterior to become cold.

It is a principle of nature that for humans, night is the time of sleep and day the time of action. It is ideal to retire shortly after night has fully fallen (about one hour after sunset) and arise about one hour before sunrise.

Effect of Emotions on Health

The changing states of mind are part of what is called *nafs* in Tibb. *Nafs* is an Arabic word that generally refers to all of the appetites of the body and ego—for food, sex, fame, and many related things. The changing of the states of mind produces swings in mood, and these are known by the signs of the breath. If the breath is kept completely controlled and measured equally between in and out breaths, there will be stability of mind and balanced emotions. Unbalanced emotions are the result of disturbances of the balance of the breath. These changes are summarized in the following table.

The inhalation of breath is the cycle of contraction, while the exhalation is the cycle of expansion. The degree of expansion and contraction of breath affects the health. Mental events such as dreams also relate to health. For example, a person dreaming of fiery red things may be experiencing an imbalance

TABLE 5
BREATH AND EMOTIONS

Emotion	Quality of Breath	Direction
Anger	Sudden and forced	Exhalation
Delight, joy	Gentle and gradual	Exhalation
Fear, terror	Sudden and forced	Inhalation
Gloom, depression	Gentle and gradual	Inhalation

or a great increase in the blood humor. There is a well-evolved science of dream analysis and interpretation in Tibb, although it is practiced by religious savants more than by physicians.

According to Tibb, conditions of the mind, mental "diseases" in particular, are not the cause of physical ailments, but rather the result of disturbance of balance in the humors. A person muddled in his mental processes, for example, might appear to have an intellectual deficiency or some other "psychological" ailment. However, imbalance of the phlegm humor would account for the sluggishness of mental faculties and would be treated by resolving the excess phlegm humor so as to restore fluidity of mental processes. Such imbalances can be caused by thoughts, sounds, foods, and other factors, and they can be corrected with the same, or their opposites. Anyone who truly seeks the truth about health and wellness will not ignore these points.

There are five factors that will determine the particular organ or system in which the symptoms of disease appear. These are: (1) strength of the organ affected by the imbalance; (2) weakness of the organ receiving the by-products of the disordered metabolism; (3) excess superfluous matters in the body; (4) weakness of nutritive forces (poor digestion, weak liver, etc.); and (5) dilation of arteries or widening of channels carrying humors.

As noted before, there are congenital factors which are beyond the scope of self-treatment but are presented here for interest: diseases of morphology, narrowed ducts, widened ducts, increase and decrease in correct number of organs, hypertrophy, atrophy, accidents, and displacement of organs.

Now we have a composite profile of the body and its parts according to Unani traditional healing, and the basic ways in which the health is evaluated to determine how and where an imbalance of humors arises. The Tibb system considers that foods and beverages taken in as nutrients constitute the building materials of the body, including the humors. Therefore, the selection of foods for general nutrition and in correcting imbalances forms the most central part of the Tibb system of healing. I have omitted the causative factors associated with food intake and evacuation in this chapter because the subjects are so important as to warrant complete discussion. Therefore, the next two chapters will be devoted to the role that food plays in maintaining the body in a healthy state.

4
Dietetics: The Influence of Food and Drink

The Unani Tibb system places great emphasis upon diet. As Avicenna wrote, "Most illnesses arise solely from long-continued errors of diet and regimen." The manner in which foods affect the body is viewed in Tibb from a simple yet highly interesting vantage point.

There are three aspects of metabolism of food: digestion, assimilation, and residue. *Digestion* here means the initial breakdown of foods in the mouth and stomach. *Assimilation* refers to the absorption of micronutrients into the bloodstream and cells. The evacuation of *residue* implies the amount of waste products that remain after a food is completely metabolized by the body. All three of these functions must be carried out efficiently.

Although there are many complex biochemical events that transpire during the digestive process, Avicenna suggests that digestion be viewed as a process by which foods are heated or "cooked" by the body. By this is meant that the foods are altered from their state when taken into the mouth, and refined or broken down into ever-smaller nutrient parts by the process of heating. A review of the digestive process will confirm this.

Humans preserve their lives through nourishment, which they obtain through eating. The digestive processes are applied unconsciously until the food is assimilated into blood, which then carries various other biochemical components to sites in the body, and these are manufactured into tissue, flesh, organs, and other body parts. Digestion means, then, that nourishment is changed inside the body by natural heat (cooked) until it actually becomes a part of the body or is eliminated. In Tibb this process of cooking by the body is called *pokhtta*.

Food that enters the mouth first comes into contact with enzymes, which create a type of heat. The food is chewed and masticated with the teeth—another form of heat, friction from grinding. The food is then swallowed into the stomach, where hydrochloric acid (an intense heat) breaks down the solids into a semifluid mass called chyme—the essence of the food. The stomach sends this chyme via the small intestine (where additional enzymes create added heat and processing) to the site of the liver. At the liver, the finest parts are made into blood, and valuable nutrient components are carried out into the general system to participate in various chemical events that transform them into the myriad forms of the body.

Western biochemical medicine endeavors to trace each of these complex chemical interactions, and ultimately to discover when and where one or more of the biochemical exchanges are amiss. A medical pathologist, in searching for the cause of a disease, will often try to find which enzymes are functioning improperly. The pathologist can identify about twenty-eight enzymes present in each liver cell, although these same enzymes sometimes travel to far points in the body and are involved in complex processes not directly related to liver function or stomach digestion of foods. This approach might have validity if there were only twenty-eight enzymes in the cells, but there are not. In fact, a pathologist knows that more than one thousand individual enzymes have been "identified" in each liver cell, yet only about twenty-eight of these are understood definitely in terms of their functions. What the other enzymes do is not known at all.

If the one thousand enzymes were the outer limit, there might be hope. But no one knows if there are one thousand enzymes in each liver cell: there may be many thousands, or millions, or billions, or an uncountable number. The fact is, no one knows. Not at all.

Even if we assume that the one thousand enzymes are the limit, this means that with knowledge and consideration of only twenty-eight of them, Western medicine makes decisions based upon somewhat less than 3 percent of the total number of affecting enzymatic agents in just the liver! Of course, there are thousands more biochemical components that also affect sex, digestion, thinking, breathing, and every other human activity. The number of biochemical interactions are virtually limitless, and new discoveries are being announced almost daily—leading to the discarding of prior theories and treatments. In fact, not even one medicine that is in today's pharmacy was on the shelf as short a time as ten years ago.

Traditional healing, while taking some interest in these complex biochemical interactions, holds that ultimately we cannot know the total interworkings of the human body. There are many religious references to the fact that the human body has been created "infinitely more complex than the entire universe" (Hadith). Therefore, the Tibb system retreats to a comprehensible stance, which evaluates food and diet in terms of their ability to enhance or impede *metabolism*.

In Tibb, more than one single component of the food's "action" or "value" is taken into account—just as Western medical dietetics evaluates not just calories but also fat, protein, vitamins, and so forth.

In Tibb, all food substances that are consumed for the primary purpose of nutritive value (as opposed to medicinal nutrients) are called *aliment*. These aliment substances are said to possess two functions besides mere nutrition: (a) *rate of penetration*, or absorption (rapid penetration: liquids; slow penetration or absorption: roast meats and fried meats); (b) *compactness* of the substance of the digestive products in the blood, and consequent retention (this is the feature of pork, for example); or "attenuation" of the substance, meaning very rapid dispersal (as with figs and many fruits).

A great many factors and considerations follow from the above, but one of the most important is that foods should be selected that (a) are in accord with the temperament of the individual and appropriate to the season, age, climate, etc.; and (b) produce balance in the four humors.

The hot-cold dichotomy can also be explained as one factor of the considerations regarding nutritive process. Absorptive ability of foods relates to their digestibility. The power of forcefulness of the digestive energy of the person will determine the assimilability of the foods. In Tibb, the nutritive value of a food is decided by how much of each humor it produces.

The physiological value specifically relates to the hot-cold value. It is a more general aspect and the first aspect we think of, and the part that anyone can understand, as opposed to the evaluation of more complex phenomena, which a Hakim would undertake in deciding a regimen (the foregoing factors, their degree of completeness and function, are determined from a variety of diagnostic signs: pulse, urine, feces, etc.).

The hot-cold assignment is due to whether an ash is left in the tissues after oxidation or not. Thus, humorally cold foods leave more ash, and humorally hot foods leave much less. The matter of formation of ash is significant because of the risk of its lingering in the body or even becoming firmly imprisoned within the tissues.

A confirmation of the scientific validity of the Unani Tibb view of the metabolic efficiency of foods and digestion is found in recent research on enzymes. Edward Howell, M.D., is the world's leading authority on enzyme activity in food digestion. In *Enzyme Nutrition* (Avery Publishing Group, 1985), Dr. Howell's extensive research proves that 80 percent of enzyme activity is devoted to the digestion of food. Since *all* enzymes contained in raw foods are destroyed by freezing, boiling, frying, and radiation, many people consume food that has no enzyme content whatsoever.

Dr. Howell's research also reveals that when spices such as ginger, cumin, and cinnamon—the heating spices—are consumed, the production of digestive enzymes by the body *increases* dramatically.

Even more important, whenever the body undergoes fasting, enzymes normally assigned by the body to digest food are freed to conduct healing functions, such as dissolving latent tumors.

Such respected scientific research proves the value of the Unani Tibb "heating" foods and spices—they accomplish an increase in digestive enzymes, an increase in cellular metabolic function, and ensure complete assimilation of micronutrients with minimum metabolic waste.

In sum, then, by assigning a food a value as hot or cold, we mean that a heating food has the capacity to increase the metabolisms of the body (whatever they may be). Conversely, a cold food slows down metabolism. We recognize that it is the body itself that must perform the final healing, and we try to assist the body as much as possible in these endeavors. These facts can be discerned in terms of the results observed after taking in the foods, sometimes immediately, at other times over a period of time. If we had a thermometer that was measured in billionths of degrees instead of tenths, we could actually see the body temperature rise after eating a preponderance of hot foods. This idea is perfectly in accord with the laws of physics, which state that an increase in atomic velocity causes an increase in temperature.

Now, with all of the evaluations of temperament that were given in the preceding sections, one can easily determine whether a cold or hot imbalance lies at the root of disease signs.

The breakdown of nutrients as a process of the liver continues, and from this point the four humors and by-products of digestion are formed. The chart of the four humors presented in Chapter 2 may be reviewed to follow the fate of the foods through to the end of digestion and elimination.

Here is where we can begin to understand how and why disease arises. Let us assume for a moment that we have a person before us complaining of illness (the symptoms are unimportant for the moment). The very first thing we do is take the temperature, to determine precisely how well this process of heating is carrying on. Let us also assume that the patient's temperature is 97.6° Fahrenheit. Most people know that the "average" body temperature in healthy adults is given as 98.6° F. But it is important to understand just what this average means. An average is the middle point of many samples taken. In other words, to arrive at this statistical measure of normalcy, probably thousands of patients' temperatures were taken. They were then arranged on a scale from lowest to highest, added together, then divided by the total number of persons in the sample. This is how an average is derived. Therefore, according to the rules of statistics, it is also true that less than 5 percent of the total sample of patients *actually had* temperatures of 98.6°. The rest fell above or below.

Why does the temperature matter so much? We may assume that 98.6° is the actual optimum temperature for healthy functioning of the body. Lesser or higher temperatures are signs that the metabolism is disordered. So, if the reading was 96.6°, it would mean that the person's temperature was two degrees below the normal average. So what? There is a mental trick being played here, because of our decimal thinking, which assumes incorrectly that it is two degrees out of one hundred that is off. But it is actually two degrees out of the range that *sustains life*. We realize that life is carried on within rather narrow limits of temperature—95° to 105°, that if the temperature goes outside those limits for any extended time, life will end. Therefore, a temperature two degrees below normal means one that is two degrees deficient within the ten degrees that sustains life—or that the body is operating at 20 percent lowered efficiency. If you tried to operate any machine with 20 percent of its power source gone, the other parts would become stressed and overheated, and the machine would break down and wear out much sooner than if it were operating at 100 percent of its energy levels.

This example holds true for the body. The process of heating is undermined when the "heat" (called innate heat, or vital power) of the digestive process is lowered in proper intensity. What happens is that many of the foods eaten are not fully broken down into the smallest nutrient components, and this places a great strain upon the body to deal with incompletely digested foods.

The thermal function of the body is admitted by Western biologists to be situated in the liver. It is true that other glands and substances may have ancillary effects on thermal maintenance of the body. But without the liver, no one can survive for even a short period.

If we understand that each food has an inherent degree of heat or coldness—in other words, promotes or slows down metabolism—we can begin to select dietary items that harmonize all of the natural functions of the body. This is a general system of dietetics that can be learned, understood, and applied by virtually anyone—and which can be adjusted according to every possible factor of change or difference in life-style and life place. Moreover, the Tibb system of dietetics is the most widely practiced system of dietetics in the history of the world, and today remains in force for one-quarter of the world's population. It is ignorant and unscientific to assert that the combined human experience and unified results of untold billions of people over thousands of years are based upon stupidity and erroneous thinking.

What happens when the foods are not eaten according to metabolic principles? The first problem is that the foods are incompletely digested. The body responds in many ways, but the result in that superfluous matters build up in the system. This may continue for long or short periods. In due course, the body will reach the limit of excess and move into a corrective mode. This is accomplished by the strange heat we call fever, which serves to rapidly refine, or "cook down," the excess superfluous matters so that they can be eliminated by the body. This elimination is called the "healing crisis" in Tibb, and it occurs in five specific ways and no others. (A complete explanation of the healing crisis is given in Chapter 9.) One of these forms of crisis is diarrhea, which is no more or less than a rapid evacuation of superfluous (and toxic) by-products of incomplete digestion. The same thing is true of mucus and vomiting. Yet the entire approach of Western medicine is to end the fever, control the diarrhea, and stem the nausea with drugs. Therefore, the very processes the body itself chooses to correct excess are halted, and these unnecessary and damaging effluviants are turned back in upon the body, to cause further and more complex diseases to arise.

The only correct treatment of diseases is to assist the natural functions of the body. Infants and children prove these concepts perfectly. First, the average body temperature of an infant is said to be about 99.0°. This higher metabolic rate is necessary to effectively process down all of the unusual amounts of by-products that result from the child's great and rapid growth. Moreover, infants and small children exhibit vomiting, nosebleeds, diarrhea, fevers, sweating, and frequent urination—precisely the forms of healing crisis according to Tibb.

Later chapters will take up specific regimens of diet and herbs to correct imbalances after they have led to symptoms and imbalance. For now I wish to present a list of foods with their metabolic values. By constructing diet according to these principles, one can prevent a great proportion of the diseases of humankind.

A few remarks about this list will add to our understanding. The basic diet of the majority of Americans—milk, beef, potatoes, lettuce salads, refined white sugars, cheese, butter, margarine, etc.—is revealed as *all* cold foods. And cold foods lead to imbalance of the phlegm humor, first of all, and cause all of the list of complaints that are epidemic in America: migraine headache, menstrual cramps, lung and chest problems, arthritis, constipation, etc., etc. And, as the indiscretion in food consumption is continued, in time the other humors become imbalanced. When such imbalance reaches the fourth stage of the black bile humor, the diseases called cancer, arteriosclerosis, emphysema, and others arise. (The Tibb point of view on cancer will be discussed in Chapter 11.)

Moreover, if we consider those foods from the hot list—such as lamb, liver, goat, ghee, beet, lentils, eggplant, chick peas, dried fruits, nuts, honey, and spices such as cardamom, fenugreek, ginger, cumin, saffron, and cinnamon—we readily observe that these are among the *least* consumed foods in America. Even if they are consumed, it is usually part of some "exotic" experimental cuisine, not incorporated into the daily diet. These heating foods are necessary for the body to achieve and maintain a complete metabolic digestion of foods. This is the most elegant, useful, and refined manner of constructing diet and, if followed with sincerity, will provide the real basis of health for all people of all ages.

You will note that we have arranged all of the foods only according to hot and cold values, and not moist and dry. This is so because moisture is a function of heat, as heat drives off moisture. Therefore, the primary focus is on the hot-cold value of the food.

However, to facilitate use of all foods, and to use some as medicine and others simply as nutrients, Unani Tibb arranges the hot and cold foods into classifications by degrees. There are four degrees each of hot and cold, making a total of eight possible categories into which a food may be placed. Thus a food may be:

Hot in the First Degree		Cold in the First Degree
Hot in the Second Degree	or	Cold in the Second Degree
Hot in the Third Degree		Cold in the Third Degree
Hot in the Fourth Degree		Cold in the Fourth Degree

These degrees have the following effects:

First degree: Affects metabolism, but not in any way discerned by overt physical sensation. Slightest action. Water is an example of a first-degree substance.

METABOLIC VALUES OF FOODS

Heating (Garmi) Foods

Meat and Fish: lamb, liver, chicken, goose, duck, eggs, goat (male)

Dairy Products: sheep's milk, cream cheese, cream, clarified butter (ghee)

Vegetables and Beans: asparagus, beet, radish, onion, mustard greens, kidney beans, leek, eggplant, chick peas, red pepper, green pepper, carrot seed, squash, turnip, parsley

Fruits: peach, plum, lime, lemon, rhubarb, banana, red raisins, green raisins, dates, figs, olives, ripe grapes, all dried fruits

Seeds and Nuts: sesame, almond, pistachio, apricot kernels, walnut, pine nuts

Grains: thin-grain rice, basmati rice, wheat

Oils: sesame oil, corn oil, castor oil, mustard oil

Beverages: black tea, milk

Herbs: basil, cinnamon, cardamom, cloves, coriander, cumin, fenugreek, garlic, ginger, marjoram, mint, celery seed, anise seed, rue, saffron, garam masala (blend), curry powder (blend), senna, frankincense, mustard

Other: vermicelli, honey, rock candy, all sweet things, salt, all modern medicine

Cooling (Sardi) Foods

Meat: rabbit, goat (female), beef, fish (general)

Dairy Products: cow's milk, mother's milk, goat's milk, butter, buttermilk, dried cheeses, margarine

Vegetables and Beans: lettuce, celery, sprouts (general), zucchini, spinach, cabbage, okra, cauliflower, broccoli, white potato, sweet potato, carrot, cucumber, soybeans, tomato, turnip, peas, beans (general)

Fruits: apple, melons (general), mulberries, peach, pear, coconut, fig, pomegranate, apricot, orange, carob

Seeds and Nuts: none

Grains: brown rice, thick-grain rice, barley, lentils

Oils: sunflower oil, coconut oil

Beverages: green teas, coffee

Herbs: coriander (dry), dill, henna, thyme, rose, jasmine

Other: refined sugar, vinegar, bitter things, sour things, truffles, water

Second degree: Acts upon the body, causing metabolic change, but in the end is overwhelmed by the body. All nutrients belong in this category. Among the actions caused by second-degree substances are opening of pores, initiation of peristaltic action, perspiration, and stimulation of digestion. Ginger is an example of the second degree.

Third degree: Not acted upon by the body, but acts upon the body. All medicinal substances belong to this category. An example is senna pods, which overwhelm the eliminative powers of the colon and force evacuation.

Fourth degree: Poisons. Cause cessation of metabolic function. Some herbs are used as medicines from this category, but only in the most minute strengths and under the direct supervision of a physician. Hemlock and belladonna are examples of the fourth degree.

The difference between these degrees in terms of hot and cold values is that a second-degree hot substance would speed up metabolism, while a second-degree cold would slow it down. In the extreme fourth degree, the difference would become more apparent, when a hot herb would cause an increase of metabolism beyond the limits that support life, while a fourth-degree cold substance would slow down metabolism to the point of death.

Tibb Cuisine

Virtually all dietary systems, including those considered alternative or natural, evaluate foods according to the various nutrient components—proteins, fats, carbohydrates, vitamins, amino acids, and so forth. In Tibb, the food is selected according to each food's ability to enhance the metabolism of the body in general and specific organs in particular. The recipes have evolved from more than a thousand years of continuous use.

In selecting foods for yourself or your family, many factors have to be taken into account, for each person is unique and has specific dietary needs. Thus, in addition to evaluating diet in relation to the climate and humidity, season, geographical region, basic temperament, predominant humor, prevalent local bacteria or parasites, and similar factors, one should try to obtain the best and purest quality of food possible. In today's marketplace, this is no easy task.

Most foods offered for sale in a chain supermarket in the United States have been treated with chemicals and pesticides. The claim has been made that testing has proved these chemicals safe for human beings. But long-term effects may appear, as has happened with virtually every food additive initially approved by governmental agencies. Even if the small quantities added to one food, and tested alone, may be considered safe, when the cumulative effect of many hundreds of chemicals is added to the years and decades of consumption, it is fair to assume that the eliminative and detoxifying organs of the body are overwhelmed.

Besides chemicals added during processing, there are many toxic substances used in the growing of the vegetables, fruits, or meats, plus the preserving sprays used on items such as tomatoes, potatoes, apples, and dozens of other foods. Therefore, anyone seeking food of a high degree of purity must grow it at home. Possibly the greatest contribution to health that could occur in the United States would be for each family to begin growing a substantial portion of its own food according to organic principles, without chemical fertilizers and pesticides.

In particular, the meat offered for sale in supermarkets should not be considered safe for human consumption, owing to the addition of chemical drugs and other poisons used to control the growth cycles of the animals. This point has been elaborated in so many journals and articles by impeccable authorities that it needs no further comment here. Moreover, as a matter of economy, many growers feed their animals things that, frankly speaking, are garbage that is rejected for consumption for humans, and even for cats and dogs. I even knew personally of a beef-raising operation that bought candy bars that had been damaged in freight train wrecks, and used this for cattle feed—paper wrappers and all. Any animal grown on such matter cannot be considered proper nourishment for a human being.

Many people desire to have an "ideal" diet that would be the once-and-for-all perfect blending of nutrients and food groups. Such a diet is impossible to formulate, for within each household are usually found five or six persons with widely varying needs. Infants, children, teenagers, adults, and the elderly cannot be expected to thrive on exactly the same foods.

The timing of meals is important. Breakfast means literally "breaking the fast" of the previous eight to twelve hours. Breakfast can be a substantial meal of whole grain cereals and breads, fruits, eggs, cheese, and tea. The best time for breakfast is shortly after rising from sleep but after performing the toilet and any prayer or meditation practices.

The noon meal is best taken after the sun has passed the midpoint in the sky. There is no harm if it is delayed until one or two in the afternoon, but not much beyond that. This is probably the best time to take the largest meal of the day because metabolism is functioning at its highest rate for most people. Americans by habit allow the noon meal to become little more than a snack, but it is the main meal for most people in the world. The composition of this meal will depend on all of the foregoing factors and also on what kind of work one does. If you do consume your main meal at noon, it is best to take a short rest afterward, a nap of not more than forty-five minutes to an hour. This interlude will provide an opportunity for the body to digest the meal, and you will arise with considerably renewed energy to work the rest of the day without becoming sluggish.

The evening meal should be taken just after sunset and should include meat or vegetable protein, wheat or other whole grains, little or no fruit, and little sweets. It is best to conclude all eating at least two hours before sleep.

By adjusting the mealtimes to the rising and setting of the sun, one is conforming to the cycles of nature and the motions of the stars and planets, all of which have an effect upon human physiological functions. The sun may rise as early as 4:00 AM in the summer and as late as 7:30 AM in the winter.

Another important consideration is to eat foods in season. You may be able to obtain all manner of foods throughout the year, but your body will accommodate these foods best if they are eaten mainly in the season when they are harvested. It upsets the temperaments to eat strawberries in winter, for example, for it is an early summer fruit. Likewise, cucumbers—a cooling vegetable— should be avoided in winter. The natural cycles of the region in which one lives support the biolife that is suitable for people living there. Eskimos seldom, if ever, eat bananas! The monoculture of America's nationwide distribution system, along with methods of preserving foods, means we can buy and consume virtually any food on earth at any time. While this may seem to be a boon and accomplishment of technology, eating foods out of season confuses the temperaments and burdens the metabolism.

Also, whenever possible, one should eat foods grown in the locality in which one lives. This means that residents of California should not eat New York apples. The Hakims say that the onions, potatoes, and other root vegetables from one's own region contain antidotes for all of the bacteria and viruses that are common in your town.

The most important law regarding diet is this: never eat unless there is true hunger. When a true and ready appetite appears, the meal should be taken soon afterward and not delayed, or the stomach will fill with putrefying digestive gases and digestion will be spoiled.

There is no greater harm than to eat to full satisfaction after going a long time without food. This places an unbelievable stress on the digestive powers and clogs up the channels through which the humors are dispersed. Many heart attacks occur after eating an overlarge meal.

After eating, it is best to take some light activity such as walking. This allows the food to move into the lower part of the stomach, where digestion can be carried on more readily. This is especially important to do if one has the desire to lie down or feels sluggish. Mental excitement, emotion, excessive exercise, and sexual intercourse all hinder digestion.

The amount to eat in a standard meal depends upon the general condition and activity of the person. A normal, healthy person should eat enough without producing a feeling of heaviness or a sense of tightness in the solar plexus area. After eating, there should be no rumbling of the stomach or sloshing of the food on movement. Nausea, sour belching, and a lingering taste of the meal are signs that the meal was too heavy.

Foods that are quickly and easily digested should not be taken along with foods that are hard to digest. The food that is digested first will, being lighter, float over the top of the undigested food, trapping it. Unable to enter the blood, it will be retained unnecessarily long in the stomach and begin fermenting, resulting in gas and belching. A listing of the digestion times of many foods is given in Appendix III.

All liquids taken simultaneously with food dilute the gastric juices and therefore are not recommended with meals. Nor should much liquid be taken after a meal, for it causes the food to leave the lining of the stomach and float about. If there is a great thirst after a meal, it is best to satisfy it with cold water—the colder it is, the less will be required to quench the thirst.

When the initial stage of digestion is over (about thirty minutes), evidenced by a feeling of lightness in the upper part of the diaphragm, some tea may be taken, preferably one that aids digestion, such as peppermint. Oranges are ideal to eat after a meal, for the citric acid helps digestion and the fruit satisfies any thirst.

There are many well-considered opinions about the eating of meat, both for and against. There is no harm in adopting a strict vegetarian diet, provided that one exercises great care in selecting those foods that will combine to manufacture vital amino acids and necessary enzymes.

It is my personal opinion that it is permissible from a moral point of view to eat meat. However, as has been stated, all meats from commercial supermarkets should be shunned. This means one should raise and slaughter animals for one's own consumption. For city dwellers this poses some problems, but by checking with the best health food stores and Muslim (halal) and Jewish (kosher) meat markets, you can discover sources of pure meats. However, do some questioning of the butcher. Just because meat has been slaughtered according to religious law does not mean it has been grown without chemicals. Regardless of the source of the meat, the quantity of meat consumed to remain healthy and promote growth is not as much as people consume in the United States. Eating reasonable portions twice or three times a week is more than sufficient. In any event, eating meat three times per day in huge quantities produces disease.

Some meats should not be eaten at all. These include pork and any animal that eats carrion (already dead) flesh, such as dogs, cats, most birds of prey, snakes, and many wild animals. The easiest meat to digest is that of fowl. All fish are acceptable, but you should prefer those that do not feed off the refuse on the ocean or river floors. Lamb is the best meat, and that of a male yearling is preferred over older sheep. The shoulder cut is the most nutritious.

Try to find others with whom you can share meals. Everyone knows the dull feeling of eating alone. Organize people in your neighborhood, office, or club to prepare and eat meals together, at least once or twice a week. There is a saying in the East: "He who eats alone eats with Satan; he who eats with one other person eats with a tyrant; he who eats with two other people eats with the prophets."

With the foregoing as an understanding of the principles of Tibb dietetics, I present, in the next chapter, recipes based upon these concepts. These dishes are balanced, meaning that all of the elements of heating and cooling properties are nearly equal. Sometimes the hotter spices are present to offset cool vegetables, and vice versa. The overall effect of one of these meals, which would include bread, main dish, side dishes, and fruits, will produce the correct effects in the body. However, if one has been eating the so-called typical American diet of fast foods and many snacks, unusual effects may be felt. In such cases it is not uncommon to experience a flush of warmth or a slight fever. This is one of the effects from cumin and ginger. However, such things disappear within a day or two, and one is on the way to restoring the full functioning of all bodily systems. It is also common the first time one eats this cuisine to be excused from the table with great urgency to empty the bowels or bladder.

You will note that I do not present recipes for hundreds of different dishes. It is an unfortunate fact that most people live to eat instead of eating to live. They make eating a contest to find ever-more delicious and sumptuous meals, and seldom duplicate a meal in a whole year. However, the body will work much more effectively if a simple and basic diet is followed. There is ample variety in ten or twelve different main dishes to satisfy nutritional requirements. This cuts down on preparation time and costs less too, and the tendency to overeat is lessened.

The following chapter contains the basic recipes in the Tibb system of health. They are derived from the cuisine of Afghanistan, Pakistan, India, and other places where the Tibb system is in use for both health and medical treatment. Some very minor adjustments have been made for transposing them to the United States. All of the ingredients can be obtained easily from health food stores or from the sources listed in Appendix III.

The key to Tibb cooking is producing a spice-oil-vegetable base. It does not matter which meat or vegetables are used, for they all turn out vastly delicious and satisfying. In fact, it is no exaggeration to say that it will prove to be the most delicious food you have ever eaten, and is at once so simple and elegant that any guests will think you are a master chef, even after just a few tries at producing these recipes.

5
Foods for Health

The most impressive features of Tibb traditional cooking are its simplicity, the extraordinary deliciousness of its dishes, ease of preparation, and inexpensive ingredients.

The basic food around which the Tibb cuisine is formed is rice. Rice is an annual species of cereal grass called *Oryza sativa*, which Confucius said is "a necessary and appropriate food for the virtuous and graceful life." It is said that eating rice increases pleasant dreams and produces an abundance of semen.

While certain natural diets include brown rice, most Americans eat little rice. The average yearly per-capita consumption of rice in the United States is only twelve pounds, while the consumption in many Asian countries is as high as 400 pounds per year per person. In an informative article in the April 1984 issue of *East West Journal*, nutrition writer Bill Thomson revealed the astonishing fact that there are more than 30,000 rice farmers in the United States, who harvest about seven million tons of rice annually, but two-thirds of it is exported. Mr. Thomson further points out that of all the rice consumed in this country, only 1.6 percent is brown rice, and he estimates that just 0.3 percent is organically farmed.

My own preference and recommendation for the staple rice in the diet is that variety called basmati. Known throughout the world as the Lord of Rice, basmati is a thin-grained, slender white rice, minimally milled. You should make certain to obtain genuine Indian or Pakistani basmati rice, which can be purchased from one of the sources in Appendix III. Some health food stores and cooperatives also sell what they call tex-mati, which is a hybrid strain of basmati grown in Texas and cannot be considered equal to the genuine basmati, which is hand-seeded, hand-cultivated and hand-harvested, and watered from the snow-fed rivers of the Himalyan mountains, then sun-dried. Brown rice could also be used, but for most of these recipes, the texture and flavor of basmati is preferred, and you will not get the same results using any other type of rice.

Skillets and pots should be of cast iron or stainless steel, and implements such as spoons of stainless steel or wood. There is a special frying pan called *tawa* that is useful if you make chapatis or other quick breads on a daily basis. It is slightly concave and proportions the heat in just the right manner to give the best results. If you do not have a *tawa*, you can use a regular frying pan, but watch the heat so that the breads do not burn. Some people cook with woks, but Tibb is a slow cooking system, and the metal of woks is so thin that many of the sauces will burn. There is a special curved Indian pot, shaped just like a Chinese wok but much thicker. You can buy one at a good East Indian grocery.

Spice mixtures can be purchased from the suppliers in the Appendix, or you can make them yourself from individual ingredients from the health food store. However, even health food stores may not buy the particular quality of spices or herbs used in these blends. Therefore, for superior results, invest in the basic stock of herbs for Tibb cooking. When you buy powdered coriander, garlic, cumin, or cinnamon from the sources mentioned, you will find them much less expensive than they are at a grocery store. For example, eight ounces of powdered cumin in only about $1.50, compared with nearly twice that for one ounce in a supermarket. And these spices are really fresh and pungent, rather than the dried-out, tasteless spices sold in jars in most stores.

Ghee is a necessary ingredient in some dishes for best results. Ghee is clarified butter, which is made by boiling butter to separate the milk solids. You can buy prepared ghee for about the same price as raw butter. A little ghee goes a long way and will add a tremendous depth to your foods, especially curries. Some breads, such as parathas, cannot be made properly without ghee.

Chapatis are the basic bread I recommend to eat with the Tibb food. These are five-inch round, flat, unleavened breads, similar in size, shape, and consistency to the Mexican tortilla. Chapatis cannot, however, be made with either white or whole wheat flour, but require a special blend of whole wheat and semolina that is specific to chapatis. Many people love chapatis when they eat them in a restaurant, but are sorely disappointed when they try to make them at home from whole wheat flour. It took me some time to discover that it wasn't my or my wife's fault that we weren't getting a good result. This special flour is a must. And it is very reasonable, only $5.00 for almost twenty-five pounds, enough for all the daily breads for a family of five or six for three months. Chapati flour can be purchased from the suppliers listed in the Appendix.

You should make up enough dough to last several days (even for a week) at one time, and store it in a tightly sealed plastic jar in the refrigerator. The opportunity to eat steaming hot, delicious bread with each meal will be an ample reward for the small effort required in making these breads.

I recommend that honey be used wherever conceivably possible, and that refined white sugar be eliminated from the home and the diet, totally and forever. The single exception to this rule is that sugar is required to activate yeast when making breads. Otherwise, honey can always be substituted for sugar. Honey in and of itself is a healing substance, and the disastrous effects of refined white sugar cause a reasonable person to shun it entirely. You can sometimes obtain unrefined or minimally processed sugar in East Indian food stores. This substance is called *gur* (also known as *jaggery*) and resembles hard brown sugar. It can be used in some of the recipes in lieu of white sugar.

Salt is a necessary ingredient in cooking for health. I recommend sun-dried, unprocessed sea salt. The macrobiotic sea salt mined and sold by Niguro Miramoto (usually called Miramoto Salt) is the best in the world, but definitely expensive (up to $6.00 a pound). Read the label carefully on any salt bought in the store. Find one that does not contain sugar (yes, dextrose, or sugar, is the main adulterant in almost all salt sold in stores, believe it or not).

Some time should be expended on shopping for food and preparing and eating the meal. The cooking fragrances that fill up a homey kitchen and house send important signals to the body to conclude the digestive work of the prior meal. Even persons who work at full-time jobs will find these recipes easy to prepare, with a complete meal for five or six persons requiring not more than one hour of preparation. The secret of Tibb cooking is in the spices and proportions used, as well as in the sequence in which items are added and cooked.

Generally speaking, I recommend using a pure, high-grade olive oil for cooking and frying. While it seems a bit of an extravagance to some, olive oil is the purest oil there is, and it will not turn rancid, not even in a thousand years (all other vegetable or nut oils soon turn bitter). Olive oil contains zero cholesterol. After olive oil, in terms of preference, come peanut oil, safflower oil, and sesame oil.

Garam masala ("heating spices") is a spice blend that forms the basis of many dishes, particularly rice and meat dishes. The best garam masala can be purchased from one of the sources in the Appendix. But if you want to make your own, mix equal parts of powdered ginger, powdered cumin, powdered coriander, powdered black pepper, and powdered cinnamon with one-half part powdered nutmeg. There are quite a few different blends of garam masala, but this is a good basic one.

If you want to make a curry powder, make up the garam masala, and add to it:

1 part turmeric
1 part red pepper
½ part fenugreek
½ part black mustard seeds

Do not use ready-made curry powders. Actually a curry is a particular kind of dish and never uses a curry powder blend as an ingredient. As you will see in the recipes, the curry dishes combine all of the ingredients in a special sequence of preparation. Curry powders can never provide an eating experience comparable to these carefully crafted dishes.

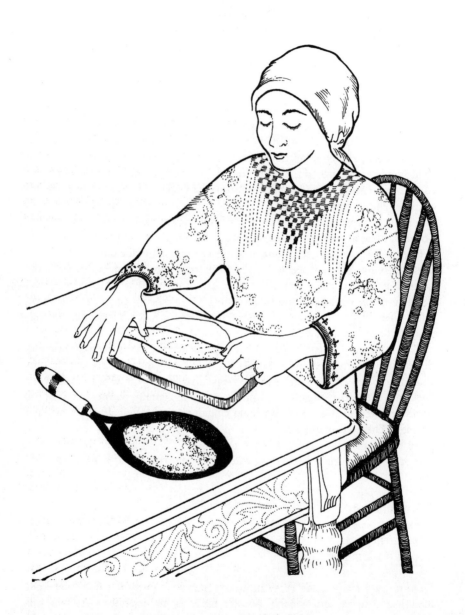

Tibb Recipes

Breads

Naun

Naun is the standard whole wheat, slightly leavened bread of Afghanistan. It is the most delicious and satisfying bread I have ever eaten. However, in Afghanistan they use a special earthen, wood-fired oven, which imparts a quality that cannot be duplicated by any other technology. Few have such an oven in America, but the following method produces an acceptable substitute. The bread takes less than an hour and can be prepared fresh daily.

1 package
(1 tablespoon)
dry yeast

1 teaspoon sugar

¼ cup lukewarm
water

3 cups sifted whole-
wheat flour

½ teaspoon salt

¾ cup cold water

Dissolve yeast and sugar in water and set aside.

Sift together flour and salt and add to the yeast mixture.

Measure ¼ cup cold water and add gradually to the flour-yeast mixture. Mix with the hand as the water is added, using a bit more water if needed to produce a smooth, firm dough (the same consistency as ordinary bread dough). Cover and allow to stand in a moderately warm place (over the pilot light is great) for 1 hour. The dough will not quite double in size, but drawing a fingernail across the surface will show small bubbles forming.

This is enough dough for about one large naun, but it is better if you make it into two, for ease of spreading out the dough and to make sure it isn't too thick, as naun should be on the thin side or it gets a little cakey and indigestible.

Preheat the oven to 500 °F, and in it preheat a large cookie sheet that has been covered with aluminum foil. Divide the dough into two balls, allow to stand for 5 minutes, and then begin to shape it into an oval, flat piece about ⅓ to ½ inch thick. The oval should measure about 7 by 12 inches, and both of them should fit onto one cookie sheet. It may help to attain the right shape if you pat the dough out first, then pick it up and flip if from palm to palm. After the naun is shaped and placed on the cookie sheets dip three fingers into cold water and make three lengthwise grooves down the center of each (if you are a female), or wet the tip of a sharp knife and make several lengthwise cuts (if you are a male).

Remove the now-heated cookie sheet from the oven and lightly brush the surface with an oiled piece of paper towel or cloth. Place the shaped naun on the hot cookie sheet and bake immediately. The time for cooking seems to depend on the type of stove, altitude, and other factors, but usually about 6 to 10 minutes is enough. Do not overcook, but remove when you see the top just beginning to show the slightest browning. Remove and immediately put under broiler for another thirty seconds. Watch so that it does not burn at this final step!

Remove from oven and serve warm or cold, cut into 4-inch squares. Naun will keep for a day or two if wrapped up tight in plastic bags. Naun is served without butter and is used for scooping up other foods. It is always served with soups.

Chapati

This wholemeal bread, along with rice, forms the basic food unit of the Tibb diet. You will need to obtain the special chapati flour (the Indian name for this flour is atta) from one of the sources in Appendix IV. Some of the better health food stores and co-ops may have it, or will order it if you use it regularly.

8 ounces wholemeal chapati flour (atta)
½ pint water
2 ounces chapati flour for rolling out

Sift 8 ounces chapati flour into a flat bowl. Make a depression in the middle of the mound of flour and pour in a little less than ¼ pint of water. Excess water will make the dough sticky and hard to handle, and makes hard bread. Mix into a soft dough.

Knead for 15 minutes by hand, or you can use a food processor. The longer the dough is kneaded, the better. Gradually add the remaining water, folding and pressing to thoroughly mix and knead. Sprinkle a palmful of water on top of the dough, cover with a damp cloth, and set aside to swell for thirty minutes. Knead the dough again for ten minutes, or one cycle through the food processor. Moisten the fingers to prevent stickiness. The dough must be kneaded sufficiently to obtain best results.

Divide the dough into ten pieces of equal size, and roll them into balls. You may now use the dry flour to prevent sticking to your fingers. Coat each dough ball with a little flour.

Flatten out one of the balls by pressing it down onto a rolling board with the palm of your right hand. Remember to sprinkle a little flour on the board from time to time to prevent sticking.

Place the flattened ball on a floured board and use a rolling pin (a special rolling pin for chapatis is called *belan*), and roll out to about a 5-inch diameter or about the size of a pancake.

Heat the griddle, frying pan, or tawa, and rub a very slight amount of grease on the griddle to prevent sticking. (When you have practiced with a few dozen chapatis, you can omit the grease.) Cook on medium heat.

The top side will dry up and small bubbles will begin to form, and gradually these will merge into several large bubbles. At this point turn the chapati over and cook the other side until brown spots appear on the under surface. Ideally the chapati should assume the shape of two saucers inverted over each other, but this will take some practice. If cooking on a gas or electric stove, you can assist this "ballooning" process by taking a kitchen cloth and pressing lightly but firmly on the places that are not ballooning up. Remove from griddle and serve immediately.

You will most often be making more than one chapati. Several pointers will help if you plan to make many chapatis. Two workers definitely helps—one to roll out and one to cook on the griddle. In any event, do not roll out all of the chapatis and stack them on top of each other uncooked. They will all stick together, and you'll have to start all over again after rolling out thirty or forty chapatis (you only do that once!). To keep the chapatis warm and fresh while cooking up a large batch, place them in a slightly dampened cloth, stacked on top of each other, after they are cooked. They'll stay warm and fresh for up to two hours. It is better if you wrap the cloth inside a plastic bag or zip-lock bag. This way they will keep for at least several days.

You should cook at least one chapati per person, although you'll probably find that people like them so much that three per person is a more realistic quantity.

There are several variations of making chapatis. The first is to roll out the chapati as above, then fry it in 2 tablespoons of oil. This will be similar to Indian fry bread. If you serve it right off the pan and coat it with butter and honey, it makes a complete breakfast all by itself.

Another method is to put a 'filling' inside and fold the chapati in half, then cook in two tablespoons of oil in a fry pan. The filling can be mashed potatoes and peas, left overs, fruits, or just about anything. These make a very quick and tasty snack or lunch.

Ravioli with Green Onion Filling

3 cups white flour, sifted

1 teaspoon salt

⁷/₈ cup cold water

1 bundle green onions

1 teaspoon salt

½ teaspoon crushed red pepper

1 tablespoon vegetable oil

2 cups drained yogurt

3 cloves fresh garlic, ground, or ½ teaspoon powdered garlic

1 teaspoon salt

½ cup vegetable oil

1 medium onion, diced fine

Combine flour and salt in a bowl. Add water and mix. Set dough aside.

Wash green onions. Cut tops into ¼-inch pieces to make 2-3 cups tops. Wash again. Squeeze with hands to remove excess water. Place in a bowl with salt and red pepper. Mix and squeeze to remove more water. Add vegetable oil, and set aside.

Drain about 1 quart yogurt to yield 2 cups. Place in bowl and mix with garlic and salt. Set aside.

To prepare meat sauce, heat oil in a pan and brown diced onion. Add beef, salt, and black pepper. When meat is browned, add tomato juice and water. Boil until liquid evaporates and sauce is oily.

To prepare ravioli, roll out half of dough into a ball on a floured board until it is very thin (¹/₁₆ inch). Cut with a round cutter (1½ to 2 inches in diameter) or in squares the same size. Put a few drained onion tops on half a circle or square of dough, moisten the edges, and seal shut tightly. The ravioli should not open during cooking. Place on tray or cookie sheet and cover until

*1 lb. ground beef,
  crumbled*
½ teaspoon salt
1 teaspoon black pepper
½ cup tomato juice
2 cups water
*1 tablespoon powdered
  dry mint*

all are prepared, repeating this process with the remaining dough and green onion tops.

Note: If this seems too much trouble, you can buy frozen eggroll sheets, which are the right thickness and shape, but read the label to make sure they are not overloaded with additives and preservatives, as most brands are.

Heat 2 quarts water in a kettle. Drop in several ravioli at a time, using a little cold water to keep the pot from boiling over. Boil for 10 minutes. Place half the yogurt mixture on a serving platter. Lift the cooked ravioli with a slotted spoon, and arrange it over the yogurt. Cover with remaining yogurt and sprinkle with dry mint.

Top with meat sauce and serve at once. (Serves 6-8.)

Split Pea Soup

*½ cup dried
  mung beans*
*½ cup dried
  kidney beans*
½ cup split peas
½ cup basmati rice
1 teaspoon salt
4 cups water
½ pound ground lamb
½ teaspoon salt
*½ teaspoon cayenne
  pepper*
*½ teaspoon black
  pepper*
½ cup ghee
1 medium onion, diced
2 cups water
¼ cup pureed tomatoes
½ cup yogurt
½ cup sour cream
*1 teaspoon–1
  tablespoon powdered
  dill weed*

Soak mung and kidney beans overnight in cold water.

Place them in a large kettle or pressure cooker with split green peas, rice, 1 teaspoon salt, and 4 cups water (including soaking water from beans), and cook until soft.

Mix together ground lamb, ½ teaspoon salt, cayenne, and black pepper. Form into balls ½ inch in diameter. (Vegetarians may omit this step.)

Heat ghee or vegetable oil in saucepan. Add the diced onion and brown lightly. Remove from fire and cool slightly.

Add 2 cups water, ¼ cup puréed tomatoes, and meat balls. Cook until all water is evaporated.

Add to this mixture the following and heat gently: all the cooked grains and beans, the yogurt, sour cream, and powdered dill weed, and 1 to 2 teaspoons salt, to taste.

Serve in individual soup plates with naun or chapatis. (Serves 4-6.)

Carrot, Almond, and Raisin Palaw

This is probably the most widely known and popular of many rice dishes. It is a dazzling dish, especially popular for wedding feasts and other important events.

2 cups cold water
1 cup dark seedless
   raisins
½ cup vegetable oil
1 medium onion, diced
1 lb. chicken parts
2 cups water
1 teaspoon salt
1-1½ teaspoons
   garam masala
4 medium carrots
³/₈ cup olive oil
1 tablespoon honey
½ cup slivered
   blanched almonds
2 cups basmati rice
1½ teaspoons salt
pinch saffron

Put raisins in 2 cups cold water. Set aside for 30 minutes, then drain off water.

Heat ½ cup vegetable oil in a kettle. Add diced onion and sauté until quite brown (but not burned).

Add and brown lightly 1 lb. halal or kosher chicken (in parts), or lamb or beef, cut into half-inch squares.

Add 2 cups water, 1 teaspoon salt, and garam masala. Cover and simmer until the meat is tender (chicken about 45 minutes, beef or lamb about 2 hours). Remove the meat from the juice and set aside. This juice will be used for cooking the rice.

Wash and scrape or peel carrots. Cut into toothpick-sized pieces. This is best done by making longitudinal slices, then cutting again along the length to produce right shape. A food processor will slice them quickly, but usually they are a bit too thin and turn to mush as they are cooked.

Heat olive oil in a small saucepan. Add honey and sliced carrots. Cook until the carrots are slightly browned and totally tender. You may add ¼ cup water to help soften the carrots. This is a tricky part of the cooking, to get the carrots to turn out right. Watch the dish closely while cooking, and stir gently but frequently. Do not be afraid to turn the heat up; you'll need rather high heat, or they'll take a very long time to be done. Cooking time is about 45 minutes, so start this early in the preparation process.

Remove carrots from oil and put in a glass dish. Put another ⅛ cup olive oil in the cooking pot and add the drained raisins. Cook, stirring constantly, until the raisins begin to balloon up and swell. Remove from heat and put in bowl with carrots.

Add almonds (or peeled pistachio nuts) to remaining oil. Cook until the nuts just begin to turn brown, but do not overcook, or the oil will turn rancid.

To cook rice, begin by boiling the meat juices, and

add 2 cups basmati rice and 1½ teaspoons salt. Add boiling water to bring the level to two inches above the rice (about 4½ cups total liquid). Add a pinch of saffron.

Cook until all water is absorbed and rice is tender. Test for doneness by removing one grain and squeezing between thumb and forefinger. Then, when rice is done, pour any remaining oil in which carrots were cooked over the rice.

Mix gently in with the rice. (Don't add the carrot-raisin mixture yet!) Put the rice into a casserole dish and put meat on top, saving some rice to cover over the meat. Set in a 300° oven for 20 minutes. To serve, put a layer of rice on platter, a layer of meat, then the rest of the rice in a mound over the meat. Finally, use your hand to spread the carrot-raisin mixture over the entire surface of mounded rice. (Serves 6-8.)

Plain White Rice (Chalow)

¼ cup diced onions
3 cups basmati rice
1 teaspoon salt
7 cups water
¼ cup olive oil
½ cup water
½ teaspon salt
¼ cup vegetable oil or melted butter

Heat oil and sauté diced onions until quite brown.

Combine in the same pot the rice, 1 teaspoon salt, and 7 cups boiling water. Cook until rice is tender. Strain and place rice in an ovenproof dish.

Mix separately the olive oil, ½ cup water, and ½ teaspoon salt. Pour this mixture over drained rice and toss gently with pancake turner or large rice server until the oil coats all the rice. Cover and place in 300° oven for 20 minutes to complete cooking.

To serve, mound rice on a large platter. If desired, pour over the rice an additional ¼ cup vegetable oil or melted butter. Accompany with a vegetable sauce or meat sauce. (Serves 6-8.)

Vegetable Sauce

1½ lbs. vegetables of
choice (cauliflower,
cabbage, spinach,
fresh peas or beans,
eggplant, squash,
etc.)

¾ cup olive oil

2 medium onions,
sliced thin

2 cloves garlic, minced

1½ teaspoons salt

¼ teaspoon black
pepper

½ teaspoon red pepper

½ cup water

Cut vegetables into 1-inch cubes.

Heat olive oil in a kettle. Add and brown lightly the cubed vegetables, onion slices, and minced garlic.

Add salt, black pepper, and red pepper. Cook slowly until vegetables are browned lightly. Then, to complete the cooking of the vegetables, add ½ cup water to sauce and simmer 5 to 10 minutes. Serve over rice. (Serves 8.)

Fried Eggplant with Yogurt

1 cup yogurt, drained
at least 1 hour

3 cloves garlic, minced

3 medium eggplants

4 cups vegetable oil

1 medium onion, diced

2 teaspoons salt

2 cups tomato sauce or
3 cups tomato juice

¼ teaspoon crushed red
pepper

¼ cup chopped green
pepper

¼ cup water

Combine and mix well the yogurt, garlic, and 1 teaspoon salt. Set aside. (This mixture is used in a number of meat and vegetable dishes.)

Wash and peel eggplants and slice widthwise. Score slices lightly with a knife. Spread slices on board or counter top on paper or cloth towels. Sprinkle with 1 teaspoon salt. Allow to stand 10-15 minutes to draw out some of the bitter juices. Wipe tops of eggplant with cloth or paper towel.

Heat 1 cup vegetable oil in kettle or deep frying pan. Fry eggplant slices until lightly browned. You will have to keep adding more oil as you put fresh eggplant slices in. Remove and set aside.

Dice 1 medium onion very finely and add to oil. Fry until browned.

Add eggplant slices, 1 teaspoon salt, tomato sauce, red pepper, and chopped green pepper. Make layers, alternating eggplant, green pepper, and sauce, so that the whole contents of the kettle are covered. Add salt, sprinkle red pepper over top, and add water to top of eggplant.

Cook slowly until eggplant is tender, about 1 hour.

The sauce will become thick. Do not stir much, or the eggplant will break up when tender.

To serve, use a tablespoon to spread out half the garlic-yogurt mixture on a platter. Use a large spatula to place the eggplant on the platter. Top with remaining yogurt mixture, and spoon some of the tomato sauce over the top. Serve with naun bread. (Serves 6-8.)

Fried Turnovers with Stuffing (Bulannee)

6 cups sifted white flour

2 teaspoons salt

2 cups water

1 lb. leeks or green onion tops

1½ teaspoons salt

½ teaspoon crushed red pepper

1 tablespoon olive oil

vegetable oil for frying

Stir flour and 2 teaspoons salt together in a mixing bowl. Mix in 1¼ to 2 cups water, and knead to form a stiff, elastic bread dough. Cover dough and set aside.

Sort 1 lb. leeks or green onion tops and wash carefully. (Other fillings can be used, such as steamed, mashed vegetable, meats, potatoes, etc.) Cut into ¼-inch pieces (there should be 4 cups after chopping or mashing).

Put leeks or other filling into a bowl and add 1½ teaspoons salt and ½ teaspoon red pepper. Add olive oil, mix, and set aside.

To prepare dough, divide and shape into balls the size of walnuts. Roll them out the same way as for making chapati bread. This recipe should yield about 18 or 20 of this size. Roll each circle out very thin on a floured board to not more than $1/16$ inch. The diameter of the circles can be from 6 to 9 inches. If they are tough after cooking, it is because the dough was not rolled out thin enough at this stage.

On each half-circle spread 3 to 4 tablespoons of filling. Moisten edges of dough, fold over in half, and seal. In a shallow pan, heat ½ cup vegetable oil for frying. When oil is hot, add turnovers two at a time and cook until well browned on both sides. Serve warm. This dish is specially suitable for birthdays, picnics, and other parties. (Serves 6-8.)

Garlic Ginger Chicken

1 whole chicken, cut into pieces
½ cup vegetable oil
¼ cup diced onions
2 tablespoons minced garlic
1 tablespoon ginger, powder or fresh
1 cup tomato sauce
salt

This dish is easy to prepare and takes just 1 hour from beginning to serving.

Prepare one whole chicken, washing and cutting into pieces.

Place in a kettle the vegetable oil and diced onion. Cook over medium heat until onions are quite browned but not burned or scorched. Stir frequently.

Add garlic, ginger, and salt to taste. Cook all ingredients in oil about 45 seconds to release volatile oils.

Quickly add all chicken pieces plus tomato sauce, salt, and water to cover chicken. Cook over low heat 45 minutes, until chicken is tender.

Remove chicken to bowl and set aside. Turn heat to medium high and cook remaining liquid until fairly thick sauce, about 10 minutes. Be careful not to burn bottom of pan.

Arrange chicken around sides of mounded rice, and serve sauce in side bowl. Serve with chapatis. (Serves 4.)

Spicy Chicken

This is for those who cannot take the heat of the Curry Chicken recipe. Rich and delicious, it does not offend by being overly spicy.

1 whole chicken, cut in pieces
1 cinnamon stick, broken into bits
3 cloves garlic, minced
8 whole cloves
2 tablespoons minced ginger root
1 tablespoon cumin seeds
2 teaspoons salt
½ cup water
2 medium onions
⅓ cup ghee or vegetable oil

Wash one whole chicken and cut into pieces.

In blender, make a purée of the cinnamon stick, garlic, cloves, ginger root, cumin seeds, salt, and ½ cup water.

Slice onions thin and fry in ⅓ cup ghee or vegetable oil until golden brown but not burned. With a slotted spoon, remove from cooking oil and add to blended mixture. Resume blending until all ingredients are smoothly mixed.

Reheat remaining ghee in pan and add the chicken and blended spice mixture. Bring to boil, then lower heat and cook for 45 minutes or until chicken is tender. (Serves 4.)

Baked Chicken with Garlic and Vinegar

This dish takes only 10 minutes of preparation, then cooks all by itself. It is tasty and hearty.

1 *whole chicken, cut in pieces*
¼ *cup vinegar*
5 *cloves garlic, minced*
¼ *cup olive oil*

Prepare one whole chicken, washed and cut up into pieces. Place chicken pieces in ovenproof dish, and sprinkle with vinegar, minced garlic, and olive oil. Salt and pepper to taste. Bake in 350° oven for one hour, or until chicken is tender and skin is crisp. (Serves 4.)

Curry Chicken

1 *whole chicken, cut into pieces*
¼ *cup olive oil (or vegetable oil or ghee)*
6 *cloves garlic*
2 *tablespoons ginger root*
1 *3-inch cinnamon stick*
2 *bay leaves*
5 *whole cardamom pods*
2 *dried red peppers (or ½ teaspoon cayenne)*
1 *teaspoon turmeric*
1 *cup tomato sauce*
1 *tablespoon lemon juice*
1 *cup yogurt*
½ *cup water*

This is a classic curry recipe, very quick and easy to prepare.

Prepare one whole chicken, washing and cutting into pieces. Place olive oil in kettle, and brown chicken pieces on all sides.

Puree in a blender the garlic, ginger root, cinnamon stick (broken into pieces), bay leaves, cardamom pods, red peppers, turmeric, tomato sauce, lemon juice, yogurt, and ½ cup water. Pour the purée over the chicken in the kettle, turning the chicken to cover with sauce.

Simmer on low heat for 45 minutes to 1 hour, turning pieces occasionally. Remove from heat when tender. Place chicken on serving platter and cover with remaining sauce. The sauce may be strained off and served as a gravy in side dish. Serve with palaw or plain rice and chapatis. (Serves 4.)

Kofta Chalow (Croquettes with Rice)

This is a simple, very tasty dish. With bread and a small salad, it makes a complete meal.

2 cups basmati rice
1½ teaspoons salt
¾ cup vegetable oil
1 tablespoon yellow
  split peas
1 lb. lamb or beef
2 cloves garlic
2 small onions
1 teaspoon ground
  coriander
1 teaspoon ground
  cumin
3 black peppercorns,
  ground
¼ teaspoon ground
  cardamom seeds
  (optional)
¼ teaspoon ground
  cinnamon (optional)
1 cup yogurt

Combine rice and ½ teaspoon salt with 4½ cups boiling water. Cook until rice is tender. Strain and place in casserole dish.

Mix ¼ cup vegetable oil with ½ cup water and ½ teaspoon salt. Pour over the drained rice, toss gently with pancake turner until rice is coated. Cover and place in 300° oven for 20 minutes to complete cooking.

Boil 1 tablespoon yellow split peas until soft. Drain, mash, and set aside.

Grind lamb or beef, garlic, and 1 small onion. Combine this mixture well with softened split peas and the coriander, cumin, black peppercorns, 1 teaspoon salt, and optional cardamom and cinnamon if desired. Shape into balls 1 inch in diameter.

Heat ½ cup vegetable oil in a saucepan. Add 1 small onion, diced, and brown lightly. Add and brown the meatballs.

Add yogurt and cook for 10 minutes.

To serve, place meatballs and sauce on platter. Serve by filling middle of rice casserole with kofta. (Serves 6-8.)

Kofta (General Meat Sauce)

1½ lbs. boneless lamb
  or beef
3 medium onions
2 teaspoons coriander
1 teaspoon salt
1 teaspoon crushed red
  pepper
1 cup vegetable oil
2 cups water
½ cup tomato sauce

Grind together the lamb or beef, 2 onions, and coriander. Add salt and red pepper. Mix well. Shape into small balls ½ inch in diameter.

Chop 1 medium onion. Fry in ⅛ cup vegetable oil until browned. Add 2 cups water, ½ cup or more tomato sauce, and meatballs. Cook until water evaporates and a thick sauce remains (about 1 hour). (Serves 6.)

Garam Masala Chicken

This is possibly the simplest and most delicious basic recipe in the world. Any meat can be used, but lamb and chicken are best. You can use soup cuts or stew meat and extend the cooking time another 30 to 45 minutes. The result is a very tasty main dish that requires very little time in the kitchen.

2-3 lbs. chicken, cut into pieces
2 tablespoons olive oil
2 teaspoons garam masala
½ teaspoon salt

Wash chicken and cut into pieces. Heat oil in saucepan and add garam masala. Add chicken or other meat, salt, and enough water to reach top of meat. Cook on high simmer for 1 hour or longer. Remove meat from kettle and set aside.

Cook remaining liquid 15 minutes on high heat to drive off excess moisture, leaving a rich gravy. Serve with rice, bread, and salad. (Serves 4-6.)

Barley and Turkey Legs

I prepare this dish to prove that ten people can be fed for less than five dollars.

3 large turkey drumsticks
¼ cup olive oil
1 medium onion, diced
2 tablespoons garam masala
1 teaspoon salt
1 lb. barley
1 teaspoon black pepper

Wash turkey drumsticks.

In a pan, heat olive or vegetable oil. Sauté diced onion until brown. Then add garam masala. Allow spices to release oils in hot pan. Then add turkey drumsticks, water to cover turkey, salt, and barley. Cook all of these together on medium heat for 2 hours, stirring occasionally. Add water as it is absorbed by the barley.

When turkey is cooked, after about 2 hours, lift it out with tongs, remove the meat from the bones, and return it to the barley. Add 1 teaspoon black pepper before serving. Serve with Afghan naun bread. (Serves 8-10.)

Stuffed Peppers

This recipe can be used to make stuffed cabbage leaves, grape leaves, lettuce leaves, eggplant, or green peppers.

½ cup vegetable oil
1 medium onion, diced
5 cups water
1½ teaspoons salt
1 cup tomato sauce
1½ lbs. ground lamb or beef
⅓ cup cooked basmati rice
½ teaspoon black pepper
1 teaspoon ground coriander
4 large green peppers

Heat vegetable oil in a kettle. Add diced onion and brown lightly. Remove from flame and cool a little.

To the oil and onion, add 5 cups water, ½ teaspoon salt, and tomato sauce. Boil gently for 15 minutes to develop flavor.

For the filling, mix in a bowl the ground lamb or beef, cooked rice, black pepper, 1 teaspoon salt, and ground coriander.

Cut off the stem and remove the seeds of four large green peppers (or similarly prepare leaves). Fill with meat filling, fasten tops with toothpicks, and place in sauce. Cover and cook slowly, turning frequently, until meat is done and water evaporated (usually about 30 to 45 minutes). Serve on a warm platter with some of the sauce spooned over top. (Serves 4.)

Cucumber-Onion Salad

This is a simple but necessary side dish, as the cucumber and yogurt will help to cool down a spicy meal. It is a side dish, and about 2 tablespoons are enough per person.

1 large cucumber
1 small onion, diced
¼ cup drained yogurt
½ teaspoon salt
½ teaspoon crushed dried mint

Wash and peel 1 large cucumber. Dice into $\frac{1}{16}$-inch pieces. Use up the whole cucumber.

Dice 1 small onion. Mix with cucumber in a dish.

Add drained yogurt, salt, and mint. Mix well, and place in refrigerator for 45 minutes before serving.

Honey Egg Custard

5 eggs
¾ cup honey
1 teaspoon vanilla
   extract
2 cups milk
½ teaspoon nutmeg
pinch ground cloves

Beat eggs. Add honey and vanilla extract. Stir to mix in honey, then add milk slowly, stirring to mix. Add nutmeg and pinch of cloves. Pour into ovenproof baking dish or individual custard cups. Place in pan of water about one-half to three-quarters full. Bake for 45 minutes or until firm to touch. Allow to cool. (Serves 6-8.)

Honey Rice Pudding

4 tablespoons uncooked
   basmati (or short-
   grain) rice
3 cups milk
dash salt
dash nutmeg
⅓ cup honey

Mix all ingredients together in a pan. Simmer 2 hours, uncovered. *Do not allow to boil.* If too thick when done, the pudding may be thinned by adding a little cream or milk. (Serves 4.)

Honey Graham Crackers

3 cups whole wheat
   flour
½ teaspoon salt
½ teaspoon baking
   powder
½ teaspoon ground
   cinnamon
6 tablespoons butter
½ cup honey

Sift together the dry ingredients. Melt butter and honey in a separate pan. Pour over dry ingredients and mix with a fork. Then form into a large mass by hand. With a floured rolling pin, roll out to ⅛ inch thick. Cut into rectangular pieces 1½ by 3 inches. Prick tops with fork. Place on lightly greased baking tin and bake at 375° for 10 minutes. (Serves 8-10.)

Dried Fruit Compote

4 cups dried apricots

4 cups dried seedless raisins

2 cups yellow raisins

2 cups English or California walnut pieces

2 cups shelled pistachio nuts

2 cups blanched almonds

Wash all of the ingredients. Into one bowl, put the dried apricots, seedless raisins, and yellow raisins. Cover with cold water to 2 inches above fruit. Cover bowl and refrigerate for one day.

In a second bowl, place the walnuts, pistachio nuts, and almonds. Add water the same as above, cover, and set aside for one day.

As the skins soften on the nuts, they should be peeled (or you can buy the nuts already peeled). Soak another day. Then combine apricots, raisins, and peeled nuts.

To serve, spoon fruit and nuts into individual dessert dishes or cups. Add ½ to 1 inch of juice to each cup. (Serves 8-10.)

6
Signs of Health and Disease

The best place to start a discussion of the signs of health and disease is with a clear understanding of precisely what constitutes a healthy human being. But when one tries to arrive at a simple explanation of what is health, almost everyone is at a loss for a definitive answer. The general reply seems to be that health is simply not being sick. But definitions of disease do abound.

Primitive cultures believed that disease was due to the evil influences of malignant ghosts, devils, magic, and spells. Many religions have taught that diseases are punishment for sins. The ancient tribes of Australia traced disease to "bone pointing." The Pythagoreans connected the origin of disease with mathematics and saw diseases as being related to odd numbers!

Paracelsus (1490-1541) stated that all disease was the result of maladjustment of three elements: sulfur, mercury, and salt. According to the doctrine of Goto (1659-1733), the universal spirits of cold, air, heat, and humidity circulated in the body and caused illness. Samuel Hahnemann (1755-1843) explained that disease was the result of weakness of the vital force of a pathenogenic matter called "psora." Others have advanced theories that disease is the result of imbalance of colors, cellular salts, psychological factors, and many other sources.

Our modern notions of disease were a distinct development of the nineteenth century. Bacteria were unmasked and claimed as the definitive causes of such diseases as typhoid, cholera, tuberculosis, and others. Stedman's *Medical Dictionary* currently describes diseases thus: "Morbus, illness, sickness. An interruption or perversion of functions of any of the organs, a morbid change in any of the tissue or an abnormal state of the body as a whole, continuing for a longer or shorter period of time."

Actually there are several subcategories of disease, such as ailments, illnesses, weaknesses, conditions, and so forth. But the most interesting point of all of these assumptions about disease is their reliance on a description of a deviation from a norm, namely health. Yet none of these systems offers a definition of health! Each system places greater or lesser emphasis upon some elements of the body and its malfunction.

Also interesting is that among the history of definitions of health or disease, a very long list of physicians and scientists have held to the view of the humoral basis of health and have stated that improper metabolism of foods leads to disease. Those holding to the humoral concepts include some of the most glittering names in medical history: Thales (sixth century B.C.), Hippocrates of Cos (460 B.C.), Aristotle (384-322 B.C.), Asclepaides (first century B.C.; he was the first to hint at the atomic variation in hot and cold foods), Galen (c. A.D. 131-200), Avicenna, Ishin Ho (Buddhist school), Theophilus Lobb (author of *Medical Principles and Causations*, 1751), Abernathy (1764-1831), Broussais (1772-1838), Samuel Thomson (1769-1830), and many others.

The Tibb system is the summation and codification of the accumulated experience and knowledge of all those who have worked within the humoral and dietetic framework of medicine and health. In Tibb, we define first of all the state of the human being in a balanced state, which is called equable temperament, or health. In addition to the general descriptions in the preceding chapters, we may add the following signs of a normal temperament:

1. The *feel of the skin* and members, within and without, gives a sensation between hotness and coldness, wetness and dryness, softness and hardness. That is, the skin feels slightly moist and warm, and has a lovely, smooth complexion and elasticity.
2. In *color*, the body is between whiteness and redness (in light-skinned peoples).
3. In *stature*, the body is neither bulky nor skinny, though generally more fleshly than overly thin. The person should exhibit an erect, tall posture and during the developmental years should be inclined to quick growth.
4. The *veins* of the skin do not bulge out, nor are they submerged below the muscle layers.
5. The *hair* is neither excessive nor sparse, thick nor thin, curly nor straight, black nor white, and grows where it should. During adolescence, the hair should tend to a tawny hue, while in adulthood it should darken.
6. *Sleep* should be balanced with wakefulness.
7. *Pleasant dreams* should be experienced, evidenced by hopeful, happy images, the scents of sweet perfumes, lovely voices, inspiring visions, and pleasant companions.
8. *Mental faculties* should demonstrate strong imagination, intellect, and memory. The emotions should remain between the extremes of anger and joy, between courage and fear, and between changing the mind and inflexibility.
9. *Perfection of functions* means that the digestion, urination, defecation, and other functions are without pain or discomfort, and the discharges are without unusual foul odor, blood, or other matter. The appetite should be exercised according to real hunger, and there should be no unusual cravings for liquids besides water. The person should easily adapt to changes in climate.
10. *Movement of the limbs* should be quick, easy, and deft.

One who possessed all of these points would be an appealing, confident, positive, and healthy human being. Such a person would bear a happy expression most of the time, exhibit modest desires for foods and beverages and all other condiments, and possess excellent digestive and assimilative powers throughout the system.

The arising of disease can be said to be the result of an excess, or plethora, which is called an "obstruction" in Tibb. Such excess is said to exist either as an overabundance of the *quantity* or *quality* of the humor.

In the first case of excess in the quantity of humor, the humors may be healthy in temperament but excessive in quantity, so that the channels bearing the humors become overburdened and overfilled. The channels run the risk of rupture; there is the pressure of backup of the humors and a choking off of life force into those areas where the excess exists. Such imbalance provides an excellent opportunity for various forms of bacteria and viral life to multiply in numbers far greater than would normally occur. Such diseases as influenza, heart attack, epilepsy, apoplexy, and others are seen as due to excess in the quantity of humors.

In the case of deviation in the quality of the humor, the natural nutritive faculties of the body become overwhelmed because the capacity of the digestive processes of the body are made inefficient. Most of the chronic and degenerative diseases, such as cancer, emphysema, and arthritis, have their ultimate origin in the unhealthy quality of humors. In all of these conditions, the Tibb physician admits to the existence of various biochemical and pathological happenings, yet in order to effect a true cure, it is necessary to treat the underlying humoral imbalance (whatever its nature) instead of killing off the excess microscopic life that is a *result* of the imbalance and not, truly speaking, the cause of the disease.

Both physicians and lay persons use the words *signs* and *symptoms* to describe various diseases. There is no difference in the significance of the terms, but to the patient they are symptoms (of pain or discomfort), while to the physician they are signs (leading to an understanding of the underlying imbalance). Symptoms in Tibb are grouped into three classes: (1) alteration of temperament, (2) organic disease, and (3) break in continuity. The signs identifying these imbalances are evaluated by means of the sense perceptions of both patient and physician—sight (jaundice, redness, whiteness), smell (foul perspiration, acetone of urine), taste (bitter, salty), touch (softness, hardness), and sound (passing gas, hoarseness, yelling of anger)—and by the quality of eliminations.

The first step in evaluation is to assess the basic obstruction of humor in terms of quantity or quality. Such excesses of humors can be observed by the following signs:

Alteration in quantity of humor: red face, full veins; tightness of skin, dull movements and gestures, full pulse, colored and dense urine, poor appetite, feeling of weight in the limbs, poor vision; dreaming that one cannot speak or cannot lift a heavy object.

Alteration in quality of humor: Sluggishness, loss of appetite, feeling of bearing emotional burdens, sensation of itching, stinging, burning, and smelling foul odors in dreams.

The specific humor that is affected may be determined from Table 4 in Chapter 3. Once the specific humor that is out of balance is identified, it is necessary to determine whether the intemperament is hot, cold, moist, or dry. The following list presents the evidences of the four primary intemperaments.

THE FOUR PRIMARY INTEMPERAMENTS

Excess of heat: (1) feelings of uncomfortable heat, (2) great suffering from fevers, (3) easily fatigued, as activity stimulates further production of heat, (4) excessive thirst, (5) burning and irritation in the pit of the stomach (epigastrium), (6) bitter taste in the mouth, (7) pulse weak, rapid, and fast, (8) intolerance of hot foods, (9) relief and comfort from use of cold foods and other cold things, (10) great suffering in summer, (11) inflammatory conditions, and (12) fatigue and loss of energy.

There are five causes of excess heat in the body: (1) immoderate movement, either of the spirit or the body (motion of the spirit means things like anger or worry; motion of the body means physical exercise); (2) exposure to actual warmth (heat of fire, sun, etc.); (3) entry into the body of "potential" warmth (eating hot foods such as onions, garlic, mustard); (4) closing of the pores; and (5) putrefaction.

Excess of cold: (1) weak digestion, (2) diminished desire for drinks, (3) laxity of joints, (4) tendency to phlegmatic type of fevers and catarrhal conditions, (5) cold things easily upset and hot things are pleasant and beneficial, and (6) great suffering in winter.

There are eight causes of cold imbalance: (1) exposure to actual cold (snow, winter air, etc.); (2) ingesting substances with "potential" cold (foods such as cucumber and yogurt); (3) excess of substances that overwhelm the innate heat (marijuana); (4) lack of nutrients that produce heat (fasting); (5) excess thickening of the residues of metabolism, which extinguishes innate heat; (6) excess of heat in the body for a prolonged period, causing destruction of the heat regulation function of the body (fever); (7) excessive motion; and (8) excessive rest.

Excess of moisture: Signs are almost similar to excess of cold, but in addition there will be (1) puffiness, (2) excessive salivation (mucus in saliva) and nasal secretion, (3) tendency to diarrhea and upset stomach, (4) desire for moist type of foods, (5) excess of sleep, and (6) puffiness of eyelids.

There are four causes of moist imbalance: (1) exposure to moistening substances (baths); (2) moisture reaching inside the body from moistening foods (fish); (3) excess intake of food and beverages (gluttony); and (4) emotional excess (life of ease and weakness of character).

Excess of dryness: (1) dryness and roughness of skin, (2) insomnia, (3) wasting, (4) intolerance of dry type of foods, while moistening foods will give comfort and pleasure, (5) suffer greatly during autumn, and (6) hot water and light oils are readily absorbed by the skin.

There are four causes of excessive dryness: (1) exposure to actual dryness (winds); (2) administration of drying substances (vinegar, salt); (3) lessening intake of food and beverages (starvation, fasting); and (4) excessive motion.

The reader may find it useful if here we present a brief overview of the temperaments according to Avicenna. He remarks in the *Canon* on the temperaments of various age groups:

> It may be summarized that children as well as grownups are balanced in respect to their heat, while the old and senile are relatively cold. Children possess a moderate excess of moisture to meet their requirements for growth. This can be observed from the softness of their bodies and nervous tissues, and easily understood from the fact that it has not been long since they grew and developed from semen, blood and the vapory vital fluid. The fact that old and senile individuals are not only cold but also dry can be observed from the hardness of their bones and dryness of their skins. This will also be clear if one remembers the fact that, after all, a considerable time has passed since they originally developed from blood, semen, and the vital fluid.
>
> Children and adults both possess about the same degree of heat. Moisture and air are, however, greater in children. The old and particularly the senile show greater earthiness than adults and children. Adults and children are both balanced, and adults more so than children. They are drier than children but not so dry as the old and senile. The senile are drier than adults in regard to their innate secretion but moister in respect to the abnormal moisture which makes their tissues only temporarily and superficially moist.

The significance of the above statements is that the innate heat tends to be hotter and moister in youth than in old age. However, in some older persons the moisture fails to dry up, and they collect more fluids in their tissues, which give rise to certain diseases, two common ones being peptic ulcer and hyperactivity.

It would be worthwhile here to pause a moment and review the basic overview of the Tibb system of health and disease.

Review of Tibb System

The human body normally exists in a state of balance, harmony, happiness, and wellness so long as the proper quality and quantity of foods and sensory nourishments are supplied and fully assimilated. The brain, heart, liver, stomach, and reproductive organs, along with various enzyme functions, all serve to sustain the metabolic functioning of the body in a state of balance. This state of balance—with no overt signs of disease, no pain, complete digestion, and no fevers, inflammations, or other signs—is called health.

There arise in the body four semigaseous vapors, called humors, which are responsible for maintaining the body fluids and digestive by-products in a state of balance. These four humors are associated with the blood, phlegm, yellow bile, and black bile, which refer to the stages of breakdown of nutrients in digestion. Each of the humors has its own characteristic temperament. Blood is warm and moist; phlegm is cold and moist; yellow bile is cold and dry; and black bile is hot and dry. Moreover, each person has one of these as the "dominant" humor, and his or her personality type may be expressed according to the humoral prevalance: blood is sanguine (optimistic); phlegm is phlegmatic (apathetic); yellow bile is bilious (peevish); and black bile is atrabilious (melancholy).

All of the food substances consumed in order to preserve life are classified according to their ability to increase or slow down metabolism, and thus will contribute to each of the humors maintaining its proper inherent temperament. When the diet, sleep and wakefulness, digestion and evacuation, and other factors are taken in excess, one or more of the humors becomes unbalanced, and the signs of disease arise and can be observed. The specific type and location of disease, its severity and duration, will depend upon the inherent strengths and weaknesses of each person's organ systems. The evidences of disease are observed by sight, smell, touch, and taste.

It is important to keep in mind this overview—a whole image of the mental, physical, emotional, and spiritual aspects of health.

Besides the overt physical and emotional signs of imbalance (disease) that have been presented above, Tibb performs a careful evaluation of the pulse and of the qualities associated with the urine and feces, and also classifies the many forms of fever and pain that occur. From all of these, the physican probes deeper to pinpoint the precise location and form of humoral imbalance.

The Pulse

According to the Hakims who practice the Tibb system, all discomfort, disease, decay, and destruction is ultimately traceable to lack of life—the diminished metabolic force that is responsible for fully assimilating nutrients in the body. The word *life* that we use in everyday language is the result of two activities working harmoniously: one is the constant life of the spirit; the other is the life that "matter" provides to give expression to the spirit.

In Tibb, we use the word *nafas* to express this concept of the primary life force. The word *nafas* also means soul, spirit, essence, and breath. The *nafas* is the breath or thread of life that runs through all human beings, and is the one element without which life could not be sustained even for a short time.

While some physicians may try to determine how a person is "breathing," Tibb's concept of the life breath/force is broader. Breath is the most important nourishment to human life, much more important than any other substance, for there is a connection between our own breath, the life force, and the light of the cosmos. In many scriptures, the word *light* (Ar. *nur*) is used frequently in connection with life. This is not merely a metaphor. The connection between light and our life, our breath, is demonstrated by the scientific knowledge of the West as well; for through the process of photosynthesis, light catalyzes in the transformation of the chlorophyll of plants into oxygen, which is then taken into the lungs as the sustaining life force. Indeed, our breath is simply another manifestation of the pure light of the sun and of the universe. Yet how unconsciously we engage in our breaths!

Realizing that breath is the carrier of the life force, we must discover a method for evaluating the efficiency of this process. The key to this is the pulse. It is worth noting that in the Tibb terminology, the words for *breath, pulse,* and *ego* are all spelled the same. In other words, the ego represents all of the various excessive appetites of the body, and the breath is the means of regulating those factors, while the pulse is the monitor over this process. The intimacy of the interrelationship of these factors is conveyed by using the same word for all three.

In determining the relative harmony of this life force within the body, the Hakim performs an evaluation of the pulse. The system of pulse diagnosis evolved by the Chinese was studied by Avicenna, who incorporated its most salient features into the Tibb system. While pulse evaluation can become quite complex, and does require extensive personal instruction in order to master it fully, the essential features are presented here for those who want to study and begin to apply pulse evaluation.

The pulse is a movement in the heart and arteries which expands and contracts, whereby the "breath" of the innate life force becomes subjected to the influence of the indrawn air. Every beat of the pulse consists of two movements and two pauses. The movement is thus: expansion—pause—contraction—pause.

The pulse is felt at the wrist because it is readily accessible, there is little flesh covering it, and the patient is not embarrassed by exposing this part of the body. When feeling the pulse, the palm should be turned upward, especially in thin people. If the palm is turned downward, the readings will be higher and exaggerated in degrees of excess. If the patient is a male, read from the left hand; if a female, use the right hand. Both patient and examiner should be in a calm state, without having performed exercise or eaten within one hour before the reading.

Developing sensitivity to the subtle actions and elements of the pulse takes much time and practice. The capacity to sensitize the fingertips to the pulse variations can be enhanced by taking a single strand of one's own hair, and so that you do not see the placement of it, have someone put it between two sheets of plain white paper on a hard table top, so that you do not know the location of the hair. You must then "feel" the hair through the paper. Once the position of the hair can consistently be identified through a single sheet, a second sheet is added. This process is repeated until the hair can be felt through seven thicknesses of paper.

Technique of Pulse Evaluation

In pulse evaluation, the examiner's middle finger must be placed exactly at the junction of the carpus with the lower end of the radius. The other two fingers are allowed to rest on the artery, one on each side of the middle finger, but with the index finger nearest the heart.

For some difficult or contradictory initial diagnoses, the Hakim will utilize what is known as "two-element" evaluation. This is obtained by taking the first and second factors of the pulse. The length, width, and depth comprise the first element. The second element is obtained by comparing that pulse with one of a bird or some other animal, so that the patient's pulse can be judged against a norm in nature. There is also a "three-element" evaluation, which combines the readings from the wrist, the forefinger, and the tips of the four other fingers to arrive at a composite of the complete internal functioning of the body. However, I present here only the single-element evaluation.

These ten guides are used to measure and evaluate the condition of the pulse:

1. Quality of expansion (amount of diastole, measured in terms of length, width, depth)
2. Quality of impact of beating of the pulse against the finger of examiner (strong, weak, moderate)
3. Duration of cycle of pulse (fast, slow, moderate)
4. Duration of pause (successive, different, moderate)
5. Emptiness or fullness of vessel between beats (full, empty, moderate)
6. Compressibility of artery (hard, soft, moderate)
7. Moisture content of perspiration of pulse (full, empty, moderate)
8. Regularity (regular different, irregular different)
9. Order and disorder (ordered, irregularly ordered, irregularly disordered)
10. Rhythm (similar, different, out of rhythm)

Avicenna consulted the Chinese system of pulse diagnosis, and the similarities between the two systems are remarkable. Table 5 provides the Tibb and Chinese terminologies for pulse diagnosis.

Quality of Expansion

The quality of expansion and contraction is measured according to the length, width, and depth of the artery carrying the blood. A long pulse is one that is passing over the measuring point in a longer duration than a normal pulse beat. The cause of a long pulse in this element is an excess of heat.

A short pulse passes over the measuring point more quickly than would a normal pulse. The cause of a short pulse is lack of internal heat, often accompanied by body temperature lower than 98.0° Fahrenheit.

A moderate pulse is balanced between a fast and slow pulse; in other words, it is normal. We use the word *moderate* as opposed to *normal* when describing the pulse measures because it implies that there is neither too little nor too much of a humoral substance. Hence, the word *moderate* indicates a condition between extremes, or health.

The second factor within this classification is the width of a pulse. A wide pulse can be felt to have expanded the arterial wall beyond the normal width. Its cause is an excess of moisture in the blood. A narrow pulse is felt as being less in width than a normal pulse, and its cause is an insufficiency of moisture in the blood.

The third factor in this initial assessment of the pulse regards depth. An eminent pulse is one that can be felt as the artery rises above and presses against the surface of the skin on the wrist. The cause of an eminent pulse is excess heat. A lowered pulse can be felt as having dropped down away from the surface of the skin of the wrist and below the point considered as moderate. The cause of lowered pulse is lack of internal heat.

Thus, with this initial evaluation, we arrive at nine basic pulse types, or possibilities, according to the factors of length, width, and depth:

Length of pulse—long, short, moderate

Width of pulse—wide, narrow, moderate

Depth of pulse—eminent, lowered, moderate

The complexity of pulse evaluation is evident from this classification, because simply within this first factor, there are twenty-seven possible variations of the pulse. For the sake of interest, the twenty-seven variations are reproduced in Table 6.

Quality of Impact

There are three qualities: strong (resists the finger during expansion), weak (the opposite character), and moderate (between the two). A strong pulse is due to an excess of animal power (sexual energy, libido*). A weak pulse is due to a weakness of the animal power.

Duration of Cycle

Duration of cycle is the measure of the speed with which the pulse beat passes over the measuring point of the fingertips. It is a measure not of duration (as with the first component), but merely of speed. Fast cycle completes the cycle in a brief period of time. Slow cycle completes in a longer period. The moderate pulse is between the two.

This movement of speed and undulation is sometimes compared to the movement of waves for the last twenty yards or so before they break upon the shore. In fact, one can observe this "wave" of the motion of the arterial pulse along the forearm in some individuals who have eminent arteries.

Duration of Pause

There are three modes: successive, different, moderate. *Successive pause* means that the pulse not only moves across the measuring point in less time than a normal pulse, but also successively slows (and this slowing may run in cycles). This is not simply an opposite measurement of the quality ascertained in the duration of cycle, because of this successive nature of the variation. The cause of successive inaction is weakness of the animal power.

Different pause means that the interval between the pulse beats varies; usually it is shorter than that of a normal pulse. The cause of different pause is the presence of the highest possible degree of animating life force, which is an imbalance, not health.

The moderate state of this pulse finds the intervals between pulse beats virtually equal. It is the desired condition.

Emptiness or Fullness

The pulse is full (or "high"), when it seems to be overfull of humor and needs to be allowed out; an empty (or "low") pulse is flattened and opposite in character. The Chinese describe this empty pulse as "the hole in the flute," while Avicenna said it feels as if the artery were filled with bubbles of air, so that the fingers seem to fall on empty space. The cause of the full pulse is thickening of the blood. The empty pulse gives a "clammy" feeling at the point of feeling the pulse. A moderate state is the condition of balance between the two.

---

*"Animal power" does not precisely mean "sexual power" as it is used in current psychological and media jargon. Perhaps the Greek word *animus* would more closely convey the connotation desired, including not only sexual energy, but also willpower, concentration, emotional stability, and similar factors.

TABLE 6
VARIATIONS OF QUALITY OF EXPANSION

Length factor: long, short, or moderate
Width factor: wide, narrow, or moderate
Depth factor: eminent, lowered, or moderate

The possible variations are:

Long—Wide—Eminent
Long—Narrow Eminent
Long—Moderate—Eminent
Short—Wide—Eminent
Short—Narrow—Eminent
Short—Moderate—Eminent
Moderate—Wide—Eminent
Moderate—Narrow—Eminent
Moderate—Moderate—Eminent

Long—Wide—Lowered
Long—Narrow—Lowered
Long—Moderate—Lowered
Short—Wide—Lowered
Short—Narrow—Lowered
Short—Moderate—Lowered
Moderate—Wide—Lowered
Moderate—Narrow—Lowered
Moderate—Moderate—Lowered

Long—Wide—Moderate
Long—Narrow-Moderate
Long—Moderate—Moderate
Short—Wide—Moderate
Short—Narrow—Moderate
Short—Moderate—Moderate
Moderate—Wide—Moderate
Moderate—Narrow—Moderate
Moderate—Moderate—Moderate

Compressibility of Artery

There are three forms: the soft pulse is easily compressible; the hard is difficult to compress; and the moderate condition falls between the two.

Moisture (Temperature) of Pulse

This guide is simply measured by the sense of touch at the point of taking the pulse and by reflecting upon the temperature of the surface "moisture" of the matter being eliminated by the pores of the skin. Both hot and cold pulse are easily determined. The former is caused by excess internal heat, and its opposite by the lack of internal heat. The moderate temperature falls between these two.

Regularity

This guide synthesizes all of the preceding evaluations into one measure.

By taking all of these factors into account, one can note the general pulse condition.

The modes of equality are regular or irregular. *Regular* means that it is moderate in all of the above factors. Likewise, it would be called irregular if excessive in all of the factors. However, if it is regular in six aspects and irregular in one only, this fact is noted, along with the specific irregular pulse.

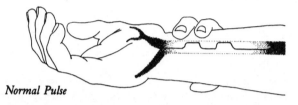

Normal Pulse

With the foregoing analysis of pulse providing the overall condition of the patient, the last two factors allow the examiner to adopt more critical measurements, which reflect the conditions of specific imbalances within particular organs.

Order and Disorder

The pulse may be irregularly ordered or irregularly disordered. These two forms are sometimes referred to as regular different and irregular different.

A regular different pulse keeps one, two, or more circulations, or cycles, without changing the pattern of the beating of the pulse. One circulation simply means the number of beats that occur within one second, and the interval between beats. For example, one circulation might be considered thus: two beats per second, with an interval of one-quarter second between beats.

The irregular different pulse has similar variations in the interval, but does not come around in a full circle to the original pulse beat pattern.

Rhythm

The final guide to the pulse derives from the concept that each man, woman, and child, while in good health, should possess a certain pulse rhythm that is appropriate for the age and emotional development of that person. If the pulse is beating in accordance with the norms, it is said to be benign. If it is out of rhythm, it is said to be malignant (though not meant in the sense of malignant tumors or cancers). Malignant pulses are of three types. A similar rhythm is that which resembles an age rhythm that follows immediately in development sequence, such as a child having the pulse rhythm of a young man.

Different rhythm is a pulse that does not immediately follow in the developmental sequence, such as a child having the pulse rhythm of an old man. The third form—out of rhythm—does not resemble any normal pattern of any developmental age. This is the ultimate kind of irregular pulse, for it signals an imminent and severe change in temperament.

The varieties of irregular pulse are classified according to distinctive names. These are summarized below.

VARIETIES OF IRREGULAR PULSE

1. *Gazelle pulse:* Expansion is interrupted and lasts for a longer duration than normal, remains at a fixed height, then quickly increases to full height. The second beat begins before the first one is completed. The cause is the heat of fever. It is commonly observed in pericarditis.

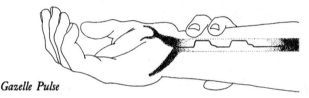

Gazelle Pulse

2. *Waving pulse:* Beats follow in a rolling manner, one upon the other, like waves. The beat is irregular in regard to largeness, degree of rise, and breadth. It seems to come too soon or late, and the force is soft. The cause is usually a weakness of the vital power. The significance of this pulse is that a form of the healing crisis (see Chapter 9) by perspiration or diarrhea is imminent.

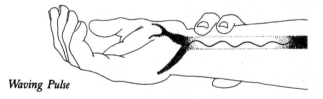

Waving Pulse

3. *Sawlike pulse:* This is rapid, successive, and alternating in hardness and softness of moisture content. The irregularity is with respect to the size of expansion, and of hardness and softness. It is caused by moisture mixed with blood humor, or excess of yellow bile or phlegm humor; or it may be caused by swelling of the nerves, which causes perspiration matter to become hard.

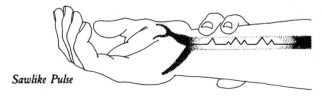

Sawlike Pulse

4. *Antlike pulse (formicant pulse):* This is similar to the wavy pulse, but more intense in the successive and soft aspects. It is the smallest, weakest, and most hurried of all pulses. It is caused by weakness of peristaltic action.

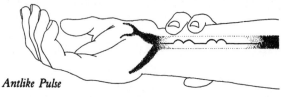

Antlike Pulse

5. *Rat-tail pulse:* This pulse alternates between excessive and insufficient dimensions. It often begins in an excessive mode, reverts to insufficient, then breaks midway and returns to excessive. It is a sign of malignancy and is caused by a very weak life force.

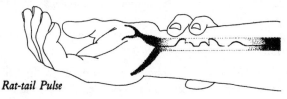

Rat-tail Pulse

6. *Flickering pulse:* Your first finger feels the pulse as small, the middle finger feels it large and swollen, and the last finger feels it small again. This signifies weakness of the arterial wall and destruction of tissues around the artery. The cause is extreme disability, often due to unresolved inflammations of long duration.

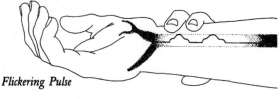

Flickering Pulse

7. *Cordlike pulse (twisted pulse):* This feels like a band of thread or cord that has become twisted. There is an evident tension. The "twisted" sensation may only be for one part of the pulse and not the second beat. The cause is due to dry intemperament.

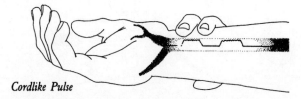

Cordlike Pulse

These are the main kinds of simple pulses, although there are many more forms of compound pulses, none of which have been given specific names. Pulse diagnosis is remarkably accurate in allowing the physician to recognize the site, severity, and intensity of interior disease conditions. However, the basic texts on the pulse run into many volumes (the Chinese classic text on the pulse is in twenty-five volumes), and I stress again that some formal personal instruction by an experienced Hakim would be necessary to verify one's impressions of the pulse.

There are several factors that provide the inherent pulse. These factors are the vital power of the heart itself, the elasticity of the artery, and the resistance, or urge, of the force of the pulse. These factors will not provide variation in the pulse, but together they are responsible for the normal pulse in any person.

There are a host of nonessential factors that may produce changes in the pulse. These include such things as age, season, changing temperament, bathing, exercise, gymnastics, sexual intercourse, pregnancy, foods, intoxicants, medicines, emotional states, pain, secretiveness, habits, and putrefactions.

We shall turn now to a discussion of the subjects of fever and pain and their significance in various imbalances.

7
Of Fire and Light:
Fever and Pain

Fever and pain are the two most common—and for most people, alarming—signs of imbalance in the body. Fever, technically speaking, can be a very slight elevation above the "normal" temperature of 98.6° Fahrenheit, or a raging, fearsome soaring up over 105°. Temperatures above 106.5° are quite rare and usually occur only in conjunction with some form of injury to the brain. Fevers are usually preceded by chills, a mechanism the body uses to prod the thermal regulators into action to raise the temperature.

Orthodox medicine divides fevers into two basic types: those of known causes and those of unknown causes. But whatever the cause, the best course of treatment is not always to cut short the fever, because this strange and unusual heat is a valuable indicator of bodily functions.

Pain is a rather different topic. Western medicine views it almost exclusively as a symptom of some form of physiological disruption of function. Of course, the pain associated with a broken bone obviously derives from the violent break in the continuity of the limb. But the other forms of pain—abdominal cramps, headaches, lower back pain, "growing" pains, and similar discomfort—are generally treated symptomatically; that is, a drug is administered to shield the body's pain sensors and bring relief. For very deep, acute pain, some palliation may be necessary. But for the slight pains of the head, back, and abdomen, Tibb has some very interesting insights into their origin. Let us now observe the Tibb perspective on these two phenomena of fever and pain.

Any fever is worthy of concern. It can be a sign of slight importance, or it may be one symptom of advanced cancer. The explanations that follow on the Tibb perspectives on fevers should be used as reference by physicians and students of natural healing. Individuals should not attempt to diagnose their own diseases from these signs.

Fever

Fever is an unnatural heat that arises from the heart, according to Tibb. Some biologists may wish to disagree, saying that the heart is merely a muscular pump with no other functions. However, scientists at Cornell University Medical College recently reported the discovery of biologically powerful substances in the heart and noted that they "probably act as hormones." Dr. John H. Laragh, a Cornell researcher, revealed that one of the substances was a compound, named auriculum, that acted as one of the most powerful diuretics known. From the Tibb viewpoint, any excessive decline in moisture would cause a rapid increase of heat: in other words, fever. Similar discoveries about unusual functions of the heart have been reported by physicians in Japan and Canada.

According to Tibb, fevers are divided into three classes. Those that originate in the spirit are called *ephemeral* fevers; those that originate in the humors are called *putrefactive* fevers; and those that occur in principal organs are called *hectic* fevers.

Ephemeral fevers have many causes: external exposure to extremes of heat or cold, or bathing in very hot or cold water; things ingested, such as heating foods, hot beverages, and hot medicines; and things that cause excessive motion, either of the body (sports) or of the spirit (anger and grief).

Ephemeral fevers are often emotion-related and are generally classified according to their mental signs, such as mental, angry, joyous, painful, fainting, hungry, solar, heating, water, and so on.

The ephemeral fever usually lasts only twenty-four hours, and the temperature is consistent, not rising. There is no sign of infection. The remedy is to remove the mental or spiritual cause and try to reduce food intake as much as possible, but inducing vomiting is not advised. Mild pain relievers and warm baths often prove soothing.

If an infection is present, there will often be a foul smell to the urine and feces. This kind of fever needs medical attention and possibly treatment by antibiotics. The signs of fever due to typhus infection (transmitted by animals) are excessive perspiration, nosebleed, asthma, great hunger, incessant sneezing, and fainting.

Putrefactive fevers have five causes: (1) overabundance of humors, (2) thickness of humors, (3) stickiness of humors, (4) obstruction of humors, and (5) the putrefaction that happens to humors when they remain too long without circulating and lack ventilation.

Hectic fevers also often arise from emotions—grief, worry, fear—but there are other causes that dry the body excessively while at the same time heating it. These fevers may also be caused by certain chronic diseases, very heating diseases, hot tumors, and similar conditions.

Fevers are said to be either continuous or intermittent. A continuous fever begins at one point and continues either to rise or to decline, or else it begins at one point and continues, neither increasing nor decreasing. With an intermittent fever, the temperature rises, then falls, then rises again. Continuous fever occurs when putrefaction is occuring inside the blood vessels, whereas intermittent fever is a sign that putrefaction is occurring inside one of the principal organs.

There are four general types of putrefactive fevers:

Permanent fever is due to putrefaction of blood (including bacterial infections) and is continuous.

Al-ghabb is due to putrefaction of yellow bile humor and alternates one day on, one day off.

Balgham (phlegm) is due to putrefaction of phlegm humor and appears daily.

Al-rub' is due to putrefaction of black bile humor and alternates one day on, two days off.

The alternating cycles of the intermittent fevers are due to the ease or difficulty in collecting, refining, and expelling the matter of the humors. The time between the appearances of the temperature of fever is called *rigor*. The time when the fever is apparent is called *paroxysm*. If a fever does not follow one of the three stated modes (daily, one day on and one day off, or one day on and two days off), it is because more than one humor is affected or more than one kind of imbalance or disease process is going on.

The time of paroxysm, the sudden rise of temperature announcing the fever, is also indicative of the specific humor being cleansed. The essence of the phlegm humor is viscid and difficult to dissolve and evacuate, and its paroxysm lasts generally eighteen hours. The black bile humor is even more difficult to decompose, due to its coldness, and its paroxysm lasts twenty-four hours. The yellow bile humor is between these two, and its paroxysm lasts about twelve hours.

TABLE 7
ORIGIN AND TYPE OF FEVERS

Type of Fever	Origin/ Cause	Duration/ Cycle	Paroxysm (With Fever)	Pause (Without Fever)
Ephemeral	Spirit/Emotions	24 hours only	24 hours	None
Putrefactive:				
Blood	Blood Humor	Continuous	24 hours	None
Phlegm	Phlegm Humor	day on/night off	12 hours	12 hours
Yellow Bile	Yellow Bile Humor	1 day on/1 day off	24 hours	24 hours
Black Bile	Black Bile Humor	1 day on/2 days off	24 hours	48 hours
Hectic:				
Tertian	Cold Yellow Bile	7 days	12 hours	36 hours
Quatrain	Corruption within principal organs	72 hours	18 hours	54 hours

The nature of the paroxysm is altered by the strength of the patient (the stronger the patient, the shorter the paroxysm), the nature of the residues being eliminated (the thicker and colder, the longer the paroxysm), and the constitution of the patient (the hotter the constitution of the patient, the shorter the paroxysm).

Hectic fevers are of three types: (1) those due to reduction of moisture in small vessels; (2) those in which moisture is fully dissipated and the heat fills the empty spaces caused by the absence of moisture; and (3) those in which the moisture of the organs is used up by the fever and the heat of the organs themselves adds to the fever.

It is important to know the *origin* of the cause of a fever. Fever is said to originate in the spirit, the humors, or the principal organs. Thus, if it originates from causes that heat the spirit (e.g., exposure to hot external temperatures), spreads from the spirit to the organ moistures, and then, after drying them up, heats the principal organs, it is still called emphemeral fever, because that is its point of origin. Likewise, if its course originates in a moisture that putrefies, then heats the spirit, then attacks the principal organs, it is called putrefactive fever, for that is its origin. The cause will be found at this point of origin, even though some treatment may be used to alleviate symptoms that arise in other parts.

Hectic fevers are called either tertian or quatrain. The whole cycle of the tertian fever lasts forty-eight hours, with the interval (period without fever) lasting approximately thirty-six hours and the paroxysm lasting twelve hours.

A pure tertian fever usually does not last more than one week. This is usually caused by the yellow bile humor becoming too cold and moist. If there is constipation, the superfluous matters are inside the veins and not in the principal organs. Food should be withheld as much as possible on the days the fever returns. If the person feels cold and trembles, give him or her oxymel (1 teaspoon honey with 1 tablespoon vinegar) with warm water. This will help purge the yellow bile. If the person vomits, it is a sign of healing. When the fever comes down, put the person's feet in a warm-water bath and massage them, which will help the fever descend from the head. Diuretics may be given, but no laxatives. If there is an abundance of mucus, use less cooling herbs and foods, but if the phlegm is "salty," use only cooling herbs and foods.

The quatrain fever has a cycle of seventy-two hours, the paroxysm lasting eighteen, and the pause lasting fifty-four hours.

There is no one specific treatment for each of these fevers, because each person would have to be evaluated in terms of age, temperament, vitality, season, and so forth. However, it is very useful to identify the origin and type of fever so that one can coordinate all diet and herbal medicines so as not to confuse the body in what it is trying to accomplish.

A general advice for returning fevers is to reduce food and water, especially cold water, on the day the fever returns. Avoid all fruits and foods that produce flatulence, and everything that is hot and dry in temperament. The humor should be purged, according to the signs of imbalance or the features of the fever (see Chapter 9).

Part Two, the Formulary, provides specific details of treatment for various imbalances, including regimens for extended chronic illnesses that exhibit one or more of these types of fevers.

Pain

Pain is usually thought of by physicians as a sign or signal of some "deeper" causative factor. But to the *patient*, it is the primary ailment. In fact, pain is the symptom that most often causes a patient to seek help from a physician.

The symptom of pain may be the cause of a disorder, because persistent pain impairs vitality; in this sense, pain is a disease.

Most people suffer predominantly from two kinds of pains: those of the abdomen and of the head. Western medical texts list almost forty different diseases of which headache is one of the main symptoms. But headache can also be a temporary sensation due to fatigue or stress. (I will exclude discussion of pain associated with accidental injury, for its causes are self-manifest, and emergency medical treatment is indicated in every case.)

Pain can be a symptom of conditions varying from a slight change in mood to terminal cancer of the colon. But the sensation of pain frequently appears long before an organ or internal system is degenerated to a terminal state. Yet most people try to dodge the signal offered by pain, masking it with aspirin and other remedies. This is unfortunate, because often years and years pass during which these signs are covered up, while the disease expands and ultimately becomes difficult to cure; and even if it can be, the procedures are gruesome.

According to Tibb, pain is a sensation produced by something contrary to the course of nature, and this sensation originates in one of two circumstances: (1) a very sudden change in temperament or the bad effects of an imbalanced temperament, or (2) the resolution of an imbalance—that is, a return to health.

To explain it another way, I might give the example of a person who has had properly balanced humors for years, but whose temperament, owing to a radical change in diet, changes to a hotter or colder character. The sensitive faculties of the body become aware of this change: this is "pain." There is no pain except as the sensation of an opposite force. A temperament that is always unbalanced (chronic) does not produce pain. This is so because, over time, the improper temperament thoroughly destroys the healthy temperament, so that it acts as if it were never there and becomes "used to" the intemperament. Therefore, it neither experiences pain nor becomes aware of it (because there must be a contrariness of forces for pain to be felt).

The hot, cold, moist, and dry temperaments of the whole person, as well as the specific parts (see Chapter 2), provide a very useful index to understand the nature of imbalances—both their immediate causes and the preexisting dietary indiscretions that led up to full-blown disease states.

The reason some people suffer more pain than others, often during a similar or identical illness, is due to the relative strength or balance of the innate temperaments of the body parts, and the strength of the force that opposes it. A hot intemperament can cause pain by its own energy, as can a cold intemperament. But a dry intemperament causes pain only as a secondary matter, and a moist intemperament is painless. This is so because heat and cold are active qualities, and dryness and moisture are passive ones. According to Galen, pain is due to one thing only: loss of the proper continuity of temperament. In order to experience the sensation of pain, there must be a rapid coming together or rapid dispersal of particles—the fact of this motion accounts for the painful sensation. For example, viewing some object of extreme blackness can cause pain to the eyes, as can viewing an object of severe whiteness (such as sun-drenched snow). In both cases, it is due to the very compacted nature of the particles of color. The effect of heat is the opposite—the rapid dispersal of particles, which causes pain. This is true of all forms of pain perceived by the senses of touch, taste, smell, and sight.

There are fifteen kinds of pain identified in Tibb. These are listed below, with the causative feature of each.

KINDS OF PAIN

1. *Boring* pain is caused by retention of gross matter or gas within the folds of a "hard" organ, such as the colon. The retained matter constantly rubs and pushes against the organ, "boring" it.
2. The pain of *compression* is produced when fluid or gas is confined in too small a space and causes a squeezing or compression of the tissues.
3. *Fatigue* pain is caused by excess labor, gaseous substance, a humor under tension (overabundant humor), or a humor of ulcerative properties.
4. *Corrosive* pain derives from material being trapped between the muscle fibers and their sheaths, stretching it until it disturbs the temperament of the muscle fiber and the muscle itself.
5. *Dull* pain is from an overly cold temperament, obstruction of pores so that the vital force cannot penetrate into a member, and distension of the cavities of the body.
6. *Stabbing* pain results when a humor enters between and separates membranes. In some cases the whole body is affected; in others only one member is affected.
7. *Heavy* pain is due to an inflammation in an organ that has few or no pain sensors, such as the lung, kidney, or liver. The weight of the inflammation

added to the organ causes it to drag against adjacent organs and tissues, which experience the pain.

8. *Incisive* pain is due to a humor of sour quality.
9. *Irritant* pain occurs when a humor is changed to a harsh or rough nature.
10. *Itching* pain is due to the bitter, sharp, or salty nature of a humor.
11. *Relaxing* pain is caused by matters accumulating and stretching the muscle, not the tendons. The pain is due to the belly of the muscle being more lax than that of the tendon.
12. *Throbbing* pain is due to a hot inflammation.
13. *Tension* pain is produced by a humor overstretching nerves or muscles.
14. *Pricking* pain is due to matter entering into an organ for a time, then rupturing it.
15. *Tearing* pain arises when a humor or gas enters between the bone and the periosteum, or from cold which strongly contricts the periosteum.

The main effect of pain on the body is that it causes weakness and interferes with the normal functioning of organs. In particular, the lungs are constricted and unable to perform complete oxygenation. The breath becomes either too fast or unnatural in rhythm. Severe pain, such as that of distension (incisive pain), disperses the breath. Any pain in the area of the heart will also disperse the breath. The temperaments become cold because the vitality is lost.

Most temporary pains are due to one of two factors: (1) corrupted or overabundant humors, which causes stretching of the tissue fibers or adds excess weight to the organ, or (2) accumulations of gas in the viscera of the stomach, the membranes of nerves or organs, the sheaths of muscles, the subcutaneous muscles (as between the muscles and loose skin), or the internal muscles, such as those of the thorax. Such gas may be dispersed quickly or over time, depending upon the amount of gas, its quality, and whether the affected part is dense or light in structure.

There are three approaches to the relief of pain. The first is to do something contrary to the cause of the pain—that is, to remove the cause. The second is to use an agent that counteracts the corrupted humor, soothes the body, induces sleep, or dulls the sensitive faculties and lessens their activity. Agents that accomplish this include inebriants, milk, and massage oils (saffron, rose). The third method is to use some agent that completely dulls the sensation in the painful part. All narcotics and sleep-inducing drugs are used in this approach. The first method is the most certain to produce relief.

In sum, pain is caused by either a sudden change in temperament or a loss of continuity of function. The first class of causes is due to the arising of a hot, cold, moist, or dry intemperament. The second class of causes is the result of deposits of matter or the effect of gas or inflammatory conditions.

When considering the three choices of treatment, the least favored is to destroy the sensation of the part feeling pain. This destruction of sensation can be accomplished only by making it extremely "cold" or by exposing it to toxic agents (narcotics), which interfere with its functions.

A basic formula for alleviating pain is to make a poultice of dill seed and linseed oil and place it over the painful part.

In addition to dill and linseed, other substances that create relief by soothing include chamomile, celery seed, bitter almond, and anything that is hot in the first degree, especially if combined with some glutinous agent such as prunes, starch, saffron, marshmallow, cardamom, cabbage, or turnip. These can be made in decoction (tea) form. The useful oils are rose, violet, saffron, sweet almond, and sandalwood. Laxatives and other forms of elimination must be encouraged, for they will help draw away the cause.

The most powerful herbal anesthetic medicine is opium. Less powerful agents are deadly nightshade (belladonna), lettuce seed, snow, and ice water. Some herbal agents are unavailable without prescription, and even if obtained, must be used under a physician's direct supervision and should never be self-administered.

One should always be alert for obvious, external causes of pain that may have been forgotten, such as recent falls (e.g., during epileptic attack or drunkenness), improper posture during sleep, or straining during heavy work. If no such cause can be uncovered, look for the signs of excess in one of the humors.

A pain may originate from an external cause and then become internal. Drinking very icy water will cause pain in the stomach and liver area. In such a case a full regimen of adjusting humors is not required. A good warm bath and a restful sleep are sufficient. Or one may have indulged in eating too many hot peppers, and a headache resulted. A glass of cold water is enough.

The remedies selected for pain must be appropriate to the particular condition. Colic may be cured by evacuating the contents of the lower intestine, but the pain may be so severe that more immediate relief is necessary. On the other hand, very rapid relief may be provided only by creating a worse injury than what one was trying to cure. This is the unfortunate result of treatments with many biochemical medicines.

Judgment and sense must be applied in selecting a course of treatment. If a pain is allowed to increase, it can cause death by destroying innate heat and vitality, interruption of the heart, and so forth. So a judgment must be made of the potential harm that will result by making the organ insensate to pain. For example, the bowels may not be able to function. In this case, one should make the organ insensate, for the immediate danger of death from extreme pain is averted, and other methods may be used to evacuate the bowels.

A general principle is that internal remedies for pain should not be excessively cold in temperament. All narcotics are extremely cold. Such agents not only decrease the innate heat but also increase the amount of superfluous matter and solidify it and enclose it, making it quite difficult to refine and expel.

Other methods of relieving pain include walking around for an extended period. The motion softens the tissues and relaxes the body. Music, especially if it is agreeable and softly inclines one to sleep, is a powerful pain reliever. Being intensely engaged in an activity one finds engrossing helps reduce the severity of pain.

We have now examined all of the fundamental principles of the Tibb system of healing, including the basic temperaments, the humors, the process of digestion, dietetics, and the major signs that indicate the body is well or ill. In the next chapter, I present the evidences of a metabolic efficiency as reflected in the eliminations of the body.

8
The Cycle Completed: Elimination

There is a simple yet stunning way to think of health, and that it is in relation to the three basic functions of the individual cell. Each cell must (1) take in nutrients and (2) metabolize those nutrients; and (3) the by-products of this metabolism must be carried away. So the simplest way to think of disease is as a condition in which one or more of these three cellular functions has become disordered. Either the nutrient substances are wrong and harmful, or they are not being metabolized correctly, or the by-products are not being carried away efficiently.

We have examined the quality and quantity of foods and nutrient substances and many factors relative to the measurement of the life-force functions of metabolism. Now we shall discover the significance of the signs of the elimination of the by-products of bodily metabolism.

It is in the West that perhaps the greatest aversion to and embarrassment over bodily wastes is encountered. Virtually no one cares to discuss urine and feces, much less to *look* at them! Nonetheless, there are important signs to be found in these substances, which after all are simply a product of one's own natural bodily functions. And, in health at least, they are no more offensive than what is being carried around within the body at all times. In the East it is the custom to squat while performing the toilet functions, and to use the hand and water for cleansing afterward. While this may seem peculiar to some Westerners, it does afford each person a direct knowledge of the by-products of digestion—and the chance to take corrective action at the very slightest and first signs of disorder. Every physician will agree that one of the most important factors in treating disease is to seek advice at the very earliest signs of imbalance. Too often people are unaware of the signs because they have never observed their bodily wastes.

Before proceeding with an explanation of urinalysis, it would be worthwhile here to quote from the British medical doctor O. Cameron Gruner, who translated the first book of Avicenna's *Canon* into English. He was trained in Western orthodox medicine, yet he remained firmly convinced of the enduring value—even superiority—of the diagnostic modes employed by our predecessors. Dr. Gruner writes in the *Canon:*

For the detection of changes in the composition of the urine, the ancients were restricted to the evidence afforded by the color, odor, and what may be called "texture." The evidence was apt to be [considered] fallacious because wide difference of composition may produce similar appearances, and differences of appearance do not always denote noteworthy changes of composition.

On the other hand, the limitations in the utility of these simple observations were balanced by the relatively vague conception of the bodily functions. The whole outlook on disease was lacking in detail without being basically incorrect. Thus, many diseased states were ascribed to defective digestive processes, a fact often overlooked today. . . .

To say that the whole body is concerned in digestion is, broadly speaking, correct, especially if we realize that the term digestion covers what we call metabolism. In the Canon, digestion is viewed in two aspects: (1) that which begins in the alimentary canal and ends in the liver; (2) that which is called "maturation," which concerns the digestive products in their course through the body and ending in tissues. If such maturation is not completed, surplus substances appear, and may undergo sedimentation. The phenomena of disease are attributable to this defective maturation. Consequently, the business of diagnosis and prognosis comes to be a matter of assessing the efficiency or otherwise of maturation.

The study of the urine is therefore directed to this assessment, its different physical properties being noted, both in health and under various unhealthy conditions. Translucence, opacity, separation out into visibility of various substances, the appearance of gaseous matter (in foam), and changes in odor—all these are interpreted in light of the two-fold division of digestion: that culminating in the liver, and that culminating in the tissues.

This basis of study is reasonable, and it is not right that they should have been superseded as is the case in modern times. . . .

Dr. Gruner then makes note of the insufficiency of modern laboratory analysis, which excludes the dynamic aspects of the *patient*, who after all is the repository and site of the processes that are disordered. Dr. Gruner continues:

So if we visualize in a practical form everything that is relevant, we must not forget the dynamic aspect of the matter. Changes are going on hour by hour, and the laboratory cannot keep pace with them. Consequently, we shall in the end make use of the self-same data which Avicenna relied on entirely, and we learn from him to scrutinize the urine—not merely to find such things as albumin, blood or pus or casts—but deliberately to know: (1) Is there any insufficiency in the digestive process in the pre-[liver] stages? (2) If not, is there any [liver] insufficiency, and in what direction? (3) If so, or if there is trouble in the tissues at large, arising out of an abnormal condition of one or more of the humors—which one is at fault? In what way is it at fault? Is it entirely morbid or not? (4) What is the degree of vitality of the patient (Avicenna included "innate heat" in this)? Is the vitality increasing, or failing, or inactive?—recovery from illness, or its duration, or succumbing to illness is often primarily a matter of vitality. . . .

Such fundamental questions the modern practitioner (even in cities) can still answer from the simple data used of old, and combine them with the intimate study of the pulse, to realize the nature of the processes in the organs and tissues of the sick from day to day, and feel himself actually armed with that *real* insight (into the state of the particular patient) which relatives and friends sometimes incorrectly assume him to have.*

Let us now consider this illuminating science of urinalysis as formulated by Avicenna. Although mastery of urinalysis requires study with an experienced Hakim, many aspects of urine can be noted and evaluated by the layperson.

Healthy urine is of medium consistency; is lightly tinted, tending to the color of straw; and has a moderate, not offensive odor. If sediment is present, it should be white and light.

The urine alters during the progressive stages of life. In infancy, it is like milk, thus nearly colorless. In childhood, it is thicker and coarser. In adolescence, there is more fire in the constitution, so the urine is more colored. In adulthood it tends to be white and tenuous, and also thicker due to the quality of excess matter being ejected. In old age the urine becomes whiter again. If it becomes very thick, it may indicate the formation of stones.

The urine of females is thicker, whiter, and less clear than that of males. If the urine of males is shaken in a beaker, it becomes cloudy, and this cloudiness ascends to the top of the beaker. The urine of females, when shaken, usually develops a circular foam on top. If urine samples of a male and a female are mixed together, a network of filaments forms almost immediately, which is also true of urine specimens taken immediately after intercourse.

In pregnancy, the urine is quite clear, and there is a light "cloud" on the surface. The color is close to that of chick peas, or yellow with a hue of blue or iridescence in it. There is also present a sort of "tinted cotton" in the midst of it. If there is quite distinct rainbow tint, it is a sign that the initial stage of conception has begun. When the rainbow tint evolves to an overall reddish tint, it means that the impregnation is complete, especially if the urine becomes cloudy when shaken.

There are two general points to consider initially with respect to the urine. First, when the urine is clear at the time of passing, then turns opaque on sitting, this means that the resolution of nutrients is difficult, that the digestive powers are having difficulty refining the food. Second, when opaque urine is passed, then becomes clear after standing, this means that the digestive powers have successfully matured the nutrients. The clearer the urine becomes, and the more rapidly the sediments fall to the bottom, the more complete the digestion.

The diagnostic features in the Tibb methods of assessing the urine are (1) quan-

---

*O. Cameron Gruner, *The Canon of Medicine of Avicenna* (New York: Augustus M. Kelley, 1970).

tity, (2) odor, (3) color, (4) foam, (5) texture, (6) clearness, and (7) sediment.

It is necessary to obtain a proper specimen of the urine to be evaluated, and for this certain precautions are necessary. The procedure for collecting a urine specimen are as follows:

1. The specimen should be collected in the early morning, and the patient should have slept through the night. It is not suitable to take the specimen the night before and keep it until morning.
2. The person must not have taken food or drink before taking the sample.
3. The diet the night before must not have included any of the following (which will affect the color of the urine): saffron, cassia, any potherbs, salted fish (causes dark urine), and intoxicating beverages.
4. The patient should not have taken any medicines that purge any of the humors.
5. The patient should not be under excessive stress or in an unnatural mental state from anger, wakefulness, or excessive labor. Vomiting will alter the color of urine; sexual intercourse will render the urine oily. Avicenna notes that urine must be collected and evaluated within one hour of taking the sample, although other physicians say it is all right up to six hours.
6. The vessel in which the sample is collected must be clear glass or crystal and must be clean.
7. The urine sample must not be exposed to extremes of heat or freezing temperature, nor to direct rays of the sun, nor to wind. The sample must be viewed in indirect light, as the direct rays of the sun will create false perceptions of the color and sediments.

Generally speaking, reading the urine of children yields little information, and that of infants even less so, because their nutrition is derived solely from mother's milk, which imparts very little coloring matter to urine. Moreover, babies sleep longer hours, which eradicates evidences of digestion.

The primary objectives of examining the urine are to determine the state of the liver, the urinary tracts, and the blood vessels. The most precise and useful information obtained is that concerning the functional capacity of the liver.

Urine felt inside the bathroom usually feels cold; when felt outside the bathroom, it feels hot. The actual temperature is actually invariable, but because the air temperature in the bathroom is warm, it causes the urine to feel cold.

There are two components of urine: the fluid, watery part, and the part that precipitates and separates from it. The two factors examined with regard to the water part are its consistency and its color.

The precipitates are three: (1) cloudiness, which is what separates at the upper part of the vessel; (2) the suspended part, which separates at the middle; and (3) the precipitate, which settles at the bottom.

The kinds of consistency are also three: thin, thick, and intermediate.

Evaluation of the Fluid Parts of Urine

Colors

There are six colors that are significant: white, yellow, fiery, bright red, dark red, and black.

The color white may be translucent, as with glass, or milky. There are eleven degrees of whiteness, each of which is associated with a different imbalance:

1. Mucilaginous: excess of blood humor.
2. Waxlike: liquefaction of fatty tissue.
3. Greasy, soapy: liquefaction of blood humor; may signify diabetes, active or latent.
4. Musty whiteness, tinted with blood and pus: ulcers discharging into the urinary passages.
5. Musty whiteness, not tinted with blood: great excess of crude, nonmatured matter; stones.
6. Like semen: inflammation arising in blood humor; disease associated with blood humor.
7. Lead-white, no sediment: bad.
8. Milk white, in acute diseases: ominous.
9. Sudden change from red to white in the course of a fever: the patient will become delirious.
10. Whiteness persisting in a person apparently healthy: absence of digestion in the veins, and in diabetes.
11. Whiteness like buttermilk, in acute fevers: may signify lifeless fetus, or wasting of entire body.

Generally, whiteness indicates that the imbalance is due to an altogether cold intemperament, but digestion remains sound. Urine often is white at the onset of a disease and gradually darkens as the disease takes its course. Urine is also white during the waking state. If urine is dusky during daylight hours, it signifies some digestive imbalance. The physical cause of the white color is the inability of bile to mix with the urine or an overabundance of phlegm mixed with the urine.

Yellow color is found in varying degrees: straw yellow, lemon yellow, orange-yellow, flame or saffron yellow, and clear reddish yellow. The last four indicate hot intemperament. A straw yellow color is due to a small amount of bile mixing with the urine; flame yellow is due to a large amount of bile mixing with it; and reddish yellow is from an even larger amount of bile. Urine tends to saffron yellow in maladies known as very hot and burning. The clearer the urine, generally, the more digestion going on. In certain diseases the urine may be tinged with red because of blood in the urine. Gradual loss of blood via urine is a critical sign because it usually means some form of internal hemorrhage.

It is even worse if the urine thins out and takes on an offensive odor. However, the presence of small amounts of blood in the urine may be a favorable sign in certain types of extended fever conditions.

In jaundice, the urine frequently turns a deeper and deeper red until it almost appears black. This is a good sign that detoxification is occurring. If the urine is white or pale red, it means the jaundice is not subsiding.

Fasting almost invariably causes the urine to become deeply colored and bitter-smelling.

The color green in urine ranges from that of the shade of pistachios to leek green and emerald green. A light green tint to urine usually indicates lack of internal combustion. If observed after great physical labor, it means there is an internal spasm. Some physicians say that a rainbow green indicates poisoning, and that if there is sediment in the urine, there is hope of recovery, while no sediment indicates that the poisoning is likely to be fatal. Green the color of rusted brass is a sign of impending death due to complete extinguishing of the innate heat.

"Black" urine actually refers to the density of red coloration to the point of utter darkness. Such coloration of the urine means there is high oxidation taking place, a great internal cold, imminent death, a healing crisis (detoxification), or evacuation of superfluous black bile humor.

Dark coloration of urine is a good sign in acute diseases if it occurs at the time expected in relation to the healing crisis (generally in the middle of the crisis). Dark urine at the onset or end of a fever disease is an ominous sign. The appearance of dark urine in the elderly is always a bad sign, for it can only indicate massive destruction of organs. In women who are experiencing childbirth, dark urine may presage convulsions.

Thinness of urine is the result of either indigestion or obstruction. Denseness of urine is a sign of the maturation of the humors (meaning that a healing crisis is imminent) or indicates that a thick humor is being eliminated and is mixing with the urine. A balanced consistency comes from a balanced quality, quantity, and maturation of the humors.

It must be noted that urine can be thin on expulsion, then later thicken or remain thin. If it is thin and remains thin, the pathenogenic matters are not yet ripened and ready to expel.

The list below summarizes various types of urine, with respect to color, transparency, thickness, clearness, and so forth, and the conditions indicated by such signs.

TYPES OF URINE

Dense when evacuated, and remains dense: Humors are at the height of their ripening.

Dense when evacuated, later clears and thins out: Ripening of the humors has abated, and the humors have begun to separate.

Thin white urine: During health, this indicates weakness of life force and temperament (common in old age). During illness, it indicates different conditions; in chronic diseases, it means that pathogenic matter has not yet ripened.

Thin, yellow urine: Nature is weak and unable to ripen pathogenic matter, which means it cannot thicken the urine; the weak start of ripening explains why the urine turns yellow.

Thin, bright red urine: nonmaturation of the disease, or lack of nutrients in young adults, or a strong heat in the body, from which excess bile is generated, as in fever or sleeplessness or by excessive heating of the body.

Dense, dark urine: abundance of blood, as in continuing fever.

Dense, black urine: dominance of cold, combustion of blood, or evacuation of black bile.

Opaque urine, with sandy sediment: stones.

Opaque urine with pus and bad odor, and scaly particles separating out: rupture of an abcess.

Color of washings of raw meat: unhealthy blood flowing from liver. If the feces are also this color, it indicates the presence of an inflammatory mass within the liver. If prior to the coloration of the feces and urine there was shortness of breath and dry cough, along with stabbing pains in the chest, it is a sign of a rupturing abcess in the chest or in the area of the aorta.

Urine resembles pus: This may be of benefit to a person who never exercises, as it purges the whole body. The substance is not actually pus, but morbid matter resembling pus. Actual pus in the urine appears only after the bursting of an abcess. In this case the urine is not only thick but also dark.

Cloudy urine: loss of vitality.

Color of chick-pea water: present during pregnancy and in persons with chronic inflammations.

Foam

The characteristics of the foam are significant. The foam that arises in urine is due to moisture and gases forced into the urine as it is emitted. A reddish or dark foam is seen in jaundice. Large bubbles indicates thickness or stickiness. Numerous bubbles indicate thickness and excess gas. If small bubbles are present for an extended time in kidney diseases, the illness will not be resolved quickly.

Evaluation of the Sediments

There are four things observed in the sediments of urine: color, position, consistency, and the time when it is observed.

The significant colors are white, black, red, yellow, and dusky.

Position means that the sediment might be situated in the upper part of the vessel, it might be suspended in the middle, or it may form in the bottom.

The *consistency* is evaluated with respect to whether it is whole or broken, smooth or rough, flaky or not, whether it resembles crushed wheat, and whether it is granular, like bran, like grains of vetch, sandy, bloody, or like pus.

With respect to *time of observation*, one considers whether the sediments are present during the whole of the illness or only on certain days and not on others, or only a long time after the illness has begun.

The most favorable sediment is that which settles on the bottom of the glass and is white, smooth, and uniform during the whole course of the disease.

The successful, complete progression of digestion can be learned from whether the sediment is floating on top, suspended, or on the bottom. Sediment remains suspended due to air captured within the organic matter that nature does not ripen and digest. If air is not dissolved during digestion, it remains enclosed in the interior of the nutritive substance. If there is abundant unresolved air, it causes the sediment to rise to the top and become a cloud.

A floating residue, when cloudy, indicates a weak and ineffective power of metabolism. A settled residue indicates complete and total maturation. A suspended residue indicates a condition between these two.

It is necessary to distinguish among white sediment, raw urine (as opposed to ripened urine), and pus, all of which are similar in appearance. White sediment results from a complete fusion of particles in such a way that there are no distinct particles in it. Rawness of urine can be known by the presence of small, distinct particles resembling sand. Pus is known from its stench. The following list gives the various natures of the sediments and comments on their significance.

SIGNIFICANCE OF TYPES OF URINARY SEDIMENT

Sediment is white, smooth, observed on some days, not on others: Indicates that natural process cannot continue to ripen the pathogenic matter in the body.

Sediment is white every day and not smooth: Natural force has failed to effect a complete maturation in one effort. This condition is worse than the preceding one because it means that the first residues have not been ripened and will be joined by additional superfluous matters.

Sediment is dispersed, broken, and not smooth: A thick air has been generated in the chyme, causing it to be cut and dispersed and digestion to be interrupted.

Residue settles at the bottom of the vessel, is not smooth: This condition is unfavorable if it persists, as it indicates that air is so thick and abundant that the natural forces cannot thin it and dissolve it.

Red sediment: Indicates indigestion, caused by blood that has not been fully ripened; thus indicates long duration of disease, since disease only ends if the digestion and ripening of blood are completed.

Dusky sediment: Shows dominance of cold and diminishing of natural force.

Yellow sediment: Very intense heat and malignant, destructive disease.

Black residue: Either excessive heat consuming the matter in the body or intense cold solidifying and blackening the matter of the body. If residue is dusky at first, then turns black, it is due to cold. If it is first yellow, then black, it is due to heat.

Oily urine (either in color or consistency, or both): Generally indicates melting of the fat, either of the kidneys or from other organs. If oily only in color, melting is at the beginning stage. If oily in consistency, melting is on the increase. If oily in both regards, melting is at its peak. One can distinguish between melting of kidneys as opposed to other organs of the body because if the fat of the kidney melts, it is eliminated in one mass, rapidly, and it floats like fat on top of the urine. Fat from other organs is discharged bit by bit, slowly.

Sediment resembling grains of vetch: From degeneration of the tissue of the kidneys or of other organs. If this form of sediment is accompanied by a high, quick fever, the disease is in the whole body; if there is no fever, it is only in the kidney.

Flaky sediment: From loss of surface cells of principal organs or peeling of the surface of the bladder. If there is fever, it is the external surface of the internal organs; if no fever, it is the inner surface of the bladder. If the flakes are brown, like the scales of fish, they are a very bad sign, for they mean that the mucous linings are being sloughed off, usually a consequence of terminal illness.

Branlike residue: Means excess heat has acted on vessels to the extent that degeneration has reached into deep inner parts; also indicates scabby disease in the bladder. Fever indicates that the disease is in the whole body; if there is no fever, the disease is exclusively in the bladder.

Sediment resembling crushed wheat: Effect of excess heat has reached degeneration into the depths of principal organs; also may indicate lack of combustion of blood. The residue resembling crushed wheat that results from degeneration of the principal organs is white, whereas that resulting from combustion of blood is red.

Thick red urine with red sediment: Indicates abundance of blood, nonripening of superfluous matters, and chronic disease but ultimate healing. If long-standing, indicates inflammation of the liver.

Thick red urine with white sediment: Indicates that blood is abundant and little resistance is offered to the ripening of humors; the disease will last long, but not too long.

Blood and pus in urine: Indicates with certainty the existence of an ulcer, in either the kidneys or the bladder, in one of the two ureters, or in one of the organs above them. Pus coming from the kidneys and bladder persists for a long time, whereas pus coming from the organs above them lasts only one, two, or three days.

Sandy sediment: Stones are forming either in kidneys or bladder.

Blood passed in urine, but only once: Indicates that a vessel has ruptured in the kidneys. (Neither the bladder nor ureters contain vessels of enough size that much blood could flow from them.)

Pus in urine with smooth white sediment: Indicates that there is a hot tumor in the bladder that has ripened.

The Alvine Discharge

The contents of the stool are called the alvine discharge and are evaluated in terms of quantity and consistency. It is first useful to have an idea of the nature of the healthy stool. The stool should (1) be held together and not loose; (2) have watery and solid parts mixed about equally; (3) be soft and tending to honey in consistency; (4) be easily evacuated; (5) be of a color nearing yellow (stools the color of the food eaten means that digestion is incomplete); (6) have an odor that is not offensive, yet not be entirely odorless; (7) be passed without audible sound or gurgling of gas; (8) be passed at the times normal for a healthy person, and (9) have a bulk nearly the same as the food consumed.

Quantity. The quantity should not be greater than the food eaten. If there is more in bulk than the food eaten, it means there is an overabundance of humors. If less than the amount of food eaten, it means there is (1) diminishing of humors, (2) retention of the food in the colon, or (3) weakness of the expulsive power.

Consistency. Moist feces indicate defective digestion or obstruction at some stage of digestion, so that insufficient water is absorbed from the food. Frothy fecal matter indicates mixing of gases with the humors, or very great internal heat.

Dry stools result from very great physical labor, internal heat, drying foods, or an extended time in passing through the colon. When the feces are both hard and dry, it is due to lack of bile or a delay in the colon with excessive moisture.

Color. White stool signifies an obstruction of the passages carrying bile and is seen with jaundice. If there is also an offensive odor, it may mean that an inflammatory mass has ruptured. It should be noted that a healthy person who seldom exercises often passes odorous matter, which acts as a natural purgative to the system.

A very red color of the stool reveals the crisis point of a disease.

Dark or black stool means high oxidation, maturing of a disease caused by imbalance of the black bile humor. There may be a silvery sheen to the stool from the passing of black bile humor. The passing of black bile in the stool or vomit is a bad sign. The passing of pure black bile matter from the anus usually indicates impending death.

Blackness of the stool can also be caused by the presence of blood in small or great quantities, which is a sign of diseases of the liver, intestinal ulcer, or rupture of internal vessels.

Green stool indicates diminished innate heat. The green coloration is due to a peculiar form of bile.

Intensely yellow stool, if occurring at the beginning of a disease, is a sign of an imbalance of the yellow bile humor. If at the end of a disease, it is a good sign, as it indicates that the body is eliminating harmful substances.

Multicolored, pus-filled, very sticky stool are all very grave signs of degeneration of the internal organs.

A bulky shape indicates the presence of intestinal gas. If the feces are passed through rapidly, it means there is an excess of bile in the gallbladder and a weak retentive power. A long term of passage of feces is a sign of poor digestion, coldness of intestines, excessive moisture, too much sleep, and flatulence.

Now that we have a comprehensive view of the signs of the body that indicate imbalances, let us consider the modes of treatment that lead to relief and the restoration of balance to the body.

9
Restoring the Balance

There are many forms of disease. The current texts of orthodox medicine identify more than twenty thousand names of diseases. It is fair to assume that no one person (or even a team of people) can possibly hold all of the various symptoms of all diseases in mind when evaluating a patient. This fact has led to the creation of medical specialties, in which a physician trained in one aspect or body part will diagnose and treat that aspect or part only. This is equivalent to a veterinarian's claiming that he only treats horses' ears and cannot be concerned with their hooves!

The first important point in considering potential treatments or therapies is that as many as 80 percent of all signs, symptoms, maladies, and conditions are not signs of disease, but rather evidence of the body performing its own self-cleansing role. Dr. Lewis Thomas, physician-philosopher and former head of the Memorial Sloan-Kettering Cancer Institute in New York City, stated in an interview for the *New Yorker* that every honest physican will admit that 80 percent of his patients' ailments will get better by themselves. This may seem puzzling, but when the Tibb principles are understood, it becomes clear that the symptoms associated with nausea, most fevers, diarrhea, sweating, frequent urination, and most nosebleeds, are all, during youth and middle age, almost invariably signs of *health*, not disease. Even though medication may be prescribed, most of these complaints would get better by themselves even if nothing was done. This means that physicians spend an undue part of their practice misprescribing for ailments, while at the same time being prevented from concentrating upon more serious cases that require more time than they are accustomed to giving. For the patient, it means that almost all responsibility for knowing about one's own body and health has been lost or abandoned. For if patients were responsible and educated about the normal processes of health, they would not require medical treatment nearly as often as they seek it today—usually with less than satisfactory results.

Let us understand precisely what is happening when the body sends forth those signals of so-called disease.

The first sign, a universal sign at least, of disease, is fever. If a person has a slight flushing of the cheeks, the dull throb of a headache, a warmish forehead, these are sufficient to call in sick at the office or take a day off from school.

But sometimes the fever is truly severe, soaring up over 100°, and the person is laid flat by the exertions of the body. Most people call a doctor at this stage because they have no idea what is going on, and the feelings they experience are intense enough for them to realize if they become any *greater*, there is reason to be concerned about the continuity of life.

In the first place, we become panicky because we are totally ignorant of these processes, and any unknown event creates awe and fear in human beings. If we had knowledge of what was happening to us, we would not become so alarmed. Hospital workers, nurses, and doctors seem so maddeningly blasé when an alarmed and terrified mother arrives at the emergency room with a feverish and vomiting baby. The signs that caused the late-night flight to the hospital are apparently not so formidable to those trained and accustomed to dealing with illness.

Mothers who have raised more than one child can attest to this. The first baby is cuddled and coddled, and the slightest whimper sends the mother with ashen face to the side of the infant, peering into its eyes and face as if to discern the very presence of an actual germ crawling across the infant's skin. Or, when the baby is teething, the crying is accompanied by vomiting, diarrhea, fevers—so much so that the mother trundles the baby off to the well-baby clinic, only to discover that the doctors have no idea what is wrong and insist on performing tests to discover what is "causing" the symptoms. More often than not, after a great deal of probing and furrowing of brows, the baby and mother are ultimately returned home, with medicine to relieve symptoms and an admonition to watch the baby closely. But the next day, the signs have passed. Doctors often say it is something "going around."

The reality of the matter is that when anyone has a fever, it is either due to a bacterial or viral infection or, as I shall illustrate, the body is trying to process superfluous by-products of digestion on the way to a healing crisis—that is, the elimination of such substances and the restoration of health.

There is no known effective treatment for viral infections. As stated in the standard physicians' diagnosis manual: "Several hundred different viruses may infect man. Many have been recognized only recently, so their clinical effects or even relationships are not fully delineated. . . . Such viruses are found in all parts of the world. . . . In theory, most viral infections can, by some means, be recognized; in practice, diagnosis remains difficult."* The manual goes on to state that even with such acute, life-threatening diseases as viral meningitis, the actual causative virus is identified "even in the best of circumstances" in less than half of the cases. For all forms of virus listed in the *Merck Manual,* under the headings giving proposed therapies, every entry states "None."

Merck Manual of Diagnosis and Therapy, 12th ed. (Rahway, N.J.: Merck Sharp & Dohme Research Laboratories, 1982), p. 170.

Physicians have no treatment except for oral administration of iodine, called Lugol's solution. As recently as the 1940s, the general public could buy Lugol's solution of iodine, and this was a common home treatment for sore throat and strep throat—painting the throat with iodine. But Lugol's is now a prescription item.

Now, it is true that viruses can cause fevers, but usually the body, if healthy, will fight them off. If the innate heat (vital force; immune system) is weakened, this process can become complicated, and organs and systems may be damaged. But in any event, physicians cannot do anything to treat the cause, the virus infestation. Their treatments are aimed at preventing complications from arising—that is, a secondary infection from bacteria, which can occur when the body is in a weakened condition (in Tibb, we would say that the humors are in a state of intemperament). This is the logic employed, at any rate, when administering penicillin for croup. Croup is caused by a virus, and penicillin has no effect on its cause. But the reasoning goes that the penicillin acts as a preventative against any *other* disease that might arise in this weakened condition. Of course, many physicians give penicillin for flus and other conditions that are not affected by antibiotics.

Now, if the fever is caused by bacteria, we have an entirely different matter, for, as the world knows, antibiotics will definitely kill bacteria. However, the common scientific knowledge of today has elaborated the problems associated with bacterial strains evolving their own defensive mechanisms that can sidestep these killer medicines, creating ever-more-virulent strains of bacteria.

According to Tibb, the reason so many people are afflicted with the symptoms usually associated with viral infections, or influenza and the common cold, is that the body's own self-healing and cleansing mechanisms are trying to eliminate excess toxic matters from the body: this is the force behind those 80 percent who "get better by themselves."

The health industry in all its myriad manifestations has so conditioned people to believe that all diseases are caused by bacteria and other germs that people have a very difficult time accepting that these are not truly the cause of disease after all. Please reread the first chapter and the discussion of the evolution of the concepts of causative agents of disease, and ponder over the fact that the bacterial theory of disease has come into prominence only in the past fifty years, and may not be the prevailing accepted medical theory even ten years from now.

In the chapter on food, it was explained that food is the source of heat, the fuel for the body. The body's digestive processes are also a continuous effort to heat, or "cook," the nutrients so that they may be broken down into component parts, utilized by the body, and then eliminated completely. The secret of human health and wellness is this fact, and this fact alone: most illness results when incomplete digestion of food has occurred over a short or long period of time.

"The stomach is the home of disease" is a statement of the essence of medicine, made by the Prophet Muhammad (peace of God be upon him) more than 1,400 years ago. More recently, some prophetic-minded physicians have agreed with this dictum. Hippocrates believed it. Galen believed it. Avicenna established it as a law of medicine. Yet today it is ignored. Let me stress this point again in unambiguous terms. Since the body's metabolism causes nutrient substances to *become* the human body (including its disease-fighting mechanisms), the ultimate origin of most illness is in food, or diet.

Heat is necessary for the efficient life of the body. Heat is maintained in the stomach by consuming food. And all of the body and limbs receive their proportion of nourishment and heat from the source of the stomach. As the whole room is warmed by the fuel that is consumed in the fireplace, the greater the quantity and quality of wood consumed, the greater the heat in the room. So too in the body: the more food, well digested, the more heat and life force through the whole body.

The origin of disease is due most of all to the continuous reception into the stomach of food that is not suitable for the best nourishment; the stomach becomes foul, so that the food is not well digested. This causes the body to lose its digestive heat; then the appetite fails and becomes corrupted; the bones begin to ache, and the person is sick in every part of the whole body.

The overt feelings and signs indicate that some medicine is needed. But before administering any chemical, herbal, or any other medicine, the first and absolutely vital step is to cleanse the stomach and the bowels, to unclog and restore the digestive powers. When this is accomplished, the food will raise the internal heat again, and the whole nourishment will be regained. All the medicine or training or science or art that is needed to restore health in such cases (which are perhaps 90 percent of all illnesses) is to know which foods, herbs, and procedures will accomplish this restoration of the natural bodily heat, and how to administer them—just as a knowledgeable person can clear a stove, chimney, and pipes clogged with soot and creosote, so that the fire will burn properly and the whole room will be warm and comfortable.

The most common sign of illness—fever—is a strange heat the body develops in order to *make up* for this long-standing lack of heat within the body. A fever rapidly accelerates the refining of accumulated superfluous matters in the body, "ripening" them so that they can be eliminated. Tibb calls this process of elimination the healing crisis, which occurs in one of five forms: nose bleeding, vomiting, perspiration, diarrhea, and urination. Now, orthodox medicine, if confronted with the signs of vomiting, fever, aches and pains, and related symptoms, would almost invariably diagnose the common cold or some viral influenza. It is interesting to note that all of the various forms of influenza receive "political" names such as Russian flu, Cuban flu, Chinese flu, Asian flu, and so forth. These are never called "Washington, D.C., Politician's flu," or "Pentagon flu" or "British flu." There is a psychological and emotional component in the naming of diseases that, as far as I am aware, has yet to be examined by any researcher. Moreover, at certain times of year, people are actually "told" to develop these symptoms via the barrage of television, radio, and newspaper ads for remedies. If there is some suggestive, psychological aspect to disease, as many believe, then it is a wonder that everyone does not display the signs of flu and colds. In any event, millions of such cases are handled by physicians daily in the United States. And none of them receives the proper treatment.

Even though the common cold remains one of the most omnipresent ailments, it is apparently impossible to find a cure. Untold millions of dollars have been expended in searching for a cure for the common cold, without results. In truth, the cold is no more than a natural cleansing of the body, which, if blunted or stopped, causes more serious diseases, sooner or later. In fact, the high incidence of disturbing the progress of colds and so-called flus—by medicines to plug up nasal discharge, thwart diarrhea, and stop fevers—is responsible for many of the chronic and degenerative diseases of the nation. Those who have taken suppressive remedies in order to prop themselves up to attend a meeting, or to make it to work or to other functions they consider important, pay a huge price in contradicting the vital health-gaining functions of their own bodies. Over time, the blocking of exit and consequent reabsorption of these harmfully toxic matters creates chronic and degenerative disease—for which the only possible treatment is surgical removal of the affected organs, because all of the vital force of the body is extinguished.

The foregoing explanations may seem radical to some, and others will ask for confirmation, for research, for published results. My reply is, first, that Tibb and Western (allopathic) medicine do not share a comprehensible terminology, and it does not seem likely that the Tibb concepts could be framed to coincide exactly with the theories and vocabulary of Western medicine. I have worked closely with medical doctors who referred patients to me, and even when they could observe results from Tibb after their procedures failed, still they were not interested to learn the elementary aspects of the treatment methods used. Medical doctors are trained in a particular kind of scientific knowledge and practice. They will use what they have learned and by education, by custom, and by law must administer chemical drugs when confronted with particular symptoms. If they do not do so, their licenses will be revoked by their peers or they will not be able to find malpractice coverage. Even those physicians who try to gain some fundamental knowledge about nutrition in the broadest sense, and who may advise eating some vitamins, will still be compelled to prescribe drugs if the condition becomes "serious." Moreover, their entire viewpoint is to focus upon microbial causative agents, and they cannot adjust their thinking to perceive and understand that the body itself is cleaning itself out.

Second, to formulate the research protocols that would confirm these statements with clinical evidence would require millions of dollars in research funds—which no organization or individuals or agencies presently comprising the health industry would advance, because when these dietary and preventive concepts are proven true, the very edifice of the germ theory of disease, upon which the multibillion-dollar health industries rest, would collapse (a particularly disturbing possibility to those who earn their livelihood thereby and have invested their lives in training, if it transpired quickly).

In this book we are returning to the people the fundamental principles of human health and wellness, in simple terminology and language that can be understood and applied by anyone. The knowledge of food, bodily processes, fevers, elimination, detoxification, and all of the related topics once were part of the common traditional knowledge of every people in the world. Even as recently as the 1930s, medical doctors shared this knowledge with people and assisted them to regain their *own* health. It is my contention that each individual has a right and a responsibility to maintain his or her own health and that of his or her children. This is not the same as saying that every person should be his or her "own physician."

To those who wish to assert that the existence of flus and colds is a well-known scientific fact, it can be replied that the exact symptoms of flu, upper respiratory infection, and colds can be reproduced almost at will, simply by withholding certain elements from the diet and administering various foods, herbs, and spices.

My own clinical experience with Tibb includes more than four hundred cases with persons of all ages, suffering from asthma, chronic constipation, arthritis, cancer, emphysema, unknown diseases, colds, migraine headaches, and dozens of other "diseases." These patients have included people from every walk of life, including men, women, and children, homemakers, business people, police officers, nurses, students, and even medical doctors (one heart surgeon called all the way from France to learn the Tibb recommendations). And I have never had one person fail to respond to this treatment. Yet there have been those who refused to alter their diet, who claimed that they just couldn't possibly give up ice cream or chocolate bonbons or some other excess. Such people lack the desire to be well and cannot be helped by physical medicine. Their systems have become so fouled with toxins and clogged with excess that even their minds are confused to the point of preferring disease to health. Regrettably, there are millions of persons in such a condition today. It seems the surgical and chemotherapeutic treatments are the best course for them.

In the Tibb system, there are three things used in treatment: (1) diet, (2) herbal treatments, and (3) treatments administered to the body by hand. Dietary treatment means first eliminating all incorrect foods, such as processed sugar in all forms, other overprocessed foods, and excess meat consumption, and then increasing heating foods and spices and eating at regular times and in proper amounts.

Herbal treatments are used to assist in restoring the body to its proper balance. This requires first detoxifying the body of the accumulation of superfluous matters, whatever they may be. Naming such things is not so important as removing them. The process of detoxification is explained in detail in the following chapter. Treatments by hand can be accomplished by any of the modes of body work, but my own preference is for naprapathy and shiatsu massage, and also includes the procedure known as cupping.

The main purpose of herbal treatments in Tibb is threefold: (1) to ripen the excess of humoral substance, (2) to purge or eliminate the excess of humoral substance, and (3) to restore the humor to its proper characteristic temperament.

The majority of ailments and imbalances that affect people in the United States and the Western industrialized world are associated with imbalances of the phlegm humor (and specifically a cold imbalance of the phelgm humor). The following list provides a summary of conditions and imbalances associated with each humor. (The specific intemperament is not indicated, only the underlying humor that is out of balance.)

There are many interesting points to be gleaned from this listing. First, all of these many different symptoms—which would be considered separate, individual diseases by Western medicine—are the result of only four intemperaments. The significance of this fact is that if a patient presented the symptoms of swelling of the lips, backache, itching of the anus, and mental depression, virtually every physician in the West would consider these all unrelated and would treat each separately. By contrast, the Tibb physician would quickly perform an evaluation and discover that all of these signs fall under the imbalances of the phlegm humor. Then he or she would evaluate whether the imbalance was due to hot or cold intemperament and would effect the correction, using diet, herbs, cupping, and if necessary, some form of body work.

The adjustments to diet are used to correct the underlying intemperament, which has caused the humor to fall out of balance. The herbs, either singly or compounded, are used to evacuate the excess of the humoral or other superfluous matters that have arisen due to the imbalance. The herbs are also used to assist and speed the alleviation of the external and internal signs of swelling, redness, heat or cold, pain, and related symptoms. The treatments to the body assist in the expulsion of superfluous matters, relax the body, and improve harmony and digestion.

The lists of evidences of humoral imbalance in Table 8 are not inclusive, meaning that if one of these humors is out of balance, not *all* of the symptoms will occur in each person. The appearance of one or more of the symptoms will depend upon the inherent strengths and weaknesses of each person's innate organs, tissues, vitality, and related factors. But it is very rare when viewing these lists that one is unable to find one's symptoms falling primarily (or exclusively) under one of these four humors.

TABLE 8
SIGNS OF IMBALANCES OF THE HUMORS

Blood	Phlegm	Yellow Bile	Black Bile
Headache	Headache	Headache	Headache
Delirium	Lethargy	Delirium	Delirium
Lethargy	Insomnia	Insomnia	Stiffness
Weak limbs	Melancholy	Nose itching	Insomnia
Nose itching	Madness	Hard eyelids	Hallucinations
Poor vision	Forgetfulness	Boils on eyelid	Canker sores
Enlarged tongue	Paralysis	Canker sores	Diphtheria
Canker sores	Weak limbs	Dull teeth	Cancer
Swollen palate	Convulsions	Discolored teeth	Excessive appetite
Trembling lips	Muscular tension	Coughing	Swollen stomach
Loose teeth	Trembling limbs	Pleurisy	Vomiting
Tooth spaces	Continuous trembling	Feeling of "smoke" in chest	Heartburn
Slackness of uvula	Swollen eyelids	Heart attack	Swelling of liver
Diphtheria	Shedding eyelashes	Excessive appetite	Jaundice
Coughing	Conjunctivitis	Vomiting	Swelling of spleen
Pleurisy	Styes	Swelling of liver	Flatulence
Swelling of liver	Dilation of pupils	Jaundice	Arthritis
Hemorrhoids	Dandruff of eyelids	Hemorrhoids	Gripe
Constant erection of penis	Ringing in ears	Anal ulcer	Colic
Swollen testicles	Foul odor from nose	Gripe	Swelling of bladder
Convulsion of penis	Enlarged tongue	Burning urination	Excessive libido

TABLE 8: SIGNS OF IMBALANCES OF THE HUMORS CONTINUED

Blood	Phlegm	Yellow Bile	Black Bile
Cracked nails	Bad taste in mouth	Swollen testicles	Insufficient mother's milk
	Bad breath	Excessive menstural flow	Swelling of womb
	Canker sores	Yellowed nails	Varicose veins
	Swollen palate		Thickened nails
	Whiteness of lips		Skin cancer
	Swelling of lips		
	Dull feeling in teeth		
	Ulcers of gums		
	Swelling of uvula		
	Diphtheria		
	Constriction of throat		
	Asthma		
	Coughing		
	Pleurisy		
	Heart feels as if being pulled downward		
	Deficient appetite		
	Corrupted appetite		
	Severe thirst		
	Vomiting		
	Upset stomach		
	Convulsion of stomach		
	Obstruction of liver		

Swelling of liver
Swelling of spleen
Itching of anus
Gripe
Colic
Ulcers of kidneys
Constipation
Swelling of bladder
Retention of urine
Inability to get erection
Swelling of testicles
Excessive menstrual flow
Sour mother's milk
Swelling of womb
Backache
Joint ache
Arthritis
Sebaceous cysts
Pimples
Acne
Baldness
No nail growth
Boils
Scabs
Severe perspiration
Dandruff

TABLE 9
COMPOUND HUMORAL IMBALANCES

Phlegm and Black Bile: Projection of cornea
Phlegm and Yellow Bile: Lethargy and insomnia; sour mother's milk
Phlegm and Blood: Abscesses
Phlegm and Black Bile: Scrofula (swelling of glands, especially lymphatics)
Blood and Yellow Bile: Feeling of heaviness; canker

There are certain diseases, such as jaundice, that have almost two dozen caus-ative factors. And there are symptoms not present on this list. Some four hun-dred different conditions are presented in the Formulary, giving the main features of each of these ailments, arranged by the body part affected. When the specific humoral imbalance is identified, the herbal formulas for correction are provided, along with any other particular adjustments recommended.

Here are presented the herbal formulas that will ripen, purge, and rebalance each of these four humors. For long-standing chronic conditions, this general treatment is the best course. In addition, one should make appropriate adjust-ments to the diet and consult the chapter on detoxification, a procedure that will eliminate a great deal of accumulated by-products of poor nutrition and unbalanced metabolism.

By consulting the list of signs of humoral imbalance, as well as the other sections of the types of intemperaments, one should identify the specific humor that is out of balance. In the Formulary, the humor out of balance is usually stated under the section applying to each body part.

Whenever signs of imbalance occur, the main effort must be to rebalance the humor. This involves ripening and purging one or more of the humors. For example, cold phlegm imbalance requires that the phlegm be softened and ripened in order to be purged. The single and compound herbs and foods used to adjust each of the humors are given at the beginning of the Formulary.

In the case of long-standing dietary indiscretions, lack of exercise, improper habits of elimination, and other wrong behaviors, it is common to find that the system is very congested and disordered. In all chronic and degenerative condi-tions, it is advisable to conduct a detoxification program, to allow the body an opportunity to completely reform itself and to become cleansed and rebalanced, so that the improved foods eaten will find a completely efficient digestive system to process them. Therefore, the next chapter is devoted to the topic of detox-ification and the events that can be experienced during this process.

10
Detoxification and the Healing Crisis

The process I wish to describe in this chapter concerns three things: (1) how to eliminate the accumulation of toxins and excess by-products of incomplete digestions, (2) the means the body uses to eliminate these substances, and (3) having cleansed the body, how to strengthen and rebuild the four primary organs of the body: the brain, the stomach, the heart, and the liver.

In Tibb we often say there are three states of health: lack of any symptoms, or true health; various signs and symptoms of malfunction, or overt disease; and a third condition, in which one is not truly healthy, but the signs of disease have not yet become observable. It is this last that is the situation of the majority of people.

Many people are not sick enough to seek the advice of a physician, but they really aren't healthy either. They suffer from frequent constipation, aches and pains, occasional mild depression, passing of gas and sour belching, and intermittent skin rashes. There may be severe dandruff, stiff and painful joints, and several times a year a severe cold or some form of the flu. All of these people, if honest, will admit that they are not in as good shape as they would like to be. They might want to do something about their minor ailments, because they intuitively know they aren't really taking care of themselves. But, in the meantime, they take a few aspirins or some other drugstore remedy to get them past the symptoms.

As I have already emphasized, "The origin of illness is in food; diet is the main medicine." Such assertions may seem dogmatic to some, until they have a complete picture of how the body functions as an integrated mechanism. Let us review the process of digestion, with the purpose of understanding precisely how and why our metabolism weakens, then fails, permitting disease to arise.

We humans preserve our life through nourishment. This nourishment, in the form of foods, provides the fuel with which the body carries out millions of different functions and metabolic transactions. Each individual cell has three main functions to perform. First, it absorbs nutrient substances from the bloodstream, using the unfathomably complex triggers of enzymatic stimulus and molecular and biochemical interactions to arrive at the correct decisions as to which substances to draw in and which to pass along to other cells. Once the desired nutrient components are absorbed, the cell utilizes them for the purpose of building up the cell structure and repairing damage that may have been done over time, usually due to accidental injury or, more commonly, years of poor diet. Once this repair work is accomplished, there are by-products, wastes of various kinds, that must be eliminated. These are carried back into the blood-stream, whence the body sends them out by the most convenient and appropriate avenue of elimination, including sweat, tears, urine, feces, and sometimes nosebleeds or other forms of slow passing of blood, in stools, piles, or the gums.

In Tibb, the processing of the original food is broken down into two stages: (1) from entry into the mouth up to arrival at the liver, and (2) from the liver until it is utilized by the cells, or subsequently eliminated.

It is true that foods are broken down into various components, such as protein, fats, and carbohydrates, and that many complex biochemical interactions occur during digestion. While there is no objection to trying to understand these events, even in the most minute forms, contemporary research into cellular biology has become so complex that no one can understand it with any degree of clarity; there is no agreement or overview of the basic principles of proper digestive function, let alone dietary recommendations. What is worse, most people, through the indoctrinations of the media, have come to accept that it is the hospitals, medicines, and doctors which *cause* healing, and that the patient is simply a passive participant in this process. Of course, such a viewpoint is erroneous, and it is dangerous, because the people have lost control over their own lives. Let us present the features of Tibb medicine that will allow anyone to regain control over his or her own body and make the decision not to suffer illness, or greatly reduce the chances of becoming ill.

While there are other scientific modes of viewing the digestive process, let us explain it in terms of the analogy of heating and cooking of the food. The food that enters the mouth is chewed by the jaws (friction of chewing: heat) and subjected to the action of enzymes that cause chemical reactions (heat). The food is then swallowed directly into the stomach, where hydrochloric acid (heat) virtually boils the food, until it becomes a semifluid mass called chyme—the essence of the "cooked" food.

The stomach sends this essence along through the small intestine, where additional enzymes act upon it (heat), and the food then arrives at the liver. Here, some of the least choice parts are ejected to the colon and bladder to be eliminated directly. The finer, nutritious parts are processed by the liver, which applies a direct heat (vital force or innate heat) until the essence exists as biochemical particles. These are then conveyed via the bloodstream throughout the body, to become part of tissue, bones, skin, and so forth.

From the essence of the choicest nutrients, the body produces the blood humor, which surrounds and accompanies the substances of the blood, ensuring that they maintain the proper temperament of warmth and moisture to ensure health. The less choice parts of the nutrients become phlegm, which also has a humor admixed with it, to maintain its balance. The even coarser parts of nutrients become the yellow bile, and the least choice parts become black bile—both of which also have their adjusting humor admixed.

In sum, the food is altered from its original composition by the process of heating. The quality, the efficiency, of this heat is determined by the nature and quality of foods eaten. Some foods are quite high in producing the innate heat, others much less so. If a body has a low innate heat (often reflected by lowered body temperature and lower vitality), there will not be sufficient heat to completely process the nutrients at each stage of digestion. For example, if the body is low in salt, there is likely to be low hydrochloric acid in the stomach, and if a person eats vast quantities of food, the body cannot properly process the food. When one meal is piled on top of another, before the first meal is digested, the stomach has no choice but to send the incompletely digested portions along, regardless of whether it is fully digested or not. This incompletely digested food arrives at the liver in this state, so that the liver must make adjustments to accommodate such excess.

If the body cannot carry through the digestion to the fourth stage, the eliminative stage, excess mucus and bile will accumulate in the system. The mucus will spread throughout the body, eventually coating the lining of the colon, which hinders proper peristaltic action; sluggish bowels and constipation result.

Many people find that they cannot get their day going, nor have a daily bowel movement, without a morning cup of coffee. But coffee is a highly toxic substance, and the reason it moves the bowels is that the body simply treats the coffee as a poison and endeavors to speed it out of the system as rapidly as possible. But the poisons in the coffee irritate the internal nerve endings, causing one to become nervous, jittery, and often angry. The body's response to this toxic poisoning is to produce even more mucus, to coat the internal nerve endings, so that the body's proper frequency and quantity of eliminations are seriously impaired.

The point is reached when the body, in an effort to refine and eliminate the mucus and other superfluous excesses, will develop a high body temperature (fever), which will rapidly "melt" down the excesses, so that they can be eliminated. This is usually accomplished in the form of nasal discharge, sneezing, sweating, vomiting, tears, urination, or diarrhea.

If the person ignores these signs of imbalance, and instead takes remedies to end a fever and settle the stomach or stifle the diarrhea, the substances that were poisoning the body are turned back inside, and the body must now try to cope with these for even longer periods—even though it had already made the decision to eliminate them.

It may take many months, and even years, before the internal organs become exhausted from this confusing and deadly cycle. In due time, there will be even more severe signs, such as inflamed liver or gallbladder, kidney or bladder stones, arthritis, and all of the other diseases that people believe are caused by germs. The reason that germs are found to be present in such diseases is that any composite humid substance (such as partially digested foods) which is not fully processed and assimilated will undergo putrefaction, meaning decomposition by action of bacteria. The body contains billions of bacteria, even when healthy (we draw in millions of bacteria with each breath, none of which are present in expelled breath: we retain them). When digestion is impeded for long periods, the oxygen flow is seriously diminished to all parts of the body. Bacteria thrive in anaerobic (lacking oxygen) environments. When cigarette smoking, lack of exercise, consumption of alcohol, and other poor habits are added to nutritional abuse, a perfect environment is provided for bacteria and viruses to expand beyond their normal levels in the body. Thus, they can produce diseases of their own, attacking and destroying the cellular life of tissues. It is true that chemical drugs will kill many of these bacteria, but if the underlying congestion and improper nutrition are not corrected, the problem will recur—but not necessarily in the organ that was originally affected (it may have been surgically removed).

The excessive consumption of refined sugar in the United States is traceable directly to this very process. Sugar, according to the Tibb system, is cold, meaning that its net metabolic effect in the body is to slow down metabolism. Yet sugar is a high-calorie food, meaning that it gives off a great heating energy. But this kind of heating energy is not suitable for health. There is a difference between the heat produced by sugar and the heat provided by metabolically sound foods and spices such as ginger, cumin, or lamb. These foods will be fully assimilated by the liver and will produce a heat very much like that of a fully ignited charcoal briquette. Sugar, on the other hand, produces a very attenuated heat, meaning that it is too rapidly burned off, leaving a great deal of ash and debris. The difference might be thought of in this way: the heat of metabolism-promoting foods is like the warm glow of a fully ignited piece of charcoal or embers in a wood stove, providing a continuous, even, intense heat that burns everything that comes into contact with it to a fine ash. By contrast, poorly heating foods such as sugar burn from the outside, like a match held to a piece of wood, with which it is almost impossible to produce a full blazing fire, much less glowing embers.

People crave sugar because it is practically the *only* heating food in the Western diet. As noted in the chapter on foods, most Americans eat beef, cow's milk, salads, potatoes, butter, and vegetables—all cooling foods. Even those concentrating on so-called "health foods" lack this heating quality in their diet. Thus, the body, depending for its very survival on some form of heat, craves sugar. Whatever else it may be, sugar is also a very potent narcotic, and once consumed in large quantities, it is very hard to bring under control. Sugar is virtually impossible to eliminate, if one does not replace it with foods and spices high in metabolic heat (just consider the failure of reducing diets, as the weight lost is rapidly regained).

There is another problem with both refined sugar and most processed salt, which have been superheated to keep them from becoming lumpy during humid weather ("When it rains, it pours"). Such great heat of processing alters the helical structure of the molecules of the sugar and salt, so that they will not be fully dissolved in solution. If you were to dissolve a teaspoon of refined sugar or salt in a glass of water, and then examine it under an electron microscope, you could see minute shards of the part of the molecules that are not liquefied. These shards are passed into the bloodstream and cause an abrasive, slicing action on the interior walls of the arteries, gradually wearing them thin and creating weak points. The body "stuffs" these weak points with fats. When a person reaches middle age and the blood pressure increases, these weakened spots can break through and cause embolism or heart attack.

Persons who smoke a great deal of marijuana are at particular risk of destroying their health. Researchers at the University of California at Los Angeles found that the body temperature drops an average of between two and seven degrees within twenty minutes of smoking marijuana. Almost everyone who smokes marijuana reports getting the "munchies" soon after ingesting the herb. And what do they want when they get the munchies? Sugars, and almost exclusively sugars. For the body is responding to this dramatic drop in body temperature by insisting on a very rapid replacement with high-heat (but not necessarily good-heat) sugars—ice cream, cakes, cookies, candy bars, halvah, and any other sugars: all are considered superior "munchies" foods.

One of the most curious things is that when people hear my recommendations to add heating foods and spices, they refuse, stating that "Spicy foods don't agree with me," or something like that. When I ask *how* these spices don't agree with them, they report that they suffer from headaches, upset stomach, loose bowels, fever—the very signs that the body is trying to clean itself out!

We have so far in this book concerned ourselves with outlining the limits of proper health and nutrition. Yet most readers probably find themselves far off on a side road of many years of incorrect eating and other abuses of good health. It is true that healthy people, when confronted with a sign of the body's cleaning itself out, will have an easier course of treatment. When people have eaten incorrectly for years on end, a special regimen is needed to cleanse the body quickly of the accumulated toxins and superfluous matters. This regimen is called detoxification and provides the body with an opportunity to repair much of the damage that has been done over years of dietary abuse.

Detoxification

Before presenting the specific details of the seven-day detoxification program, I should first explain what you can expect to experience. The detoxification is a modified fast, a period of time in which we restrict the quality and quantity of foods introduced into the body, to allow it to eliminate excess that has built up over time. The type or quantity of such excess does not matter, for the body's own inherent knowledge will determine how much and what kind of superfluous matters should be eliminated.

The mode of elimination is called the healing crisis. In other words, when the body's food intake is reduced, the first thing it will do is try to throw out excess matter. There likely will be initial signs—within a few days (in some cases, hours)—of a slight headache, perhaps dizziness, weakness, and a queasy feeling in the stomach. All of the signs are evidence that the toxic matters are being moved out of the body.

The process has four stages: addiction (the period of buildup of toxins), growth (the period of ripening of superfluous matters), crisis (the period of elimination from the body), and decline (the period for rebuilding and repairing the body).

The healing crisis, the specific mode the body uses to eliminate the superfluous matters and toxins, occurs in one of five forms: nosebleed, vomiting, urination, perspiration, or diarrhea. The crisis may occur at any time, but usually follows a pattern of four, seven, or fifteen days, depending upon the type of substances to be eliminated. Phlegm imbalance—which is the mode of elimination for the vast majority of people—occurs on the fourth or seventh day of the detoxification program. Elimination by vomiting or diarrhea is said to be "complete," meaning that both the solid and fluid parts are eliminated, while the other three forms of crisis are called "incomplete," meaning that some of the matters still remain. In case of incomplete crisis, the detoxification must be repeated at a later time.

Generally speaking it is enough to conduct a detoxification program once per year. The ideal times are the autumn or spring equinox because the body is itself trying to accomplish the eliminations at these times, in harmony with the seasonal changes.

The central feature of the detoxification program is the following list of foods. It is important that *only* the foods on this list be consumed and nothing else whatsoever. This list is fairly long, considering that the program is called a form of fast. But there are some important features. First, there are no sugars and only one fruit, and few carbohydrates, which the body can convert to sugars. For those who believe they have no sugar problem, this diet will test their assertions. Neither are there any salad dressings listed, so you must make up your own (store salad dressings contain a great deal of added sugar or honey). This can be done by adding some chives and garlic to yogurt.

You may eat as much of each food as you like, but consume normal portions at each mealtime. You may have some salt, preferably taken as a pinch at the beginning of each meal. Do not use salt added to foods, either in cooking or at the table. Neither should you eat only one food exclusively, such as potatoes.

The principle of this diet is to provide only foods directly necessary to sustain life. The foods on the list are composed primarily (about 80 to 90 percent) of water, and are high in vitamins and minerals.

The diet is not high in metabolic heating foods, because we are not trying to induce growth or metabolism, but to eliminate toxins and repair damage. Once you have finished the program, you should resume eating according to the recipes in Chapter 5 and pay particular attention to those foods listed after the detoxification foods, which will build up the brain, heart, liver, and stomach.

I have guided hundreds of people through the detoxification program, and my experience is that most people will have their healing crisis on the fourth day. The signs of the *manner* of healing crisis can be known ahead of time. If the crisis is to occur in the daytime, the precursor signs will occur at night, and vice versa. The signs of crisis by vomiting are asthma, change in rhythm of breathing, bitter taste in mouth, cardiac pain, stomach convulsions, lowered pulse, and trembling of the lower lip.

The signs of crisis by diarrhea are intestinal pain and cramping, heaviness of body, stomach gas, backache, colored feces, and grumbling intestines.

The signs of crisis by nosebleed are dull sense of hearing, ringing in the ears, tears, nose itching, and beating of the veins in the temples.

The signs of crisis by urination are heaviness of the urinary bladder, thickness and excess of urine, bright color of urine on the fourth day of detoxification, and the crisis on the seventh day.

Signs of crisis by perspiration are lightheadedness, itching, and alternating chills and feverishness.

The correction of the body occurs from top to bottom. Thus the first sign is usually headache, the last diarrhea. In my experience, almost 90 percent of people on the detoxification program experience crisis by diarrhea.

If the body is *able* to produce a crisis, it will do so. It is very important that on the day (or night) of crisis no stimulation or herbs or other methods be used to assist the crisis. This is because we are never certain (even with definite signs) just how the body will choose to respond. At the last moment, the body may make a decision to eliminate by vomiting rather than diarrhea. If you act according to the body's initial indications, you will weaken the body's own healing forces. If you happen to act against the force of the crisis, the nervous system will become totally confused, and the crisis will end in midstride, with toxins adrift throughout the system.

This program is in no manner dangerous to people who have no serious disease. In fact, anyone in any state of health would find it of benefit. Nevertheless, those who are suffering from any degenerative disease or are taking any kind of medications whatsoever should undergo the program only with the agreement and supervision of their doctor. *Pregnant women and nursing mothers should not undergo detoxification. There should be no exceptions to this advice!*

Let us now learn the detoxification foods.

DETOXIFICATION FOODS

Vegetables: asparagus, beet, broccoli, Brussels sprouts, carrot, celery, chard (Swiss), cucumber, eggplant, endive, garlic, kohlrabi, lettuce (leaf), mushrooms, mustard greens, onion, parsley, parsnip, pepper (green, hot), potato (white), radish, spinach, squash (zucchini), tomato, watercress

Legumes: beans (green, snap), peas

Grains and flours: wheat germ, bran, oatmeal

Fruits: avocado

Seeds: pumpkin, squash, sesame, sunflower

Nuts: Brazil (for protein), piñon

Meats: It is better not to eat any meat during the program. For those who feel too weakened by complete abstinence from meat, the following are permitted, in 3- to 5-ounce portions, once per day: chicken (white meat only), lamb, turkey (white meat)

Fish: bass, trout, perch

Dairy products: butter (maximum of three pats per day), yogurt

Herbs: chives, sweet basil, dill

Beverages: green herb teas only (chamomile, peppermint, etc.)

Despite anyone's enthusiasm for the above foods, it is inevitable that after two or three days, the diet will seem bland. After five days it will be a real struggle to continue. After six days, it will be an ordeal—but that is when the benefit will be highest!

If the crisis occurs before the full seven days, there is no need to continue the program. For some people with long-standing chronic and degenerative diseases, even seven days of this program may not produce a crisis. I had one patient (an alcohol and drug addict) who required almost three months before the crisis occurred. Again, however, one should not undertake extended periods on this diet without the advice and supervision of the health practitioner or physician of choice. Most medical doctors will approve it, or at least say they don't suppose it will hurt.

Enemas

During this detoxification process, the selected foods will encourage the body to eliminate a great deal of accumulated by-products. It is *imperative* that you keep your bowels open and functioning. Usually, even if you have been constipated in the past, you will move your bowels after the first day. If you don't, or if you are constipated at any point in the seven days, you must either take an enema or discontinue the program.

The enema is excellent for removing superfluous matters in the intestinal tract, as well as relieving pains over the kidneys and bladder, and for allaying inflammatory conditions of these organs. It also relieves colic, and draws toxic matters from the vital organs in the upper parts of the body. Fever is often produced when the function of the liver is impaired by acute superfluities.

Substances to Use for Enemas

For phlegm humor imbalances, use a mixture of decoctions of beet, dried figs, dill, and honey.

A decoction is made by boiling 1 to 3 teaspoons of each substance in 3 cups of water for 8 minutes. Let it stand for 20 minutes. Cool to body temperature, strain, and use.

If there has been prolonged heat and signs of excess dryness, the formula is a decoction of marshmallow herb, fenugreek, chamomile, and 1 teaspoon each olive oil and honey.

Take the enema in the morning after arising and before eating. You may use the enema even if your bowels move some matter; more will often come out.

How to Administer Enemas
Materials

8 ounces enema formula
Enema bag, open-pour spout type, with shut-off valve
Lubricant for tip of nozzle (e.g., petroleum jelly)

Taking the Enema

1. Hang enema bag not higher than 24 inches above body entrance of hose tip.
2. Pour 1 pint of liquid, at body temperature, into the enema bag.
3. Lubricate nozzle tip with petroleum jelly.
4. Place towel or newspaper around area of buttocks in case of accidental spillage from hose or premature expulsion.

5. Lie on right side and gently insert hose tip into anus.
6. Release hose valve. Liquid will flow into colon. If too much much pressure is felt, close valve until pressure passes, then release valve and continue.
7. When enema bag is emptied of contents, close valve and remove nozzle tip.
8. Retain fluid 10 to 15 minutes (but no longer), then evacuate. If little or no liquid comes out, it is not harmful. If it happens more than once, apply a poultice of hot millet over the navel before taking an enema.

The positive effects of the detoxification program should be evident by the second day, with an improved sense of well-being, lessening of depression and uplifted mood, lightness of stomach, easily moved bowels, normal temperature, lowered pulse, and similar evidences. It is common to experience an average of between seven and fifteen pounds of weight loss during the seven-day program of detoxification. There is no special changeover diet necessary after this program. It would be a good idea not to eat to excess for the first few meals (or ever, for that matter). To introduce fruits back into the diet, eat one or two dates, with some water.

Once the harmful and toxic excesses have been ripened and expelled from the body, it is important to allow the body a time of rebuilding and rebalancing the major organs. The foods given below should be eaten as much as possible for three months following the detoxification; and, of course, one should have eliminated all improper foods from the diet.

To Strengthen the Brain. Include these items in the diet: quince, apples, orange, rose water, ginger, valerian, cloves, chicken, brains, and goat's milk. Use the following scents: rose, musk, jasmine, ambergris, 'oud (aloeswood), frankincense.

To Strengthen the Heart. Eat peaches, pomegranate, tamarind, apple, rhubarb, cowslip, mint, coriander seeds, orange, cinnamon, senna, gur, saffron, carrot, cardamom, and mint. Use the following scents: sandalwood, amber, camphor, rose, 'oud (aloeswood), hyacinth. Wear ruby and lapis lazuli jewelry and silk clothes (women only).

To Strengthen the Liver: Include in the diet: chickory, roasted chickory root, pomegranate, nutmeg, cinnamon, cloves. Liver weakness comes mainly from things that cause coldness and moisture. Therefore, include heating foods and spices. Use the scent of amber.

To Strengthen the Stomach: Include in the diet: pomegranate, quince, orange and orange peel, cinnamon, gur, senna, cloves, cardamom, and mint. Scents to use are rose and 'oud (aloeswood). Remember that every purgative weakens the stomach, with the exception of senna. Everything that strengthens the stomach also strengthens the intestines and throat.

11
Case Histories

Many factors have to be taken into account before a specific regimen of treatment is suggested for correcting any imbalance. It must always be remembered that the objective in Tibb is not to treat disease per se, but to reform the entire internal and external biotic environment—which, when accomplished, often results in improvement or cure of disease. Therefore, in presenting specific suggestions for treatment in Tibb, it is impossible to list general diseases and then give the corresponding herb for each illness.

The cases that follow illustrate the different ways in which the humors can be unbalanced, in a variety of people—men, women, and children, of all races and locales.

Many of the patients who ultimately end up in treatment with me have already exhausted the orthodox approach and often have also tried several alternative therapies. This is not to say that such therapies besides Tibb have no value, but especially in chronic and degenerative diseases, many people seek an alternative to highly toxic drugs and the devastation of surgery.

The first thing most patients want to do is explain their disease to me, giving me the name assigned by orthodox medicine, asking, for example, "Can you do anything for lupus?" (or whatever they have been told they have). My answer is always, "No." Moments of shocked silence follow. "In the first place," I tell them, "I am not interested in disease. Let's talk about health!" The first point on which I must obtain agreement is that the patient actually *wants* to get better. It is astonishing how many persons who are ill will actually refuse to get better. They have built their lives around their disease, and it is terrifying for them to imagine being without it. It is like dying.

I expect my patients to make an investment in their own health—they must be the ones to do the work of altering whatever negative habits are causing their problems, and they must also invest the time, money, and energy to become educated about certain aspects of cooking and nutrition. They may even have to purchase new clothing (if all they wear is synthetic fabrics), new cookware, and so forth. It has been my experience that anyone who has reached my office door will probably require at least one year of dedicated adjustment and work on his or her health before he or she can expect to be called completely healthy. Granted, this is more than many people will "pay" in terms of commitment. For most patients, for every year they spent getting into their trouble, they will have to spend one week getting out. This means that if a forty-year-old man has cancer of the prostate, and has lived with poor habits his whole life, it will require about forty weeks, or nearly one year, to completely regenerate his system. Natural methods are not for everyone. If a person has severely degenerated health, so much so that the vitality to recover is in doubt, the treatment of choice may lie with Western medicine, and I am not hesitant to refer doubtful cases to a medical doctor, preferably one with a nutritional approach, although these may be hard to find.

If a patient has already been in treatment with a medical doctor or other practitioner, or is taking medication at the time, I insist that these people also be involved in the treatment program, even if only as a monitor. A portion of my patients are referred by medical doctors, but even those who arrive on their own, if they are at the degenerative stages of disease, should also have a medical doctor ready to step in if an acute concern over pathology arises.

Children and people up to age fifty or so (with exceptions, of course) are the best candidates for Unani Tibb medicine, because they still have a considerable reserve of vitality in their systems and will respond to the Tibb treatments. But those who are quite elderly, or who have had a long history of treatment with drugs and whose vital organs are dysfunctional, make less ideal candidates for natural treatment. This is not meant to sound cruel, but only acknowledges the reality that the repair and growth rate of the bodies of some persons may be overwhelmed by the force of a particular disease.

The Unani Tibb Treatment

Most patients have one main complaint that becomes, or is, the focus of their "disease": "It hurts *here.*" Every form of medicine has some measures and methods to alleviate the symptoms of pain. But according to medical statistics, almost 80 percent of patients coming to physicians have nothing organically wrong with them; that is, there is no overt symptom that can be identified or treated. Yet they have come to the doctor with some complaint, often exaggerated or altogether made up.

The first step is to conduct a complete interview to determine all of the signals and signs that can be elicited from the patient, to evaluate in the broadest terms what really is happening with the patient. If there is to be a treatment resulting in cure, and not simply palliation of the overt symptom, then the entire constitutional makeup must be evaluated, including the physical body, the mind and emotions, and the spiritual side of life. I treat persons of all religions, and the cases that follow include Muslims, Christians, Jews, Hindus, Buddhists, and several who would consider themselves faithless.

During the initial interview, an important objective is to probe the memory of the patient for signs he or she might not ordinarily think significant, such as colors occurring during dreams, small itches and tics, and so forth. And, although it takes some delicacy and real confidence to get to the point of trust, it is also necessary to understand the person's sexual life. The sexual energies are among the most forceful and are at the root of many diseases, especially today. Yet almost all patients are very reluctant to speak about these things to a stranger, even one who is a physician. They may be embarrassed, hurt, modest, or nervous.

Therefore, the interview and evaluation tend to be lengthy, up to an hour. Within this time, the patients realize that I am truly interested in them, and they will, ultimately, come forth with the real problem as opposed to the problem they stated at the outset.

Of the following cases, all but two had already been through the full spectrum of orthodox medical treatments, and their disease had not been resolved. Three of the patients were referred directly from medical doctors, and the remainder were referred by other patients. All of them had faulty diets—actually abominable diets from the Tibb viewpoint—although some of them believed they were seriously committed to eating "health foods."

No system of healing can cure every disease, every time. Two of these cases did not have completely successful results. It is important to illuminate problems that arise during the course of treatment that prevent complete success.

There is a difference between what the physician needs to know and what the patient needs to know. With every case, from an evaluation by pulse I knew within minutes the nature and source of the problem and could have instituted the treatment immediately. However, it is always necessary, to me anyway, for patients to understand what has happened to them, what is happening at the present time, and how they can avoid such unpleasant situations in the future. In all but two cases the pulse reading was the primary mode of diagnosis, although the testimony of the patients as to their signs affirmed the pulse diagnosis. In two cases, urinalysis was used to refine the diagnosis. The shortest treatment period was one appointment of one hour. The longest extended over four months.

Names and certain personal facts have been amended to protect the dignity and confidentiality of patients.

Case #1

T.K.; Anglo female; married; age 36. Stated complaint: frequent urination and painful menstrual periods.

This was one of the first cases I treated with Tibb, and it was one of the most difficult and remarkable that I have had. T.K. had not been my patient before, but she had obtained my address and wrote me while I was in Afghanistan performing my initial research into Tibb during 1975.

The woman had experienced severe cramping during her menstrual periods since she was fifteen years old. The pain was so great that she had asked a physician for medication, and she received aspirin with codeine. Over the years, she had developed other problems, most notably with urination, and I say "problems" because despite several hospital examinations, no organic basis for her difficulty was ever discovered. She was unable to travel away from her home without feeling an overwhelming urge to urinate. For example, if she got into the car to make a quick trip to the grocery store, no sooner would she have the car backed out of the driveway than she would be forced to run back inside the house to go to the bathroom. She had become a virtual recluse, after trying to take a vacation one year and being forced to stop literally every few miles to urinate. She had spent more than three thousand dollars in medical fees, but the doctors could find no organic basis for her condition.* One of her doctors recommended that she undergo a hysterectomy, presumably to see if it would help. Most of the doctors she went to told her the problem was "in her head." Her husband had purchased a complete portable toilet, but this proved quite embarrassing to the woman, and she refused to be seen driving along with that bulky device in the car with her.

In her letter, she indicated that her condition had worsened. She used drugs for the pain of her menstrual periods (which she suffered through in bed seven days per month). To counteract the narcotics for sleep, she drank five or more cups of coffee in the morning to "get going." On top of this tragic cycle, she had begun drinking wine at night, initially to help her "relax" and get to sleep. But the alcohol enhanced the effects of the drugs, and it soon became apparent that she was a borderline alcoholic.

The woman's husband had a high-paying job in Washington, D.C., and they lived in a mansion in the suburbs. Yet, as she related in her letter, she was losing all sensation in her arms and legs, and she believed she was dying.

It was some months before I returned to the United States, but when I did, as promised, I visited her at home. She had been a lovely woman, a high school beauty queen, but the ordeal of the past years had wrinkled her skin. She was thirty pounds overweight. She chain-smoked. Her mind skittered from topic to topic. At the time I saw her, she was taking a combination of alcohol, Valium, codeine, Librium, and perhaps other drugs.

Besides her difficulties with urination and menstrual pain, her symptoms in-

---

*Current research indicates that she probably was suffering from interstitial cystitis, a condition difficult to diagnose and for which orthodox medicine offers no treatment. It is thought to be caused by the destruction of the elasticity of the bladder wall, restricting the capacity of the bladder to only two or three ounces as opposed to the twelve-ounce capacity of a normal bladder.

cluded migraine headaches, depression and melancholy, dizziness, loss of sensation in the extremeties, pleurisy, heart palpitations, severe thirst, swelling of the bladder, excessive menstrual flow, swollen lymph glands, insomnia, and a great deal of muscular tension and anxiety.

All of these signs, in Tibb, are related to imbalance of the phlegm humor. And an indication that it was a severe cold imbalance was that she enjoyed oversleeping and would sleep an entire day if the chance was offered to her.

The pulse evaluation revealed not only a cold imbalance of the phlegm humor but also a hot imbalance of the black bile humor. It is very uncommon to see a divergence of intemperament between humors. In other words, if one humor is excessively hot, the other humors, if also unbalanced, would likely also be hot. That one of her humors was excessively cold and another hot betrayed an extreme disorder of her metabolism. Even though her symptoms were focused upon the urinary tract, the involvement of the black bile humor could indicate that she might develop cancer in one of her organs, so degenerated had her system become.

I could not treat her away from my base office and told her that if she wanted me to help her, she would have to come to stay with me for a time. In addition, I had sent my collection of Tibb formulas ahead by air freight and would need them for her. She discussed her situation with her husband, who agreed that she should come stay near me, and about two weeks later she arrived by airline for treatment.

I had arranged for her to occupy the guest house at the home of a friend of mine, where there was plenty of fresh air and sunshine, Jacuzzi whirlpool baths, a swimming pool, and a soothing environment in general. One of my colleagues agreed to start some bodywork treatments to help unbind the tensed muscles that were packed and coiled throughout her body.

The first objective of the program was a complete detoxification. As the first week progressed, I used the Tibb formulas to purge her black bile humor, then the phlegm humor.

The first two days were the most difficult, because all of her normal reflexes of the nervous system had been anesthetized by the drugs she had taken over ten years. By the third day, she was virtually a new person, at least in terms of her outlook. After the third day, the eliminative functions of her body finally resumed on their own, and her bowel and urine functions were normal. In fact, she felt so well that she thought she could return home. I urged her instead to continue the program until she had the healing crisis, explaining that only then could we be certain that her system was at the point of being able to rebuild.

She remained on the program for three months plus one week. In this time she had rented a modest apartment and taken up oil painting, a talent she had developed as a young woman. Now she found great pleasure in reviving this creative side of her personality.

Her husband had agreed that he would quit his job in the East and move away to start a new life. When she was at the airport to return to close up their affairs and ready for their move, she thanked me for saving her marriage and her life. In the course of three months the Tibb principles had been applied to successfully rebalance this woman's entire physical and emotional life.

Case #2

G.R.; Anglo male; divorced; age 38. Stated complaint: cancer of prostate.

This case came at a very inconvenient time for me personally, because my wife had just delivered our first son two days before. I had taken a hiatus from my practice, and my wife and I were living in a cabin in the remote mountains of upstate New York. G.R. arrived one morning, walking up the side of the mountain, and insisted that he needed to be treated and would most strictly follow my advice. Well, any patient who displays such a level of commitment and motivation deserves to be helped. But after I interviewed him, I wondered if I had made a mistake in taking on his case, which was one of the most distressing I had encountered.

He seemed to me thin and slightly jaundiced, his hair turning prematurely white. His posture was such that he must have had a terrible tension within, as if he carried a terrifying secret guilt that no one could remove from him. Our interview was conducted under the shade of several hundred-year-old oak trees, as we sat perched on some old stumps surrounded by ferns.

His problem, he related, was probably cancer of the prostate. He had seen a medical doctor and been through all of the hospital tests. The overt symptoms were blood in the urine, which was much more than a trace. He related that he had all his life been virtually addicted to salt and ate almost a full one-pound container each week. He had gone prematurely bald, suffered bouts of melancholy and great depression, and in his early twenties had been hospitalized for psychiatric problems, intensified by experimentation with LSD and other drugs. He still experienced occasional hallucinations and fits of temporary paralysis. He was from a wealthy family in Connecticut and, thanks to a sinecure from his parents, had never had to work, and so never did. This idleness led to various forms of sexual excesses, which he related had begun in late childhood, when he experienced excessive sex drive. Other symptoms included flatulence, hardened and thickened nails, boils and carbuncles, and canker sores in the mouth.

Despite all of these signs, he seemed overtly rather cheerful and had a positive attitude toward his problem. He almost dismissed his physical symptoms, saying he assumed that the great salt intake all his life had bothered his kidneys. He did not agree with the medical reports that affixed the label of prostate cancer to him. He was certain the origin of the difficulty was in his kidneys.

I was not the first healer he had seen. In the city where he lived, he had been introduced to an alternative diet therapy, and had been on it for almost one year. This consisted of no meat, no salt, and plenty of brown rice and fresh vegetables. He claimed to have reduced his weight and felt that his health might be improving slightly, but still he had the blood in the urine (he carried his own test sticks).

The pulse evaluation showed a total disorder of his metabolic system, particularly his phlegm and black bile humors. Cancer is not actually one disease, but several hundred different symptoms affecting virtually any organ. According to Tibb, cancer is a disease of the black bile humor. That is, it means that all four of the humors are out of balance. Ripening, purging, and rebalancing of each of the four humors in turn are required for a cure to take place. This is not an easy procedure, because the superfluous and toxic by-products are constantly being emitted, and since the last humor that is out in the chain must usually be treated first. This means that one must try to treat the black bile humor first. But, with all of the others out, even if that humor is restored, it almost immediately is thrown out of balance again. Therefore, the Hakims state that cancer is a difficult disease to cure.

According to medical statistics, more than half of all cancer patients do not live five years. There have been reports that one out of three persons dies of cancer today, and by the year 2010 this figure is expected to be one in two.

There are some who assert that the orthodox medical treatments of chemotherapy and radiation are unsuitable for cancer. While I agree they are more radical than the period of life extended might justify, no system of healing can produce very impressive cure figures for all forms of cancer.

Dr. Ernesto Contreras operates a cancer treatment clinic in Mexico. He is a Harvard-educated medical doctor and at his clinic uses all forms of treatment—chemotherapy, radiation, surgery, laetrile, glandular injections, and many others—depending on each patient's specific needs. In 1979 he claimed an absolute cure rate of about 2 percent, the same rate as for any other kind of treatment. By "cure" it is meant that the cancer goes into total remission, does not return, and is not the cause of death (not just within five years, but not ever: that is a cure). In any event, the cure rate is approximately equal to that for spontaneous remission, in which the cancer disappears without treatment.

The Tibb philosophy is that cancer is the end stage of the degeneration of the metabolic efficiency of the body—the extinguishing of the innate heat—brought on primarily by incorrect diet and other imbalances in various aspects of the patient's life, usually occurring over a long period of time. Therefore, I do not emphasize cancer treatment as a feature of Tibb, although sometimes remarkable results do transpire. These are due, in my judgment, not to the remarkable powers of Tibb or herbs, but simply to the fact that the patient had sufficient metabolic efficiency to recover.

As I noted above, cancer is a disease of the black bile humor. It can occur with only the black bile humor out of balance, or one or more humors out of balance along with it. In this case, all four were disordered.

The therapeutic alternative diet that G.R. had been using was good as far as it went. But, again, it was composed of entirely "cold" foods, which were supplying very little vital heat for his liver to promote healing. My suggestion, therefore, was for him to undertake the complete seven-day detoxification program, which I agreed to supervise and administer to him. He took a room at a nearby motel and visited town to buy the herbal supplements he would need.

He did beautifully. He was disciplined and followed the program perfectly. Within four days he had provoked his healing crisis, and a substantial amount of toxic matter was eliminated in a diarrhea crisis. Immediately after the detoxification program, I explained to him the principles of Tibb dietetics and cooked a complete meal to demonstrate cooking techniques for him. He was amazed at how delicious the food was.

I also provided this patient with a fourteen-day supply of a special formula made of Tibb ingredients obtained from Hakims in India. It contains twenty-two different ingredients and will rebalance all four humors, if it is possible to do so. The regimen we had performed together apparently had the proper effect, because the blood in his urine had disappeared for the first time in almost a year. The man left in very good spirits, promising to report back to me with his progress. That was almost four years ago, and he still stays in touch with me and reports that none of his symptoms has ever returned.

Cancer is a disease that exists in a nonmanifest (hidden) form for a considerable time, and then becomes manifest—as evidenced by swelling, tumors, bleeding, and other symptoms. During the period of its growth, it is difficult to detect with certainty, because even Western scientific diagnosis of "precancerous" growth does not always ultimately manifest as cancer.

According to Tibb, cancer is a fourth-stage degenerative disease. Cancer should be rare in any society that bases its dietetics on the Tibb principles. The Hakim that I studied with in Afghanistan had seen only two cases of cancer in more than sixty years of practice. He had no explanation for the high rate of cancer in the West, but said it was "probably" due to eating pork and drinking alcohol—two substances that greatly corrupt the black bile humor.

The Tibb treatment for cancer, when it does occur, consists in trying to manage the growth of the tumor, to keep it stationary and prevent its increase and avoid ulceration. If it is discovered early enough, it may be cured with herbal means. But when it has become well developed, Tibb has no effective cure. There is an important distinction here—when I say that the cancer is well developed and it will not cure, I am speaking of its being well developed in a person who has lived and eaten according to Tibb throughout his or her life. For one who has never done so, a radical revision in diet may provide an opportunity for the body to respond and effect a cure. Certainly there are cases on hand of persons from Western countries who achieved a cure by dietary regimen. But such cases are not great in number, and many do not respond. If there was any such thing as an absolute cure for cancer, people would find it and use it, regardless of who approved of it and who didn't. It would be known.

The Tibb herbal treatments, which are not for self-administration, include red clover, fleawort, orpine, wall pepper, houseleek, black hellbore, gillflower, purslane, frankincense, foxgrape, lettuce, aloeswood, myrrh, and oxymel. Most of the herbal applications are used not to effect a cure but to treat external tumors. It is advised to avoid surgery if at all possible, for many cancers are spread when disturbed by incision.

Cases #3 and #4

G.J.; Anglo female; single; age 25. Stated complaint: irregular pituitary.

J.A.; Hispanic male; age 7. Stated complaint: childhood asthma.

These two cases are presented together because they illustrate the great symptomatic range that occurs with a single humoral imbalance.

The twenty-five-year-old woman had a long list of complaints: nausea, abdominal pain, flatulence, dizziness, headaches, difficult breathing, coughing up phlegm, eyestrain, sore gums, and dental problems. Although physically attractive, she exhibited a disturbing lack of self-image and was concerned about being "overweight," even though her weight was normal. She admitted to periods of confusion, not being able to "make up her mind," as well as being forgetful. She had been examined by a doctor, who diagnosed what she described only as "irregular pituitary." She was seeing me to determine if there was any Tibb treatment for vaginal discharge—a very common complaint with young adult single women. She did not believe her pituitary and other symptoms were interrelated.

The pulse evaluation revealed the lack of vital heat, which had created a classic cold imbalance of the phlegm humor—all of her symptoms were typical of phlegm imbalance.

My recommendation for this woman was to conduct a seven-day detoxification, to purge her system of the buildup of mucus. She performed the diet well and within four days began excreting gross amounts of phlegm. Within a day she reported a heightened sense of well-being and improved concentration and general mental state. Following the detoxification diet, she began eating the Tibb foods, which provided a high metabolic heat. Within a few weeks, she reported that the vaginal discharge had abated and all of her other symptoms had disappeared.

The second case in this cold phlegm category is that of a young boy who was brought by his mother, who reported he had suffered from asthma "since he was born." She had taken him to an allergist but felt that there had been no change in his condition. Having been raised in a traditional culture in rural Mexico, she felt that diet and herbs could play an important role in health and was interested to learn the Tibb perspective for her son.

The list of signs besides asthma included insomnia, muscular tension, dilation of the pupils, chronic constipation, and the very telling sign of a sensation in the chest as if the heart were being "pulled" downward. The mother was particularly concerned because her son had lost almost ten pounds in the past several months—an unnatural and unhealthy sign for a boy his age.

The boy went on a modified detoxification program for one week, and the results were so remarkable that his mother continued it for another two weeks, after which time all of his symptoms of asthma had disappeared. We added a supplement of tincture of lobelia, to cut and eliminate the phlegm, while at the same time supplying a high degree of heat to soften and refine the mucus.

Although these two cases are widely separated in age, sex, cultural situation, and even symptoms, they both had the identical humoral imbalance: excess cold of the phlegm humor. The treatment in such cases is usually quite straightforward: a brief detoxification to refine and eliminate phlegm, then adjusting the diet to include more heating foods.

There are two keystone signs of the cold phlegm imbalance, which occurred in these cases: forgetfulness and the sensation of the heart being pulled downward. After I had asked the woman a few questions and had an idea that the phlegm humor was affected, I asked her, "Do you seem to be very forgetful much of the time?" "Yes!" she exclaimed. This is the type of sign that would frequently be overlooked or ignored in most systems of medicine, yet it is a common sign of phelgm humor imbalance.

Case #5

G.A.; Anglo female; age 30; married. Stated complaint: inflammation of the gallbladder; possible gallstones.

This woman's husband called to describe his wife's symptoms, and to ask if I would take her case. She had been suffering extreme nausea and violent stomach cramps for the past several nights. At first, he explained, she thought it was merely indigestion, but last night she had been awakened at two in the morning with gastric pains worse than before, and vomited for several hours. She had two small children. I agreed to see her that morning.

During our interview, she related that she had eaten a chicken dinner the night before, but nothing unusual. She thought it was her gallbladder, she said, because she had had a similar attack several years before, but not as severe as this one. At that time a medical doctor had diagnosed "gallbladder problems."

She also reported lower back pains, spells of dizziness, sporadic painful joints, and what she described as "occasional" constipation. She also had hemorrhoids and acknowledged that she was somewhat overweight, which she ascribed to continual nursing of her small children. She described the pain in her stomach and abdomen of the night before as being as severe as that of childbirth. The other interesting symptoms she revealed were a bitter taste in her mouth and that she was often thirsty. She expressed concern that she might be prediabetic. I always ask patients what *they* think is causing their problem. She believed it was probably her gallbladder.

Her blood pressure was normal; her temperature was 97.6°—low but not alarmingly so (it was early in the morning). Her pulse evaluation revealed a hot imbalance of the yellow bile humor, and all the symptoms that she had experienced were indicative of a yellow bile humor imbalance. That could have accounted for her gallbladder problems, but the rhythm of her pulse indicated that something else was going on. "Is there any possibility that you're pregnant?" I asked. She was almost stunned and quickly answered, "No." Despite my repeated questioning on this point, she adamantly stuck to her denial: "Impossible."

From all of the outward signs, I would have agreed with her assessment of some form of inflammation of the gallbladder, probably gallstones. But from the information of the pulse, I thought she was pregnant. I advised a mild cleansing diet and gave her the formula for purging the yellow bile humor. That would end the gallbladder spasms—if that was the cause. I sent her home with the formula and a diet sheet, which she pledged to follow. She was to report back in two days.

She called two days later to report that she had made an appointment with a medical doctor because she had had another severe attack. Her husband agreed, she said, that they should "get to the bottom of this, whatever it is." I asked her if she had taken the formula and followed the diet. Yes, she said, and the pain and nausea had gone away completely that night. But, she confessed, she just didn't have the willpower to avoid all of the foods she liked ("I guess I just love cakes and chicken skin too much").

What this woman really needed was a complete detoxification. But she did not have the determination to do it, and it is not recommended to do the detoxification when pregnant or nursing. Therefore, she would have to keep her appointment with the medical doctor, I reasoned.

I didn't hear from her for another week and so called her husband to check on her situation. He related that the doctors had said that x-rays had revealed no gallstones, but nonetheless they said that she had a gallbladder problem and recommended immediate surgery. I explained to him my suspicions about her being pregnant. He was even more astonished at this assertion than she had been, but promised that he would take some time to arrive at a decision.

Two weeks later, I received a call from the patient, who rather sheepishly informed me that her test had just come back positive: she was pregnant. So she had decided to put off the "gallbladder" surgery until after the delivery!

I gave her the formula for a pregnancy tea, which is as follows:

1 part spikenard
1 part blue cohash
1 part red raspberry herb
1 part peppermint (for flavor, nerves, and digestion)

Steep ½ teaspoon of each in 1 cup water for 5 minutes. Drink one cup in evening before retiring. For the last six weeks of pregnancy, add ½ teaspoon of squawvine herb.

This case is interesting because it highlights a fact that arises quite often: the early signs of nausea and discomfort of what is termed morning sickness are frequently mistaken for signs of disease. The female body, when pregnant, prepares for the unique events of carrying the baby by performing its own natural kind of detoxification, in the form of vomiting, urination, nosebleeding, and diarrhea—the signs of morning sickness. Perhaps some women may not be prepared for a pregnancy at that period in their lives, and so avoid thinking of the obvious.

The fetus shares a common circulatory system with the mother, whose body treats the fetus as a "new" organ and will dump its own toxic and superfluous matters into the fetus. This is confirmed by the fact that Anglo babies are almost always born with blue eyes, which are said to "change color" within a few weeks after birth. According to the science of iridology, the eye nerves of infants only develop sufficiently at the age of several weeks, to reflect the changes in their organs—the deposits of toxic by-products that have built up over the blue pigmentation and collected during pregnancy. According to iridology, the mixture of the yellowing of mucus with the natural blue of the eyes results in the "changed" green color, which many times reverts back to the original blue following detoxification.

This case also demonstrates the usefulness of the Tibb analysis, which revealed her state of pregnancy considerably in advance of confirmation by other methods, and spared her and her unborn child the very great dangers of undergoing surgery during pregnancy.

Case #6

A.H.; Anglo male; married; age 28. Stated complaint: methadone addiction.

This case also shows the value of detoxification. The young man came to me requesting to be guided through the detoxification program, because, he said, he had been addicted to methadone for almost six years. His daughter was nearly eight years old, he related, and he knew that as she got older she would soon be able to intuit his addiction, and he was ashamed to have her arrive at this realization. He had been addicted to heroin for seven years prior to the methadone, which he was taking under medical supervision. He had tried several other times to get off the narcotic substances, and confessed that he believed that methadone was more addictive than heroin.

The reason that most people have trouble ending their dependence on addictive substances is the extremely low vitality of the liver, resulting in a cold imbalance of the phlegm humor. In this man's case, I put him on the detoxification diet but added certain spices high in metabolic value. If the heating spices are not added at the earliest stage, the patient will crave sugars and carbohydrates. It is particularly a hallmark of heroin addiction that the diet often consists almost exclusively of sugars.

With severe cold imbalance of the phlegm, the peristaltic action of the colon is usually dulled or nonfunctional. Therefore, we utilized coffee enemas to assist the initial stages of elimination. Within one week his bowels were functioning normally.

I would have preferred that he end the methadone while undergoing the detoxification because there is nothing gained if the substances are continually being replaced as they are eliminated. But he was not emotionally prepared for this drastic step. I added to his regimen a series of breathing and sound practices that helped to relax and balance him, and also advised a series of seven yoga postures.

He had been on the program for about thirty days when he met me on the street one morning, looking as if he had tears in his eyes. I asked him what was the matter, and he said, "It's over. I woke up this morning, and knew that I was through with the drugs." I congratulated him and advised him to keep up the basic detoxification diet for several more months, because the cells and organs of his body needed more time to complete the cycles of elimination and regeneration.

This case seems almost too simple, in light of more than a decade of drug addiction. Yet, when the key factor of the metabolic heat is understood, often what seem to be impossibly difficult cases are resolved with little effort.

Case #7

N.R.; Hispanic female; single; age 27. Stated complaint: severe chronic constipation.

This patient was a registered nurse who came with a problem that had defied her own knowledge of healing, as well as that of the physicians she knew and worked with. She was severely constipated, having only one bowel movement every ten to fourteen days. As she sat in my office, she was crying as she explained that the odor of feces actually came out through her skin. In the past week, she had left work several times early in the morning, because the odor had become noticeable to her co-workers and she was too embarrassed to stay at work.

Many physicians claim that there is no such thing as a "proper" or "normal" number of bowel movements per day. While it is true that some people process their food more quickly than others, it is also true that almost all food is fully metabolized by the body within four to six hours, sometimes much less. Watercress, for example, is digested within an hour. Some nuts may take up to six hours. But, generally speaking, the food has served its functions and is ready to be expelled within six hours. This means that even if a person has one bowel movement every twenty-four hours, the wastes are actually remaining in the body up to three times longer than they need to. Poor metabolic heat and excess mucus in the bowels often create the conditions for constipation. Most people take a morning cup of coffee to stimulate the bowels. But for many, over time, the bowels become more and more sluggish, until serious diseases arise. Infants, it may be noted, usually move their bowels six or more times per day: they are healthy.

The woman told me that she had tried every kind of remedy, but to no avail. I asked her about her diet, because there had to be some rather radical imbalance for this condition to arise. She related that she had been housesitting for a friend the past eight months or so and, for the sake of convenience, had cooked a steak on the outdoor barbecue almost every day, and this comprised her entire diet.

She also complained of other signs and discomforts: migraine headaches, depression, dizziness, muscular tension, dandruff, flatulence, bad taste in her mouth, severe perspiration, lethargy, and insomnia. Her skin was slightly jaundiced, and her pupils were dilated—a sign often found with drug addicts. I asked her if she ate much sugar (a narcotic), and she admitted that she did eat candy a great deal. So that was her diet, candy and steak.

The pulse evaluation revealed all four humors out of balance. I gave her the diet sheet for eating according to Tibb principles, and even gave her a spice blend of heating herbs so she could eat the very next meal using them. I also gave her the formula for purging the black bile humor. She went home to try out this advice, which seemed very strange to her with a background in hospital medicine.

The next day at noon she came into my office with a beaming smile. "Did it work?" I asked. "Did it ever!" she exclaimed. She never returned, and I assumed that she had no further problems with her bowels after applying the Tibb diet principles. Then, by chance I ran into her at a gas station almost six months later, and she confirmed that her health—and bowels—had been in perfect order since applying the Tibb principles of diet.

Case #8

N.R.; Anglo female; married; age 22. Stated complaint: epilepsy; amenorrhea.

This is another case in which a chronic condition responded dramatically and quickly to the Tibb principles. It was truly an accident that N.R. came to be treated with Tibb. It was her husband who had come to me for detoxification guidance. He was not ill in the usual meaning of the word, but he had used drugs for a period of several years, and even though he no longer used them, he wanted to cleanse his system to attain a high level of wellness. He took the instructions for the detoxification and the various herbal supplements and went home to start the program. During the detoxification, I request that patients call me daily to report various readings of the pulse and body temperature, which are reflectors of how the body is progressing. The next afternoon he called with his readings. They were all as expected. Then he said, "And here's the readings for my wife." "Your wife?" I asked, incredulous. "I though *you* were doing the detox." "Well, she decided we both might as well do it. " I dislike people doing the detox without first seeing me, because they may have some condition, such as pregnancy, that would contradict doing a rapid elimination. In any event, I asked for her readings, and was alarmed when he told me her pulse was thirty-two. "Thirty-two?" I asked with disbelief. "Yes, thirty-two," he answered calmly. I told him that he shouldn't become overly alarmed, but that, frankly, she was on the verge of being a medical emergency. I instructed him to have her eat a half teaspoon of salt so that her blood pressure might rise. If there was no increase in her pulse within ten minutes, I told him to have her go to the nearest emergency room.

I waited until he called back. "Is fifty any better?" I told him it was all right, but that I wanted to see the woman immediately. They arrived in less than thirty minutes, and she explained her medical history.

She had suffered from epilepsy since birth and had even kept a record of the date of the occurrence of each seizure she had had since age eleven, and carried these dates in a small book. In addition, she reported that she had never had a menstrual period. If she had not entered into the program accidentally and without my knowledge, I would not have accepted her as a patient. But now she was in the middle of the program, and I decided she should proceed, so long as she agreed to notify her medical doctor if her pulse dropped again.

This woman also exhibited dilated pupils, a sign of excess cold of the phlegm humor, which was confirmed by pulse diagnosis. She needed the formula to ripen phlegm, which she took for seven days, at which time she experienced the healing crisis by diarrhea without adding the phlegm purgative. There was nothing else to do, and so I asked her to call me if she experienced any notable signs.

Three weeks later she called to report that the "usual" date for her seizure had arrived and passed, and she had not had a seizure on schedule for the first time in eleven years. But she was even more excited to report that she had had the first menstrual period of her life.

I followed her progress over the next nine months, until the couple moved away from the area. Her menstrual periods occurred again, although irregularly, and she experienced no further seizures during the nine months of my follow-up.

Case #9

W.P.; Anglo female; single; age 25. Stated complaint: vaginitis.

This was an interesting case, and an important one, for it illustrates that sometimes mental factors play a more important part in illness than physical causes.

This woman was committed to healthy living and was very careful about the foods she ate. She was young and did nothing I could discern that would cause her to be ill. Yet she complained of recurrent vaginitis. Sometimes this can be caused by infection or something as simple as wearing constricting nylon underwear that prevents the free circulation of air.

The strange thing about her case was that the *only* complaint or symptom that she reported was the vaginitis. It was unique in my experience that not even one other sign, however slight, accompanied this imbalance. I was even more curious after reading her pulse, which showed that she had no imbalance of any humor: they were all normal. Yet she did have the signs of vaginitis. Therefore, the cause had to be sought in some aspect of the mental or spiritual realms. She was single. I asked her if she lived alone. She cast her eyes downward as she replied that she lived with her boyfriend. "Do you have plans to get married?" I asked further. She began to cry and let forth her account of the turmoil she was suffering at living with this man, who refused to marry her. All she wanted, she said, was to get married and have a family, but she doubted that he would ever consent to doing so.

I urged her to return home and inform her boyfriend that either he was moving out or she was. I explained that her emotional conflict over her sexual lifestyle, plus the anxiety over becoming pregnant without being married, could account for her physical signs. She left without promising to do as I said, but seemed somewhat relieved having gotten all of this conflict off her chest.

I didn't hear from this woman again and forgot about her until one day a year and a half later. I spotted her from across the street in a busy shopping section. I decided to walk over and speak to her. As I approached, I realized that she had gained twenty or so pounds and was nursing a small baby. She recognized me immediately and greeted me with a warm smile. "Whatever happened to you?" I asked her. She nodded down at the child at her breast. "Any more trouble with vaginitis?" I asked. She shook her head and said, "No, I've got him instead," unable to take her eyes off the infant. "Does this have any-thing to do with the man who wouldn't marry you?" I asked. "I did exactly what you told me to do. He's my husband now. I was afraid I'd lose him, but I didn't. That was the best advice I've ever gotten."

Vaginitis is the most common nonspecific female complaint among unmarried women in this country. It is my opinion that the extremely difficult emotional choices that confront women in today's confused life roles are sufficient cause of this and other diseases. For example, if a woman lives with a man without being married to him, she must face several possible eventualities—none of them pleasant, and all carrying a destructive impact on her health. If she is sexually active with the man, she may become pregnant. Contraceptive pills, the IUD, and other methods are harmful to women. If she elects not to use one of the available methods of birth control, she runs the risk of having to submit to an abortion; or she may have the child, but usually with the prospect of a very dif-ficult life as a single parent. All of these options are degrading to women. In my practice, I do not hesitate to advise women to refuse to submit to the con-temporary lifestyles of arbitrary sexual encounters. This may seem like an ar-chaic attitude to some, but most women agree with me.

In fact, many of the so-called untreatable diseases are, from the Tibb per-spective, creations of an emotional imbalance that upsets the internal biotic environment sufficiently for diseases to arise.

The sexual urgings and energies of humans are among the most profound and strongest of all natural instincts. Every action in the body sets off a complex chain of physiological responses, and there are various by-products and waste products of those stimulations which the body must deal with. For example, it is common today for all elements of the media to stimulate the sexual appe-tites of people to an unusual and even abnormal degree. While there is nothing at all unnatural about sexual urges, it is not uncommon for a young man to have his sexual energies stimulated and encouraged up to sixty or seventy times per day. This means that the signals from his mind and emotions are engaged with sexual thoughts—from magazines, newspapers, television, and provocatively dressed women. Now, despite receiving these many dozens of stimulations—most of which are transferred to his sexual organs to create some greater or lesser degree of arousal—the chances are great that he is not going to carry any of these initial stimulations through to the complete release of orgasm. This means that the metabolic by-products of such stimulation are left as residues in the body and have to be eliminated. Yet the body is not constructed to deal with this excessive degree of sexual stimulation and thus must deal with it in other ways. According to Tibb, such symptoms as those associated with genital herpes are often due to the body's discharging these highly toxic wastes through the skin (of the penis) rather than processing them through the normal avenue of the liver and colon.

Western medicine takes the position that some drug may be discovered to prevent these substances from being eliminated. Yet, if this is done, there will arise another site for the elimination; or if the substances do not find an avenue of exit, they will damage and destroy one or more internal organs.

The true cure of such diseases lies in creating a positive balance of sexual energies, rather than the hypersexual environment of contemporary society, which is not healthy for men or women and which has led to the increasing sexual abuse of children, sadomasochism, and similar perversions.

Cases #10 and #11

B.R.; Anglo female; single; age 36. Stated complaint: vaginitis; alopecia totalis.

B.W., C.W., L.W.; Anglo males; ages 1, 3, 4. Stated complaint: external otitis (discharge from the ears).

These cases are presented together because, despite a wide variety of signs, they all represent an imbalance of the phlegm humor—and moreover because in each case the humors became unbalanced for similar though unusual reasons.

The woman came to me stating that she had recurrent vaginitis and wondered if I knew any herbal treatment for it. As we talked, she revealed that she was a health enthusiast. She had become interested in an alternative health program, an essential feature of which was total abstinence from meat and dairy products and a high intake of concentrated green vegetables. She had been on this program for almost four years.

She wore a large head scarf and asked me if I didn't consider it strange that she didn't remove her head covering. Actually, I spend considerable time in the East, where women wear head coverings at all times in public, so it didn't seem all that unusual to me. Suddenly she tore the scarf from her head and revealed her completely bald head. Then I noticed that her eyebrows were also missing. She then related that she had alopecia totalis, a condition in which all of the hair of the body stops growing. This drastic condition had obviously affected her self-image, for she wore very masculine clothes and had a rather gruff, unfeminine manner.

She reported the usual range of signs indicating imbalance of the phlegm humor: headache, depression, dizziness, and vaginal discharge; and I could observe more signs—whiteness of the lips and muscular tension. Her overt signs were the baldness and shedding of eyelashes. And I at least considered her eating of only green vegetables to indicate some degree of corrupted appetite.

I spent several hours that afternoon explaining to her the principles of Tibb—specifically how the lack of internal metabolic heat results in incomplete metabolism. I also urged her to consider the Tibb point of view that meat is a source of protein, and that with her exclusive diet of vegetables, she was not properly combining foods to produce protein in her body. Considering the fact that hair is nothing but inert protein, it seemed to be a reasonable assumption that her dietary approach had led to her condition.

She also had irregular menstrual periods, sometimes going six or eight months without a period. She agreed to the detoxification program, although this is one of the few cases in which I didn't think it was justified. She needed protein, but she wasn't prepared to eat meat. I did urge her, as a compromise, to add the Tibb cooking spices to her foods: garam masala on rice and added as a condiment to salads. At least that would provide some internal vital heat. But unless she altered her diet, in my judgment she would not be able to regrow her hair.

She reported back after three weeks that she had had a regular period but no signs of hair growth. I again urged her to reconsider her diet and to add those elements that would provide her body with vital protein. She soon left town, and I had no further record of her improvement.

The three boys in case #11 are unrelated to this woman's case except that they also all had signs of a cold phlegm imbalance, and it, too, was the result, in my judgment, of incorrectly applied dietary experimentation. Their mother brought them to me because they all were discharging pus and fluids from the ears. One of the boys also had inflamed eyes, and all three were wracked with coughs. Two of them had a severe thirst, for twice they asked for something to drink while I was seeing them. As for their bowel habits, the mother wasn't sure, but the oldest one said he often didn't have a movement for three or four days.

Of course I inquired about the diet she was feeding the children, and she related that they were strict vegetarians who ate no dairy products or salt. The youngest child, a year old, had been on mother's milk until it "went sour," and now she had taken him off milk as well. "Humans don't need milk beyond one year of age," she explained confidently. "If this diet is supposed to be so healthy, why are all of your children sick?" I asked. I was astonished and told her frankly that I didn't think that small children could survive on such a diet. She scoffed at me.

The woman was from out of town, and had made a special trip just to see me. I realized she was quite disappointed at my advice. I decided to invite her to have dinner at my home because I knew it would do the children good, and perhaps over the dinner hour I could make some progress in gaining her acceptance of the Tibb dietary principles.

Meat is served several times a week at our home, and this night there was a lamb dish in a spice gravy. The moment they sat down, all of the children began demanding to have some of the meat dish. I glanced at the mother, indicating by my look that she should let them try it. She didn't try to stop me from serving them, and within a short time all of the meat was consumed by the three boys.

Within two minutes the two older boys leaped from the table, ran for the bathroom, and moved their bowels. I asked the mother to check the diaper of the infant. He also had evacuated his bowels.

Undoubtedly the mother was impressed at this undeniable demonstration of the relation between food and bowel movements, at least. I gave her some literature and asked her to reconsider her dietary ideas. She seemed to be somewhat open to my suggestions by then. But later, after they had left, I confessed to my wife that I believed those children had a very unhealthy future ahead of them.

There are probably a hundred different dietary "theories" being advanced today. Especially in the field of alternative medicine and natural diet, the opportunities for ignorance and abuse are severe. Some of the dietary programs may work in some cases, but too often a person has success with a diet and then tries to generalize that one experience into a *system* of dietetics. This is one of the reasons why Tibb is so worthwhile, because there is an uninterrupted period of almost two thousand years of successful application of its principles to people in all parts of the world.

Several of the popular alternative systems today advocate the elimination of milk and milk products—including cheese and yogurt—from the diet. Now, it may be true that Americans consume too much milk, or that there are additives in milk that render it undesirable or unsafe from the standpoint of purity. But this is not the same thing as saying *all* milk is bad. All health and dietary systems I have ever studied agree that milk is a good food, the most complete individual food there is. A reasonable amount of yogurt as a side dish or a slice of cheese or a glass of milk a day—it seems to me ignorant and unscientific in the extreme to assert that these moderate quantities are the cause of diseases. To deprive young children, even infants, of a rich source of nutrition is wholly irresponsible.

It is surprising how easily people will adopt an experimental diet or regimen, supposedly to relieve disease or improve health. The fact that orthodox medicine has turned its back on all forms of alternative health systems, particularly the dietary approach, means that there is no unbiased examination of these approaches. It is frequently the case—as with the woman who altered her diet in a radical manner for four years—that simply changing the diet back to its original form will not result in an immediate readjustment of the body. Such radical dietary approaches create changes in the body that may take years to effectively rebalance, if it can be done at all.

Before taking up any dietary approach, one should investigate not only the diet but its practitioners carefully, to ascertain the rationale underlying the recommendations. Any dietary system that has no recorded history, and for which there is no experience beyond a few people, should be undertaken only with great caution.

Case #12

G.B.; Anglo male; age 52. Stated complaint: post-heart attack.

Many people think an alternative natural system such as Tibb might be worthwhile to try for diseases that are not serious, but for *real* problems, one should see a medical doctor. I agree that acute problems, especially injuries, need prompt medical care; but Tibb medicine has often provided a real cure after drug-oriented medicine has failed. This is such a case.

The patient was referred by a medical doctor who had treated him for the past several years for a variety of complaints. I called the doctor to discuss the case, and he told me, "I've heard good things about you, and I'm impressed with your methods, which seem very well grounded to me." I had treated another of his patients for an inflamed pancreas, and the Tibb formulas produced results within forty-eight hours. The doctor told me then that his only alternative would have been surgery.

The patient had spoken only briefly to me to set up the appointment, and I really did not know the details of his case, so the doctor filled me in. "He's being treated for hypertension, right sciatica, renal stones, obesity, a sugar problem—preliminary diabetic—and depression. I'll tell you, he's got the thickest file of any of my patients, and I don't say that with any pride." The patient had explained to me on the phone that he was taking several drugs, including one for his heart, which were causing him to become forgetful. His sex drive had vanished, and he felt like dying. "There's no point going on like this, thinking every step is your last," he said dejectedly. I asked the doctor about his heart condition and what drugs he was taking. "His status is post-heart attack. He's had three major heart attacks in the past eighteen months, and the next one will probably be fatal, in my opinion. I've got him on Inderol, Levathyroid, Diazide two and one, and Corgard; he'll have to be weaned off that. I told him last week that we'd have to increase the Corgard because his blood pressure was up again—a hundred and ninety over one-twenty. He's a walking dead man going around like that. I hate to sound pessimistic, but I don't think there's hope for him. I wish you luck, and keep me posted," he said, and hung up.

The patient arrived for his initial consultation looking very much like the hopeless case his physician had described to me. His skin was ashen, his gait shuffling, his eyes deep-sunk and weary. "You must be a glutton for punishment," he said as he looked at me. "Not me," I replied; "you're the one who's going to do all the work!" He fidgeted in his seat and perked up, seeming interested.

We spent almost three hours conducting the Tibb interview, and I elicited a long list of complaints: headaches, lethargy, melancholy and depression, dizziness, bad taste in the mouth, canker sores, corrupted appetite, sciatica, inability to get an erection, kidney stones, overweight, diabetes, hypertension, aching joints, baldness. He seemed almost satisfied as he added ailment after ailment to the list.

"It's very simple," I told him, causing him to sit back with shock. How could it be simple, all those diseases?

"Simple?" he questioned. "Yes, you're going to die," I replied evenly. "You mean you can't help me either," he said with total resignation. "No, I can't help you—but perhaps you can help yourself. And for you to do that, this man—this overweight, impotent, depressed mess sitting in front of me—is going to have to die." He was beginning to understand as I went on, "A new person is going to be created, someone who may have your name and features, but one who is healthy. And for that to happen, the sick one is going to have to go!" His body jiggled with a hearty laugh, and the tension subsided for the first time in three hours.

I established a strict Tibb program for him. I put him on a daily diet of a total of 771 calories, yet with almost 75 grams of carbohydrate and 42 grams of protein. He wasn't ready yet for the heating foods, not until his system had cleaned out. At my initial physical examination, his blood pressure was 170 over 110, and his weight was 219 pounds at a height of five feet six inches.

I also added various nutritional supplements to assist the detoxification process: potassium (to prevent the body from pulling potassium from his heart muscles), iodine (to help strip out the mucus), lobelia (for internal heat and elimination of phlegm), niacin (to flush the head with blood, to cleanse), an herbal combination to relax and induce sleep, a digestive enzyme, and the Tibb formula to ripen phlegm.

I gave him a booklet explaining the healing crisis and told him that we could predict the exact day and time of his healing crisis. He left the office in an excited and enthusiastic mood. He went on the program immediately and called to check in every six hours, day and night. He was using a pure oil of jasmine, applied to an acupuncture point on the ear, as a remedy against his severe depression. That was working as well.

I had promised his medical doctor that I would keep him informed of the progress of the program, and he asked that our patient come in for a complete run of blood tests, "just to make sure nothing's going haywire." On the third day of the program, the patient went into his healing crisis and called me in a hoarse voice to report his condition. He had a fever and diarrhea and was discharging vast amounts of mucus in his stools and through his nose and chest. "My God, if you hadn't predicted the exact moment of this thing, I'd swear I had caught some upper respiratory infection," he said weakly. He was due to go to the doctor for his blood workup that morning. I urged him to keep the appointment. He went in and allowed the nurse to draw his blood, then stopped by my office afterward, having told the nurse to call him there if anything urgent showed up. An hour later, she did call, excited and nervous. "Doctor wants you in the hospital right now. Your blood was the worst it's ever been." I took the phone from him and asked to speak to the doctor. I explained quickly and calmly to him that the blood was showing all of the toxins that were passing out of his body. His blood pressure was better, having dropped several points in just three days. If he did not pass through this crisis, he could not continue with the program. I could only hope the doctor would agree with my explanation, despite the alarming signs. "It's up to the patient," he finally answered. I put my hand over the receiver and held a quick conference with the patient, who raised his fist in a sign of victory. "He wants to proceed," I informed the doctor. "All right," he said. "But he's going to have to have the blood work done again tomorrow. If it isn't any better, he's going to be admitted. Okay?" I agreed.

I sent the man home with instructions that he take no food for the rest of the day, if he could do without it. I also advised him to take a coffee enema every two hours, even through the night. The coffee, a stimulant, travels up the hemorrhoidal portal vein and stimulates the spleen, gallbladder, and liver to detoxify.

The next day he reported to the doctor's office at 10 A.M., left his blood sample, and again came to my office to anxiously await the results. "I feel great, I feel great," he kept saying, as if fearful of the signs in his blood. The doctor called sometime later, full of wonder. "I don't know what the hell is going on in his body, but his blood is better than it's ever been. It's normal. Whatever you're doing, keep it up."

And we did. His weight began to drop, and his blood pressure along with it. We discontinued the drugs one by one, until after three weeks he was down to only one-half tablet of Corgard a day. He wanted to drop that too, but I advised him to wait, because too-abrupt withdrawal from this drug can be fatal.

By the end of the fourth week, his weight was 201 pounds and his blood pressure was 132/78—and he was off the drugs. He was eager to go show his doctor what had happened. I was also interested in the doctor's reaction.

After his appointment he came to my office and reported. "What did he think?" I asked.

"He asked me what had happened. I told him I was healed."

"Did you tell him how? Did he ask?"

"Nope."

I advised a special formula for improving hardening of the arteries. He could make it up himself; it was composed of equal parts of millet flour, dried dill weed, chamomile, and valerian root. I had gotten the formula from the Hakim I studied with in Afghanistan.

When he had completed the month program, I invited him to allow me to cook a full meal for him—a reward, I called it—since he had been on a very strict diet for more than a month. So I spent a half day fixing a complete four-course meal according to the Tibb diet, and we later ate the meal. He tentatively sat down and surveyed the array of tempting dishes. "This is healthy? Anything that looks this good *can't* be good for you!" We all laughed.

I have since left the town where I treated this man, but have had contact with him from time to time. He has managed to maintain the progress he made and confesses that only when he deviates from the Tibb diet does he feel any return of his old symptoms. He still takes one-half tablet of Corgard when his blood pressure starts to climb.

Case #13

R.J.; Anglo female; married; age 34. Stated complaint: pain in the side; blood in urine.

This was a complex yet very interesting case in which, using the Tibb diagnostics of urinalysis, we were able to uncover the origin of a long-standing ailment in time to save the woman from an unknown danger. She had experienced a pain in the upper right quadrant of her abdomen, just over the liver, for more than eight years. It had begun as a slight irritation, then a dull throbbing. For the past few years she had "learned to live with it." Several medical doctors had been consulted, one of whom diagnosed it as "arthritis of the rib." The latest physician had detected blood in her urine during an examination for the cause of the pain. He was a practitioner of homeopathy, besides orthodox medicine, and had prescribed potentized remedies for several months as part of the treatment. The woman came to me when the quantity of blood in her urine began increasing and her doctor urged her to submit to x-rays and injection of traceable dyes to try to determine the source of her problems.

During the Tibb interview, she revealed many of the signs of a yellow bile humor imbalance: swelling of the liver, nervous tension, swelling of the bladder, blood in the urine, vomiting, pleurisy, and heartburn. She confided to me with much apprehension that she thought she might have cancer somewhere, because her father had died of it.

There were several other indicators uncovered by my probing questions: a prickling sensation in the upper part of the stomach, a recent loss of weight, and severe vomiting and gastrointestinal distress. In fact, the past several nights she had been awake all night vomiting. Gallstones, bladder stones, and kidney stones had been ruled out by prior diagnosis.

The pulse evaluation showed all four humors were out of balance, which meant one of two things to me. Either she probably already did have a cancer that had not yet manifested, or she had some other condition that required urinalysis for confirmation.

As I looked at the urine sample, the signs were unmistakable: a slight rainbow hue and the "cotton cloud" sediment. After I had finished examining the urine, I returned to the room where she waited.

"Is there any chance you're pregnant?" I asked. She blushed and answered quickly, "No, definitely no, not a chance." Now I was puzzled, because I was certain that the disturbance of the all four humors, along with the characteristics of her urine, meant she was pregnant. Still, she repeated her insistence that she couldn't possibly be so.

Even though she denied being pregnant, I believed it best to have her do only a mild cleansing rather than a complete detoxification. I provided her with the black bile humor purgatives, on the theory that if her black bile humor was purged, perhaps the others would come into balance on their own. She was quite constipated.

I told her to continue reporting to her medical doctor to monitor the blood in the urine—which, incidentally, I did not observe even a trace of in my tests. Yet a more sophisticated test may have revealed a very slight amount that I could not detect.

She called several days later to report that the pain in her side had completely gone. She was more than a little astonished. I repeated that she should visit the doctor again, just to make certain the blood stopped as well. A few days later, she called again to report sheepishly that her test had come back positive. "The blood is still there?" I asked. "No. I'm pregnant," she said with a laugh.

It is not rare in my practice to see women who believe they are experiencing some kind of illness, when all that is happening is that their bodies are conducting their own natural form of detoxification in order to prepare for carrying the fetus. According to all of her Tibb signs, the problem was not in her bladder but in her liver, which I reported to her. If the black bile humor was unbalanced with cold, it would account for the pain in her rib. I advised her to eat according to the Tibb dietary principles during her pregnancy, and the last I heard she was carrying her second baby near to term and had suffered no complications.

II
The Formulary

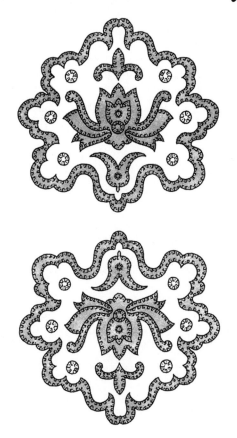

Principles of Herbal Therapeutics

The herbal recommendations in the Formulary are from the original texts of Tibb and therefore have already taken into account all relevant factors of dosage, quantity, force of the herb, the nature of the organ being treated, and so forth. Nonetheless, herbalists and those studying the Tibb system will be enlightened to learn the Tibb methods of selection and compounding of herbs.

In Tibb, the application of herbs is divided first into two general categories: internal application and external application.

A corollary principle is that nothing that is done, especially the giving of any herbs, should stir up or impair the body in its natural functions. It is much more difficult to quiet the stirring than to stir the quiet. Whenever possible, one should treat by nutritive herbs and, if compelled, by medicinal herbs—and at that, one should not go beyond using single herbs as much as possible.

Internal applications are accomplished by introducing the herbs in appropriate form through the mouth, nostrils, ears, anus, urethra, or vagina. Internal therapy is used for three purposes: (1) to evacuate something from the body, as in using senna, (2) to prevent evacuation, as with quince, and (3) to modify the temperament, as with cold water during a fever.

The purposes of external applications are four: (1) to reduce the flesh, which is mainly accomplished with caustics, not herbs, (2) to increase flesh, as with growth-promoting herbs, (3) to stop elimination, as with hemostatics, which stop the flow of blood, or (4) to modify the temperament, as with cold water poured on the body during fever.

There are five factors to consider in herbal treatment: (1) to determine the qualities of the herbs, (2) to determine the quantities of herbs, (3) to use the herbs in their proper indication, (4) to estimate the best time of administration, and (5) to make a suitable selection.

The qualities of herbs are determined by the kind of disease involved; that is, if it is due to hot imbalance, cold herbs are used. All single and compound herbs are determined in this manner of opposites: the qualities of the herbs should be opposite to the nature of the imbalance.

The required quantity of herb can be determined from the temperament of the person and the affected organ, the severity of the disease, and any other factors that have a bearing on the overall treatment plan. For example, if a person is naturally of a hot temperament and has a disease of a heating nature, one need only give mildly cooling herbs. This is so because the entire organism of the person will deviate only mildly from its original temperament. By contrast, if the person has an ordinarily cold temperament and if the disease is hot in nature, it will cause a much greater divergence from the original temperament of the person, and the cooling nature of the herb can and should be much more powerful than in the first case.

The other factors to be included are the environment of the person, the time of year when the disease started, and the state of the air at that time. If all of these factors are hot, then the treatment must cool greatly in order to restore balance, whereas if they are all cold and the disease is hot, the cooling should be mild.

The factors that decide the suitable time of administering the herbs are the period of progress of the disease, the strength of the patient, and other factors that may be apparent to the one evaluating the treatment. For instance, it is a general principle that at the very first or acute stage of disease, the management must be mild in nature; if the disease is long-standing, of chronic nature, the treatment should be heavy. If the illness is at its end, the treatment must be gentle, and if the illness is almost gone, then one should provide treatment for convalescence. As an example, if a person's strength is great and it is desired to evacuate his lower bowel while he has a fever, it can be done from the start without concern. If the patient is very weak, the patient must first be slowly cooled with gentle measures, and only after the strength returns is the evacuation done.

Since most of the methods of treatment in Tibb aim at evacuating some form of excess, there are general guidelines for applying herbs for this purpose. In winter, evacuate at midday, not in the morning. In summer, evacuate at dawn, and give food in the morning and up to midday, curtailing the food in the afternoon and night.

The proper indication of the herb means that one has considered the strength of the patient, the situation of the affected organs, and any other elements of influence. For example, if the patient is strong, one may perform an evacuation in one application, but if the patient is weak, it should be done in several small steps.

One should also consider the situation of the diseased organ. Thus, if a person suffers from diarrhea and an ulcer in the upper colon, the small intestine, he should be treated with oral medicines. But if the ulcer is in the lower colon, he should be treated by introducing the herbs via enema.

The selection of herbs depends also on the strength and temperament of the patient. For example, a person of strong temperament and great strength should be fed foods low in bulk but high in caloric value, like lamb. A weak person should be fed foods high in bulk but low in caloric value, like green vegetables.

The treatment should always first be attempted with nutrient herbs and foods. If there has been a change in the temperament of the person, the food must be of a more medicinal nature. An example of this would be adding asafoetida (a medicinal herb) to a chicken dish, as opposed to cooking it in coriander and cumin (nutrient herbs). The food must be opposite to the temperament that is being corrected.

The treatment of organs within the body depends on (1) the temperament of the diseased organ, (2) the shape of the organ, (3) the position of the organ, and (4) the strength of the organ.

The temperament of the organ can be illustrated by comparing that of flesh, in which heat predominates, to that of the nerves, in which cold predominates. Furthermore, there are organs that are moderate, such as the skin. It is necessary to know what the original, or innate, temperament of an organ is, and then the treatment is aimed to restore it to that temperament. If the innate temperament of the organ is, say, cold, and a hot disease caused the intemperament, then the selection of foods and herbs must be opposite to heat.

To consider the shape of the organ means to distinguish among those composed of flimsy, loose structure (like the lungs) and those made of compact substance (like the kidneys). The liver and spleen have a consistency between these two. The flimsy, loose types of organs cannot stand treatment with powerful medicinal herbs; the compact organs can withstand powerful treatment and are not harmed by them; the third class is in a medium position regarding their resistance to powerful herbs.

The position of an organ means its specific location in the body as well as its relation to other organs. The information about the specific location of an organ is needed to choose herbs that work at the proper site; and the relation to other organs is important when considering the avenue through which toxic matters will pass in being evacuated. If the organ is very close to the point of administration of the herb, it can be treated with just enough of a dose to achieve the desired effect. If the organ is remote from the point of administration, the force of the medicine must be increased so that it remains potent enough by the time it reaches the organ being treated. For example, if we wish to treat the esophagus, we can use the precise potency and dose to treat that organ, because the herb is swallowed directly to the site of administration. If we wish to treat the lung, the medicine has to be strengthened because it has to pass through and across many structures before reaching the lungs.

To illustrate this point further, an herb used to treat the lung has to cross the muscles of the chest, the bones of the ribs, the membrane lining the ribs, and the membrane that binds and wraps the lung. An herb taken orally must thus take the following course: penetrate into the mouth and go to the esophagus, the stomach, the pylorus (the opening into the intestine), the jejunum, and penetrate the vessels between the liver and intestine, then into the vessels on the concave side of the liver and those on the convex side. It then penetrates into the large vessel called the vena cava, into the heart, and finally into the lung.

This being the case with herbs given to treat the lung, herbs applied as poultices or any external treatment may lose their force before reaching the lung. And any internal treatment also may lose some force by traversing so many parts of the body on the way to the lung.

The first consideration related to the strength of the organ is whether it is one of the primary organs (brain, heart, stomach, liver, reproductive organs), because these are the point of origin of forces for the rest of the body. Care must be taken not to give herbs that very quickly alter the temperament of such organs, especially if they cool them. Precautions are taken in such cases by mixing the medicinal herb with others that mediate the effects of abrupt cooling or weakening of these organs—such as mixing with an astringent herb or having the patient smell sweet oils, which assist in maintaining the temperament and force of the organ.

The sensitivity of an organ needs to be known so that very hot, caustic herbs are not administered to weak organs. The weaker organs need to have the doses administered in small portions over a longer period of time.

In review, then, the considerations of herbal treatment are these:

1. The temperament of the organ
2. The range of action of the herb
3. The amount of the herb to be given
4. The place or location of the organ
5. The position of the organ in relation to those near it
6. The degree of sensitivity of the organ

These factors are assessed in relation to (1) the nature of the disease, (2) the cause of the disease, (3) the strength of the disease, (4) the temperament of the body after it deviated from its natural state, (5) the natural temperament of the patient, (6) the age of the patient, (7) the habits of the patient, (8) the present time of the year, (9) the area of the country in which the patient lives, and (10) the state of the air of the environment at the time of the illness.

Herbs and foods that enter the body act in one of three ways. Those entirely overcome by the body are called *nutrients*. Those which entirely overcome the body are called *medicines*. Those which first overcome the body but are finally overcome by the body are *medicinal nutrients*.

The herbs that are given in the following sections are both nutritive and medicinal. The best way to get herbs is to grow them and cut them fresh or dry them under proper conditions. A surprising number of herbs can be grown easily indoors or out, and will do quite well with a little morning sunlight.

Many health food stores carry fairly complete lines of dried herbs, although these are mostly stocked to use in conjunction with the prevalent herbal methods of two or three common herbal books. Some of the Tibb herbs are a bit harder to find. See Appendix III at the end of this book for sources.

Compound Herbal Formulas

Although it is advised and preferable to use a single herb whenever possible, there are reasons that compel one to devise compound herbal formulas. These reasons are due partly to the nature of the illness and disease, partly to the state of the organ being treated, and partly to the nature of the herb.

There are fourteen practical reasons for the use of compounded herbs:

1. The first reason for compounded herbs concerns the extent of the imbalance of the humor; that is, if there is no single herb with enough force to restore balance, it is compounded with others that are stronger (or weaker) in the component desired. Thus, the tendency of the humor to continue in the direction of further imbalance is opposed.
2. The strength and acuteness of the illness may be such that no single herb is sufficient against it. The herbs are compounded so that the ingredients have a synergistic action and effect.
3. Sometimes there is a variance between the action of the single herb and the nature of the disease, as when a single herb works in opposite actions at the same time, like ripening chest phlegm and hindering the growth of tumors. One would compound in order to avoid aggravating one or the other of these conditions, since the desire is to treat them in sequence, not at the same time.
4. Some herbs have such strength that they have toxic or poisonous side effects themselves. In such cases, a compound is devised that annuls the toxic effects.
5. The affected organ may be far from the site of administration, and herbs are added into the compound that speed the herb to the site of action.
6. The strength and importance of the diseased organ must be taken together. Usually an herb to dissolve a tumor is compounded with one to ease the symptoms.
7. Distasteful herbs are compounded with those that improve their flavor.
8. Excessive strength of an herb may be reduced by compounding with herbs of opposite effect.
9. An herb may be added to prevent harm from the treating herb, as in adding peppermint to senna to prevent cramping.
10. Sometimes a single herb is simply inadequate.
11. Additional herbs may be added to enhance or extend the time of action of the treating herb.
12. There is always a difference between herbs and their doses and usages. Sometimes the effects of both may be desired.
13. Sometimes in order to use an herb effectively, it is necessary to mix it with other ingredients, as in adding oil and wax to powdered herbs to use as an ointment.
14. The destructive properties of an herb may be destroyed by mixing it with other herbs, as by mixing saffron with yogurt.

Calculation of Amount of Compound Herbs

In the calculation of the weights of each herb to be included in a compound, there are seven simple determining factors to be considered:

1. Strength of the nature of the herb
2. The effect of the herb
3. Its benefits
4. Its usefulness, alone or with other herbs
5. Distance of the affected organ from the stomach
6. Which herbs in the compounded formula weaken its effect
7. Ill effects on other organs.

All of the single and compound formulas given in the Formulary have been selected with all of the various factors already taken into account. Therefore, one should try to apply them as closely as possible to the directions given. One need not discern all of the foregoing factors in adjusting the compounds or single herbs. Usually a fairly wide range of alternatives is provided, and these each will work with safety and effectiveness.

Those suffering from a serious illness definitely need proper medical advice and supervision by the physician of their choice. Sometimes the body has become so disordered or degenerated that natural methods are not sufficient to keep pace with destructive changes occurring within the body. In such cases, the use of chemical drugs with drastic effects and speed of action may be a necessity. Ideally, medical doctors would possess all of the technical expertise they do have *plus* the knowledge of Tibb. I recommend that people seeking treatment look for a naturopathic physician or an open-minded medical doctor to provide perspective on the various events the body will undergo in its efforts to restore itself to health.

Directions for Herbal Preparations

Once you have determined a formula you wish to use and have obtained the herbs, it is important that the formula be prepared properly. For the purpose of convenience, I have used some terms which apply to the fixing of herbs, such as *infusion, pomade,* and *tincture*. Rather than give a complete set of instructions for preparation in each case, this "shorthand" gives a one- or two-word directive that applies to any herb used. In addition, different directions are sometimes given, owing to the ability of one process to extract one active principle from the herb, while a different action will remove another element. For example, an infusion of lobelia will give a mildly sedative effect, whereas a tincture of lobelia can produce an emetic effect. Below are some of the most commonly used concentrations.

Capsules These are made simply by taking the herb in powdered or finely ground form, and placing it in a gelatin capsule. These are available in sizes from 00 to 4, with 0 and 00 being the sizes most often used for herbs. Capsules make herbs with an acrid taste or unpleasant oils more palatable. After making capsules, be sure to keep them in a safe container, accurately labeled, including the date of preparation. Gelatin capsules contain beef and pork tissue. However, an all-vegetable capsule may soon be available.

Conserve (Sweetmeat) A conserve is a soft mass of herbs mixed with sugar or honey. I usually recommend gur (also called jaggery, or raw Indian sugar). Date sugar works as well. Sugar burns at a higher temperature in the stomach than does honey, but the medicinal property of honey is consumed faster than that of sugar.

To make a conserve, such as rose conserve, gather fresh rose petals and add sugar in the amount of three times the weight of the petals. Mash it together with a mortar and pestle until congealed. If honey is used, roll the mixture in a little orris root powder to keep it from sticking to your hands.

Decoction Many roots and barks, as well as some stems and flowers, must be boiled for some time before their active principle is extracted. The proportion usually is 1 teaspoon of the dried herb to 1 cup of water. Always use stainless steel, glass, or porcelain vessels to make decoctions. A coffee percolator may be used to make a decoction. If none is available, boil the substance for 2 minutes, then simmer for 20 minutes covered. Let cool, and add honey or other flavoring if desired.

Essence Obtain 1 dram of the essential oil of the herb, and add 4 drops of it to 1 pint of pure water. This is sometimes very expensive for true natural essential oils (pure amber, for example, costs approximately $400 per pound), and so synthetic oils are often sold as "natural." Of course, synthetics do not have healing properties and can be used for aromatic purposes only.

Fomentation Dip a cloth in an infusion or decoction and place it over the area to be treated.

Infusion Take one-half to 1 ounce of the herb (leaves, flowers, root, or bark) and pour 1 cup boiling water over the herb. Let it stand for 3 to 5 minutes. Strain. Infusions should be consumed or applied while fresh, and the portion not used should be discarded. The infusion is usually the weakest form in which an herb will be used.

Jujube A paste made of equal parts of gum arabic and sugar.

Mother's milk Mother's milk has natural antibodies and is the most complete food, capable of sustaining the life of an infant for several years. You can of course obtain fresh mother's milk directly from a nursing mother, if available in your family. If not, the local chapter of La Leche League can usually supply frozen mother's milk.

Oil This must be made from the part of the plant that contains the particular oil desired. The best oils of peppermint, for example, come from the leaves. The most aromatic oils are usually derived from the blossoms of flowers. The basic ratio is 3 or more ounces of an herb to 1 pint of olive oil, which is the recommended base because it does not easily become rancid and can be kept a long time. Never use mineral oil, as it is not safe for internal consumption. Heat the herb in the oil at about 140°F. Afterward, strain and bottle. Another method is to simmer up to 1 pound of the herb in 1 pint of water until the oil is extracted—usually 4 or more hours. (Consult Appendix III for sources of essential oils.)

Ointment See Salve.

Oxymel This is a standard preparation in the Eastern pharmacies. It is made simply by mixing 5 parts honey to 1 part vinegar.

Pomade See Salve.

Plaster Bruise the leaves, root, or other part of the herb and place between two pieces of cloth. Moisten slightly and apply to the surface you desire to cover.

Poultice The purpose of a poultice is to apply heat, draw out toxins, and soothe an inflamed area. Some work by producing a counterirritation, some draw blood to the area, and some relax and soothe. Simmer 2 ounces of the herb in ½ pint of water for 2 minutes, then pour the entire solution (without draining) into cheesecloth. Apply the herb poultice directly to area, covering with cheesecloth and a second layer of clean cloth.

Salve The base for a salve (also called *ointment* or *pomade*) is usually almond oil, coconut oil, wax, or petroleum jelly. You can also mix some of these together to make a more readily absorbed salve or to slow down absorption. Petroleum jelly is not soluble in water and is recommended when it is undesirable to allow rapid absorption, such as for application to any of the mucous membranes.

Begin with 2 pints almond oil or other melted lubricant. Add about 1 pound of the herbs in their natural state, 1½ pounds vegetable lard, and 2 ounces beeswax. Place in a stainless steel, earthenware, or glass container and put into the oven for 3 to 4 hours at about 150°F. Check the herbs from time to time to see that they are still submerged and not turning brown or brittle.

A stronger ointment can be obtained by using more of the herb, which is also required if dried herbs are used (increase to 1½ pounds of the herb). You will be able to tell when the active principle has been extracted by the dark color of the oil base. Cool, strain, and put in wide-mouth jars or bottles for use.

A quick method of making a salve is to take one part each of almond oil, honey, and beeswax and add one part of the remedy you wish to use. Heat the lubricant, and mix in the finely powdered herb. Let cool until it gels, and apply. Another method of making salve is to boil the herb in water for twenty minutes. Strain off sediment, add fresh herbs, and repeat the boiling process (cover while boiling). Strain again. Add the resultant decoction to ½ pint of olive oil and simmer until all the water has evaporated. Strain again. Add enough beeswax or resin to solidify. Melt over a low flame and keep stirring until thoroughly mixed.

Suppository This is a preparation of herbs mixed with a suppository base such as cacao butter or glycerinated gelatin and molded into special shapes for insertion into the rectum, vagina, or urethra. The suppository bases are solid at room temperature but melt at the temperature of the body. Suppositories should be stored in a refrigerator, especially during the summer.

Suppositories are made in the following sizes and shapes:

Rectal—tapered, about 2 grams
Urethral—pencil-shaped, pointed on one end; 7 cm in length, 2 grams
Vaginal—oval, 5 grams

You can purchase the base from a pharmaceutical supply house or pharmacy, or make your own by lightly heating one of the bases mentioned above and adding the recommended amount of finely powdered herb. Dosage varies according to age, sex, condition, and similar factors.

Syrup A syrup is a thick liquid preparation made by dissolving sugar into water, decoctions, infusions, or the like. To make a syrup, first make a decoction (or other liquid base) and settle off any sediment. Then, to every pint of herbal liquid, add 1¾ pounds of gur or honey. Place in a stainless steel pan and heat (there will be some scumming, which can be taken off as it cools). Cool and store for later use.

Tincture To 1 ounce of powdered herb, add 4 ounces of water and 12 ounces of cider vinegar. Let stand 2 weeks; shake several times every day. After 2 weeks, add 1 teaspoon glycerin, stir thoroughly, strain off liquid, and seal in bottles. If the herb is weak in medicinal power, the original amount of the herb may be increased from 1 ounce to 2 or 4.

Water A water solution in which herbs are soaked is a weak infusion. These can be made by placing ½ pound of the herb, blossom, or green part, or other vegetable in pure water in direct sunlight for 4 hours, preferably from mid-morning until after the sun has passed its zenith in the sky. Properties for healing are extracted from many grains and seeds in this way. If you can't make a pure water for any reason, an infusion is an acceptable substitute. This is the manner in which the Bach flower remedies were originally made.

Notes on Preparation While it may seem time-consuming to make a tincture, for example, it should be done if that is what is called for in the remedy. If you don't have time to make a tincture (2 weeks), most herbs are available in ready-made tinctures from health food stores, botanical firms, or homeopathic pharmacies. Remember that it is important to use the herb as recommended, for there is often a difference in the properties, depending on how it is prepared. For example, a weak infusion of hops will extract aromatic properties, while a stronger infusion will extract the bitter tonic principle. A decoction will extract the astringent properties. People using herbs for the first time are often disappointed when they "don't work." Each preparation will give a specific result: an herb will not yield the same properties from an infusion as from a decoction.

Dosage Most single and compound herbal preparations given in the formulary are accompanied by proper instructions for dosage. It is very difficult to give an exact dosage to be followed in every case, as each person has a different body, so these that follow must be taken as an average. The rule adhered to by the great herbalists of all times is to begin with the smallest dose first and work toward gradually larger doses, *if needed*. The dose is also to be altered depending on the age of the person. A child of ten usually will require half the adult dose; a child of five can generally be given one-quarter of the adult dose. It is wise to give nervous, high-strung persons smaller and more frequent doses. Also, in applying diuretics, it is better to begin with small doses, so that the kidneys are not forced when in a weakened condition. The instructions for preparing the various forms of medication are given in the Formulary. Follow them carefully.

Dosages

Capsule Dosage in capsules is completely dependent upon the age, sex, general health, and nature of the condition. A general rule is to give capsules as follows:

Number 0:   Three, three times per day, with meals.
Number 00:   Two, three times per day.
Number 4:   One or two, five or six times per day.
Number 2:   Two upon waking up, two at bedtime.

Conserve (Sweetmeat) Use amount specified in Formulary, or 1 tablespoon with tea after meals.

Enema The ratio for most herbs is 1½ tablespoons to each pint of water (do not give more than 1 pint at a time for children or 1 quart for adults).

Essence Dose is variable. Consult Formulary.

Fomentation The cloth should be wet enough with the fomentation so that the fluid does not run off the body; keep damp and change every half hour to hour.

Infusion One cup three times per day is the general rule, although there is great variation in dosage of infusions.

Oil Oils are quite potent and should not be overdosed. One to three drops is the quantity limit for internal consumption. Externally, you may wish to dilute a pure flower essence with a less expensive oil such as olive oil for massages and similar applications.

Oxymel One mouthful as a gargle, or as directed.

Plaster Make up to one-half-inch thick and large enough to cover the affected area. Plasters build up heat, so they must be used with care and in consideration of the general state of the person.

Poultice If the herb is not too expensive or potent, use profusely.

Salve Use enough to cover the area, but not so much that residue is left on the skin.

Syrup According to size and age, 1 teaspoon to 1 tablespoon.

Tincture The Formulary recommends various doses. One ounce of tincture is equal in strength to approximately 1 ounce of the powdered herb, so 3 drops will be equal to ½ cup of tea. Unless used to provoke vomiting (lobelia), or unless otherwise directed, always mix 1 teaspoon of tincture with at least 1 cup of water.

Methods Without Ingestion

We must remember at all times that the stomach is the seat of disease. When digestion fails, disease follows sooner or later. It is for this reason that we may desire to use a method of correcting a part of the body without sending substances into the stomach, which may further disturb an already imbalanced metabolism. A review of the wide range of methods of correcting balance without ingesting anything follows:

1. Remedy is smelled, wet or dry.
2. A soft and sweet-smelling remedy is put in a bottle for inhaling the vapor.
3. Remedy is dropped into the nose.
4. Remedy is sniffed into the nose.
5. Remedy is dropped into the throat.
6. Ground substances are put on the teeth.
7. Remedy is dropped into the ears or other orifices.
8. Remedy is rubbed on the body as oils, washes, or salves.
9. The body is warmed by steaming.
10. Alternating warm and cool compresses are applied to the body.
11. Wet substances are rubbed on the body.
12. Liquid is injected into the intestine, anus, bladder, or womb.
13. Remedy is shaped and inserted into the anus or vulva.
14. Remedy is ground in water and used to bathe the eyes.
15. A tampon is soaked in an herbal preparation and inserted into the anus or vulva.
16. Remedy is ground and poured on wounds.
17. Substances are burned and the vapor is inhaled.
18. Herbal preparations are poured into water for a sitz bath.
19. Herbs are boiled for a foot bath.

Cupping

The operation of cupping cleanses the skin of affected parts and draws healing force to the area. Cupping is less effective with heavy, thick-skinned persons. It should be known that cupping does produce some weakness in the member to which the glasses are applied. Cupping should not be done on persons over sixty years or under three years of age.

Proper Time to Apply Cupping Glasses

Avicenna advises against using cupping glasses at the beginning of the lunar month because the humors are then congested and difficult to move. The best time is the middle of the month, when the moon is on the increase and the humors are in a state of agitation. The sixteenth and seventeenth days of the lunar month are best. The three hours after sunrise are the best time to apply the glasses. Cupping should not be done after taking a bath, except in the case of thickened blood. Then it should be done one hour after bathing.

Methods of Cupping

There are two methods: wet and dry. In dry cupping, the glasses are applied to the skin with heat from the flame used to dispel air from the chamber of the cup. Wet cupping requires making a scarification of the skin, so that a small amount of blood is drawn. The use of wet cupping serves as a substitute for venesection, in which larger quantities of blood are let out. Both wet cupping and venesection were originally used as a prophylactic measure. Exercise and adjustments to diet make wet cupping and venesection of less use than in former times.

Purposes

There are several purposes in cupping: (1) to draw inflammation away from deep parts toward the surface and make it more accessible to medicines; (2) to divert inflammation from an important organ to a less important one; (3) to infuse warmth and blood into an affected organ and to dispel humors from it; (4) to alleviate pain.

Precautions

Cupping should not be done over the breasts in women, as it will interrupt the menstrual flow. Other sites and conditions to avoid are all bony prominences, sites prone to cramps, areas showing any superficial blood vessels, varicose veins or much hair growth, tumors, and lymph nodes. Cupping should never be done on pregnant women or infants. Cupping on the nape of the neck is said to induce amnesia.

Technique

Have the person lie down on an examination table or a firm bed, in case of fainting during treatment. If the person feels unwell during the procedure, discontinue immediately. Select cupping sites or swollen spot.

Length of Application

The cups may be applied for 10 to 15 minutes, or until the site under the cups begins to appear reddish. The place of application may afterward become inflamed. To avoid this, soak a cloth or sponge in moderately hot water and place it around the base of the cup after it is sealed onto the skin.

Equipment

A small, medium, or large cupping apparatus is used, made of glass, bamboo, or plastic. Use the larger cups on healthy young people; use smaller ones for the elderly, weak, or chronically ill.

Application

Hold a small ball of cotton saturated with rubbing alcohol or olive oil in a pair of forceps or large tweezers. Ignite the cotton and quickly apply the flame to the inside of the cup, then remove and extinguish. The cup is instantly placed over the selected spot, and the cup will attach itself firmly to the skin because of the atmospheric pressure outside. This method is quite safe and painless. Some practice may be required to affix the cup properly. It may assist adhesion to apply olive oil or petroleum jelly to the lip of the jar prior to application.

TABLE 10
POINTS OF APPLICATION

Site	Indications
Nape of neck	Heaviness of eyelids, itch of eyes, bad breath.
Between the shoulder blades	Pains in upper arms and throat; to relax cardiac orifice of stomach
Over the two posterior neck veins	Tremor of head; and for conditions of the head (face, teeth, ears, eyes, throat, nose).
Legs	Cleanses the blood; provokes menstrual flow.
Under the chin	Teeth; throat; cleanses head and jaws.
Inner thighs	Inflammatory masses in upper part of thigh; pustules; podagra; piles; bladder; uterus; renal congestion.
Front of thighs	Inflammation of testicles; leg ulcers.
Behind hips	Inflammatory conditions and ulcers of buttocks.
Behind knee (popliteal space)	Aneurysm; chronic abscesses; septic ulcer of leg and foot.
Over ankle bone (malleoli)	Suppressed menses; sciatica; podagra.
Over the outer side of hips	Sciatica; podagra; piles; inguinal hernia; tissues within hip joints.
Over the buttocks, towards anus	Draws humors from whole body, from head; benefits the intestines; cures suppressed menses.

Removal

After 10 to 15 minutes, press the skin around the edges of the cup to remove it. When air enters from the outside, the cup will fall off by itself. Do not use pressure on the cup, or the skin may tear. A meal may be taken one hour after cupping is done.

Adjusting the Four Humors

The entries in the Formulary often advise "adjusting" or "purging" one of the humors. Chapter 9 may be reviewed for a discussion of humors. Although physical signs and symptoms may be present, the basis of the Tibb treatment is to *restore balance* to the underlying metabolic process: the humor. This rebalancing of the humors is called "adjusting." It requires one first to ripen the humoral substance (a process known as "coction"), then to purge it. Laxatives (used for the ripening stage) cause elimination of the contents of the stomach and intestines. Purgatives (used for the purgative stage) eliminate what is in the veins and deeper parts of the system. Each humor ripens at different intervals, which are given below. Pregnant women and infants should not be given purgative medicines. The maximum dose of purgatives for adults is four times. More than this is harmful.

The single herbs and formulas are commonly used ones, although adjustments can be made after a complete evaluation of the patient.

Blood Humor

The blood humor becomes changed in four ways: (1) an increase in quantity, (2) thickening, (3) softening, and (4) infection. Whenever the blood becomes changed from its balanced condition, it must be adjusted.

The *increase in quantity* leads to excess of heat. This is called "boiling" of the blood humor. The formula that cools down excessive heat of the blood humor is composed of chickory seeds, lettuce seeds, coriander seeds, red rose petals, lemon juice, sandalwood syrup, oxymel, and all foods and herbs that are cold.

Mixing of phlegm and black bile with blood humor is the cause of *thickness*. Foods and herbs that throw off black bile will soften the blood humor. Phlegm laxatives, diuretics, and acid foods are advised.

Softened blood humor is caused by moisture and phlegm. Therefore, phlegm purgatives should be given (see the following section, on phlegm adjustors). Second-degree hot and dry herbs and foods are advised.

Infection means that putrefaction is occurring due to bacteria, viruses, or other causes. Every humor that is infected causes fever, and fever is the main sign of infection. Cold and dry foods and herbs are advised. Infections must be watched carefully because they can increase dramatically in a short time. Treatment with antibiotics may be advised for bacterial infections. Infections may require medical treatment.

The method of purging the blood humor involves letting out small amounts of blood, called venesection. This is a surgical procedure that is not widely practiced in the West. Bleeding gums and hemorrhoids are a form of spontaneous venesection. Nosebleeding may occur as a natural consequence of adjusting the blood humor. It is interesting to note that the taking of blood samples, donating blood, and loss of blood during surgery are all types of venesection that may in themselves have direct, though unintended benefits. The blood humor, being the first to arise in the chain of metabolic process, is the easiest to correct.

Phlegm Humor

Every imbalance of the phlegm requires a period of nine days to ripen, in order that the excess may be expelled easily. Thus phlegm that is thick must be softened, that which is soft must be thickened, and so forth.

Imbalance of phlegm occurs in five forms and can be determined by the "taste" of the phlegm in the mouth and nose: (1) blood is mixed with phlegm (sweet); (2) burning bile is mixed with phlegm (salty); (3) moderate heat corrupts the phlegm (sour); (4) a small amount of black bile mixes with phlegm (coarse); (5) excessive moisture dominates phlegm (tasteless, clear). The last item is the coldest imbalance of phlegm.

Single substances that ripen phlegm include anise, cinnamon, valerian root, black raisins, cardamom, garlic, and ginger. The formula to ripen phlegm must be decided after evaluation of the signs.

One often-used formula for ripening is composed of ¼ teaspoon sebestan (capers), ¼ teaspoon cowslip, ½ teaspoon anise seed, 1 teaspoon mint. Boil in 2 cups water for 10 minutes and strain. Give ½ teacup portion as tea, three times per day for nine days.

Another ripening formula is composed of two or three senna pods and 1 tablespoon of the soft part of a fresh cucumber. These two are soaked for one hour in 1 pint rosewater or plain warm water. Drink 1 teacupful. The gripping of senna pods can be moderated by adding 1 teaspoon of sweet almond oil.

After the phlegm is ripened, it should be purged. The following formula may be used: ¼ teaspoon each of hyssop, violet flowers, and ground fennel seed. Place these herbs in 3 cups water and add ¼ cup black raisins, 2 chopped dried figs, and 1 teaspoon licorice root. Boil down to 1 cup. Add ½ teaspoon each of fresh cucumber pulp, rose petals, and gur (raw sugar). Boil 10 more minutes, and filter. Add 1 teaspoon sweet almond oil. The dose is 3 teaspoons in the morning, taken once.

Another formula to purge phlegm is composed of 1 teaspoon powdered ginger and ½ teaspoon sea salt. Mix in 1 cup warm water, and drink. One dose is sufficient.

Keeping the phlegm humor in balance can be accomplished by including these foods and spices in the diet: anise, cinnamon, valerian root (as tea), raisins, cardamom, garlic, and ginger. If there is foul odor to the mucus, do not give herbs, because it means a healing crisis is under way. If there is fever, the person should use only cooling medicines, such as oxymel and syrup made from rose petals.

If the purgative is successful, the person will move the bowels within 1 to 6 hours. Afterward, give sweet basil, honey, and rosewater as a cold drink. If the person continues having bowel movements and it turns to diarrhea, give yogurt and cooked rice.

Yellow Bile Humor

Yellow bile becomes unbalanced in five ways: (1) soft moisture mixed with it; (2) thick moisture mixed with it; (3) corrupted black bile mixed with it; (4) hot black bile mixed with it, called thick yellow bile; (5) excess of heat, called burning yellow bile. The last two are quite similar. The greater the signs of heat, the more cold herbs and foods should be given, two or three times daily.

Yellow bile takes three days to ripen, unless it is very corrupted, in which case five or more days are needed. The single herbs that ripen yellow bile are quince seeds, chickory, cucumber seeds, coriander seeds, sandalwood, lettuce seeds, and camphor. These must be given according to the needs of the individual, after evaluation. If there is coughing, do not give seeds of quince. Instead, give syrup of chickory and purslane.

A simple formula to ripen the yellow bile is to soak 2 teaspoons dried leaves of coriander in 1 cup water for 1 hour. Strain, add a little honey, and drink. Cold fruits such as watermelon and sour things like vinegar are excellent adjustors of yellow bile. Women and children should be given moderate amounts of cold things.

The formula to purge the yellow bile is composed of violet, plum, rose, and tamarind or senna pods. Some of them work immediately and some later. They can mixed together, according to the signs of the imbalance and strength of the patient.

A well-known formula to purge the yellow bile is made of 1 teaspoon pulp of plum, $\frac{1}{8}$ teaspoon sebestan (capers), $\frac{1}{2}$ teaspoon each of fumitory and senna leaves, $\frac{1}{2}$ teaspoon chickory seeds. And 1 teaspoon sweet almond oil, and boil in 2 cups water for 5 minutes. Cool, strain, and drink 1 cup. Repeat if necessary.

Black Bile Humor

Black bile requires fifteen days to ripen. Single herbs and foods that ripen black bile include sebestan, cowslip, melon seeds, figs, raisins, and moisturizing foods. Oxymel is also very effective to ripen black bile.

Black bile that has been corrupted for a long time can be ripened by making a decoction of $\frac{1}{2}$ teaspoon each of cucumber seeds, chickory seeds, cowslip, and barberry root. Put these in 2 cups very hot water, and add 1 tablespoon oxymel. This remedy should be taken during the daytime.

The single most effective black bile purgative is an infusion of senna pods (four or five pods to $1\frac{1}{2}$ cups water); drink 1 teacupful. This and other purgatives should ordinarily be taken only once. A compound formula to purge the black bile is made with four senna pods, to which is added $\frac{1}{8}$ teaspoon each of valerian root and anise seed, and one stalk of chopped celery. Boil in 1½ cups water. Cool, strain, and drink once.

Another formula specific for black bile purging is made of 4 senna pods, and ½ teaspoon each balm mint, anise seed, rose petals, and ginger root. Boil in 1½ cups water. Cool, strain, and drink ½ to 1 cup. A single dose is sufficient.

Inhalations for Hot and Cold Imbalances

Since the humors are subtle, semivaporous substances, it is often advisable to use vapor inhalations to assist the rebalancing process. Imbalances are almost always either *primary* hot or cold in nature and can be determined by the signs.

For hot imbalances, this mixture is useful: sandalwood powder, vinegar, rosewater, and fresh coriander leaves. Mix them together in a large basin of very hot water. After the water cools down enough so that it does not scald, put the feet in the basin and sit for 15 minutes, letting the steam rise from the bath.

A similar mixture for cold imbalances is made by mixing castoreum, cinnamon, cloves, musk, sweet basil, and saffron. Aloeswood incense is excellent to burn for cold imbalance.

Brain Purgatives

Some entries in the Formulary advise "purging the brain." This is done by mixing ½ teaspoon each of chamomile and marshmallow herb. Boil in 1½ cups water for 5 minutes. Cool, strain, and drink.

Things that strengthen the mind and remove throbbing of the temples and fainting are aloeswood, sandalwood, musk, and camphor. These should be burned as incense. For mental diseases, this formula is advised: equal parts of chamomile, leaves of celery, fennel seed, common dill, and cumin. Boil in water and drink as tea. These same herbs may be added to the bath with great effect.

Excess of Moisture

For imbalances of excess moisture and hectic fever, use pumpkin, cucumber, purslane, lettuce, watermelon, violet, and barley. Boil them together in 1 quart water. Then add this to a bath, and have the person sit submerged to the neck for 1 hour. Afterward, give massage with violet oil. Foot massage is more effective for removing headache than any medicines.

Strengthening the Organs

The foregoing formulas will adjust the humors to their proper temperaments. However, in the case of long-standing dietary indiscretions, lack of exercise, improper habits of elimination, and other wrong behaviors, the vital organs may have become weak or degenerated. The following foods, herbs, and spices will provide the necessary metabolic force and nutrients to assist in rebuilding these organs.

To Strengthen the Brain Include these items in the diet: quince, apples, orange, rosewater, ginger, valerian, cloves, chicken, brains, goat's milk. Use the following scents to strengthen the brain: rose, musk, jasmine, 'oud (aloeswood), frankincense.

To Strengthen the Heart Eat peaches, pomegranate, tamarind, apple, rhubarb, cowslip, mint, coriander seeds, orange, cinnamon, senna, gur, saffron, carrot, cardamom, and mint. Use the following scents: sandalwood, amber, camphor, rose, 'oud (aloeswood), hyacinth. Women should wear ruby and lapis lazuli jewelry and silk clothes.

To Strengthen the Liver Eat chickory, roasted chickory root, pomegranate, nutmeg, cinnamon, cloves. Liver weakness comes mainly from things that cause coldness and moisture. Therefore, include heating foods and spices. Use the scent of amber.

To Strengthen the Stomach Include in the diet: pomegranate, quince, orange and orange peel, cinnamon, gur, senna, cloves, cardamom, mint. Scents to use are rose and 'oud (aloeswood). Every purgative weakens the stomach, with the exception of senna. Everything that strengthens the stomach also strengthens the intestines and throat.

To Strengthen the Female Reproductive Organs Include in the diet: anise seed, watermelon, cucumber, fennel, celery, pomegranate, grapes, buttermilk, fowl, almonds, cardamom, milk, egg yolk, olive oil, figs. Scents to use are rose and sandalwood. To increase ability to conceive, add walnuts and pistachios to the diet.

To Strengthen the Male Reproductive Organs Include in the diet: lamb, saffron, honey, almonds, peas, green beans, coriander, pumpkin, dates. Scents to use are myrrh, musk, lily of the valley, violet, amber.

How to Use the Formulary

The Formulary is arranged according to the signs that affect various parts of the body. Disease names common to Western medicine are not used, unless they happen to have derived from the Tibb medical texts (such as conjunctivitis). The first thing to do is decide which is the predominate *sign* (symptom) that you wish to treat. Then turn to the section discussing that body part, and review the sections until you find the one that most closely resembles the sign you have. The signs are quite specific. For example, for the eye, there are two dozen different signs.

Once you have located the relevant signs, read the section to determine the treatment. This usually consists of (1) dietary adjustments, (2) advice on purging a particular humor, and (3) other general instructions. Sometimes a visit to a medical doctor or the emergency room of a hospital is recommended if the problem is of such a degree that immediate, drastic intervention is vital to life.

Often the section will require that a distinction be made between hot or cold imbalance as the cause. In such cases, refer to the discussion and list of features of these imbalances in Chapter 6 and decide accordingly. In most cases, the text will indicate which humor is out of balance and recommend specific herbs to make the correction. In other cases, the advice will be general, such as "Purge the yellow bile humor." In that case, you must refer to the appropriate formulas just given, or consult Chapter 9 for a complete discussion of that humor.

In making the herbal preparations, herbal apothecary terms are used, such as *decoction* (or *salve* or *poultice*, etc.). The instructions for each of these forms of herbal administration are given in the beginning of the Formulary, listed alphabetically.

It is especially recommended that you read the entire section before undertaking a particular course of treatment, because it may be that other sections contain more specific symptoms that will lead to a more accurate pinpointing of the imbalance. Moreover, a pain or event in one body part is sometimes a reflection of a causative factor occurring elsewhere in the body. The Formulary usually refers to the proper section. But it is a good idea to check the index and read the references in each section that are relevant to a condition, so that you have the most comprehensive view before undertaking treatment.

The application and use of herbs in the Tibb system are based on principles that are quite different from contemporary medical modalities of treatment. The objective of the Tibb treatment is not specifically to treat the symptoms of a disease, but rather to restore and improve the forces of the body on the most subtle levels of cellular and atomic metabolic function. Therefore, do not expect that the use of herbs advised in this book is meant as a substitute for medical treatment.

The Unani Tibb system of natural healing incorporates use of essential oils for many imbalances. Avicenna invented the process of steam distillation and was the first to distill oil of rose. In most cases, the specific oil is recommended in the appropriate subsection of the Formulary. Among the oils often suggested are rose, violet, jasmine, frankincense, myrrh, and chamomile.

There are several approaches to utilizing aromatic oils for therapy. The purpose of the application in Tibb is not to use the essential oil for its medicinal action per se, but rather as an effective method to quickly adjust the subtle essences of the humors.

It is necessary to obtain true natural essential oils, either the first pressing (called absolute or concrete) or an oil extracted into a base oil (called enfleuraged or expressed oil). The essential oils from India are considered to be the finest quality. They are called attars if unblended, and attar oils if mixed with base oils such as sandalwood or olive.

Appendix III gives sources for Tibb aromatherapy oils. Any oil made entirely of synthetics or diluted with alcohol is unsuitable for healing purposes.

The method of application is either external or internal. For external application, the oil may be used for massage in pure form or mixed with sweet almond or olive as an extender. For emotional and mental applications, apply one or two drops of the oil to a small piece of cotton about the size of the thumbnail. Roll the cotton into a small ball, and insert into the *ridge* (*not* the ear canal) of the *right* ear. The illustration shows the correct placement of the cotton ball in the ear. The cotton may be left in place for one to three hours. If absolute essential oils are used continuously for several days, an irritation may develop.

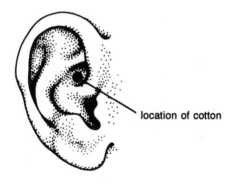

location of cotton

Placement of Cotton in Ear Ridge

Attars or essential oils may also be burned on self-igniting charcoal. A few drops ignited on the charcoal will scent a small room with fragrance for about twenty minutes.

It is very rarely necessary to ingest essential oils. They are an extremely concentrated form of the active principles of herbs, equivalent in potency and action to chemical drugs. Only two or three drops taken internally have produced adverse reactions. If a qualified practitioner or physician does advise taking essential oils internally, the dose should not exceed one or two drops of most oils. The method of ingestion is to mix with a half-teaspoon of honey. Essential oils should never be used simply as a convenient form of taking herbs. Their best purpose is to create emotional and spiritual balance, their greatest effect, on the heart.

The Tibb system approaches the subject of health and disease on the broadest possible scale and envisions the human being as an entity unified on the physical, mental, and spiritual planes of existence. One should refer to and consider all aspects of one's life—the emotional, financial, sexual, and all other factors— to try to discover how and why imbalance and disease have arisen. The full and complete cure of any disease can only happen when the causative factors have been removed and replaced by their opposites (e.g., overeating with moderate diet; anger with kindness; hate with joy; heat with cold).

Finally, it needs to be said that illness is a mechanism that is intimately connected with our own perceptions of the purpose and meaning of life, for loss of health threatens the continuation of our existence. A disease or ailment or illness is a time to discover and learn about oneself, and about God, and to reflect deeply about how one conducts one's life. Almost none of us escapes disease entirely during life, regardless of how careful we may be. As a great sage once remarked, "There are some things learned when we are sick and suffering that simply cannot be learned in any other way."

Section 1

The Well-Being of Children

Raising Children

Children are extremely delicate and elegant in body, temperature, and temperament. Their temper, as it adjusts to growth, should be kept very balanced and moderate, since it responds quite rapidly and easily to events going on about it. The reason for this tendency to moods and activities is the prevalence of phlegm in large quantities in the child's body, and the shifting weaknesses and softness of the body parts as they undergo growth.

Therefore it is necessary to keep children away from all extreme effects upon their sensibilities, such as severe anger, great fear, staying awake for extended periods, or sleeping for a long time. These things can lead not only to unhappiness for the child but also to the beginnings of disease.

It is common sense that parents, doctors, and other caregivers should be aware of what a child likes and dislikes. Things that are obviously harmful to a child should be kept away, regardless of how strenuously the child desires them; but if there is no harm in what a child desires, it should be given readily to the child, for it contributes to a happy disposition and good nature. A sense of humor should always be behind the guidance, whether one is bending to a child's desires or keeping harmful objects or activities away. Usefulness and harmfulness are of two kinds: to the body and to the essence and soul. But what is useful to the body is health itself, for if the body is always wracked with illness and upsets, the temper will be bad, because of the relation between body and the essence.

A hot intemperament is manifested in a child who is reticent to speak, is standoffish, wants to spend long periods alone, and often feels afraid. Bad morals or defective character can often be traced directly to an upset of temper in early childhood. "He's got a hot temper" is often used to describe an unpleasant adult—forceful and selfish, immature and impulsive. But the badness of temper is the result of a bad emotional environment in childhood, one that exposes a delicate child to extremes of anger, sadness, and noise. The nature of a human being is to be independent, happy, and balanced. In addition to proper nourishment of food for a balanced body, the spirit and soul must also be nourished by keeping the essence healthy. Severe anger is one of the basic causes of bad temperament and other indispositions, because it so easily throws off the balance between body and essence.

When a child rises from sleep, it is an ideal time for a bath, which should be with lukewarm water. After the bath, the child should be left free to play with other children of his or her own age, in games that are not harmful (for about an hour or a little longer) to consume the natural energy that has built up during rest. Children should not often play with others who are older or younger, because with younger children they cannot use their abilities to their full extent and because with older children they are not really qualified in skills and thus become frustrated and disposed to feeling failure. During adolescence, the child should be fed after an hour of play a light meal or snack—as much as is needed to increase growth. If he wants to play again after that, the child should not be restrained; but if the child wants to sleep, that is fine as well. After sleep, a lukewarm bath will refresh the child at a time when his mood is calm. For a daily schedule, the conditions of play and food should be considered in relation to time of day, season, climate, altitude, and similar factors.

At the age of four, a child should be taught manners and politeness, and the formal aspects of learning can begin. From the age of seven onward, the teaching of politeness should increase. It is important that the teacher be a model as well. While the influence of parents is needed and ever-present, someone outside the family can be considered for the child's instruction in morals, attitudes toward life, religious ideals and ethics, and the manner of dealing with parents, teachers, pious persons, relatives, friends, peers, and younger children. The child should be taught in a conscious way how to visit, meet, and speak with each of these societal categories and how to gather people together in meetings. According to the child's age and understanding of matters related to religion and science, things that will help him progress in more formal studies must be taught. The child should be given only as much instruction as he can hold in mind and remember without strain, so that the child does not become tired, bored, or angry. The teacher should speak to the child with kindness and mildness. If the child becomes tired or displeased, the teacher should let him go, to walk around or play for a time.

At the age of ten, the frequency of bathing a child can decrease, and teaching the meaning of disappointments, politeness, general education, and self-discipline should increase. Toward the age of fourteen or fifteen, which is nearing adulthood, the child should be introduced to mild fasting and other self-disciplines, as the phlegm which has been in his system is being used up and the extreme agility of play and the powerful exertions are being exhausted. It is at this time that parts of the body are hardening and stiffening into the bone structure and musculature of adulthood; this can be experienced as growing pains. If, during this period, a child neglects his studies, he should be punished. Children's temper is much hotter during this stage if not brought under control by mild, enforced hardships. This is the last stage on the road to adulthood, and if the child does not encounter such hardships as mild and fair punishments, in later life, when tempers and powers are weakened, the person will be prone to increases in the balance of moisture. Even at this stage, moisture can become a problem, and should be cured as the situation requires.

The foregoing brief presentation of the stages of growth of a child shows how to keep a balanced body and spirit, which will contribute to a happy, well-adjusted childhood into pre-adulthood. In some cases, either through inharmonious outside influence, poor diet, or other factors, disease occurs. The following three sections are devoted to the most common of these disturbances, with remedies given to restore balance to the child's physical and spiritual system.

Infancy

1.1 Skin

From the time of birth, the child will be exposed to many hot and cold substances injurious to an infant's sensitive skin. Therefore, an effort is made to condition the skin against this. Bathing in a salt-water solution (1 teaspoon to a quart of pure water) each day for the first several weeks will help to accomplish this purpose.

1.2 Sleeping Quarters

Babies must be placed in rooms that are airy without being too cold. Since their eyes are very sensitive to extremes, keep the drapes closed or windows covered to prevent extremes of direct light. Even a gloomy atmosphere is all right for the first month or so. During sleep, the head should be raised slightly higher than the rest of the body, and the baby should be checked from time to time to make certain that his limbs are not twisted into unusual positions.

1.3 Bathing

Hold the baby by the right hand, so that the left arm is across his chest and not hanging down over the stomach. After washing, bounce the palms of the baby's hands and soles of the feet up and down gently. Dry gently with a soft cloth, first placing the infant on the stomach, then on the back, gently singing to him all the while. Put a drop of sweet rose oil or other pleasant oil onto the pillow, and dab a little on his eyelids.

1.4 Nursing

If at all possible, the baby should be fed from his or her own mother by nursing at the breast. Mother's milk is most like the nourishment the infant received while in the womb—the menstrual nutrients—and it is these that are changed into milk after delivery. It is best suited to the baby. Infants will naturally suck at the breast if the nipple is pinched and placed between their lips. Allow the baby to nurse two or three times per day at first, but he should not be allowed to take too much. Remember that the mother has just undergone a great upheaval in her own system, and it is good to allow her a few days to recover some balance.

1.5 Strengthening the Constitution

Gentle rocking movements, humming, lightly singing, and cooing at the baby are soothing for the baby. The movement benefits the body; the melodies benefit the mind.

1.6 Inability to Nurse

Nursing problems are discussed in the Formulary. The La Leche League in your city will be glad to provide free assistance during your nursing if any problems occur. Milk can be frozen to keep up nursing even if the mother falls ill.

1.7 Test for Good Milk

Test for the proper consistency by allowing a small amount to run over the fingernail; it should be thin and flow easily. If you tip your finger upward slightly and the milk does not flow back down, it is thick. Place an ounce or two of your milk into a glass, drop a pinch of myrrh into it, and stir. The milk will separate into the liquid and "cheesy" part, which should be about equal in quantity. Breast milk should be white (not grayish or yellowish), be of good odor, and taste a little sweet (not bitter or salty), with little or no foam in it.

1.8 Diet

If the milk is thick, the mother should drink a little honey with vinegar (1 teaspoon of vinegar and 1 tablespoon of honey). Wild marjoram, hyssop, thyme, savory, and oregano should be added to foods. If the milk is thin, the nursing mother should avoid exercise for a while and eat foods that thicken, such as meat broths and bread soups. Adequate rest is vital.

1.9 How Long to Nurse

It is desirable to nurse a child for two years, if possible. If other foods are to be added to the child's diet, they should be added gradually over a period of months. This will allow any allergic reactions to be noted and enable identification of the offending foods. Weaning must not be abrupt, but should allow the child to withdraw over several months. After the first teeth appear, more substantial foods should be considered. If indigestion or flatulence occurs, all foods should be stopped for at least eight hours, and a warm, soothing bath should be given to the baby. If the infant at weaning time keeps crying and asking for the breast, make a poultice of 1 teaspoon myrrh, and add 1 teaspoon very smoothly ground pennyroyal, mix with water, and apply as a paste to the breast and let the baby suck briefly at that.

1.10 Walking

There is no rush to compel a child to sit up or walk. By forcing a child prematurely into postures for these acts, great strain is placed upon the bones and muscles of the back. Be especially careful that the child is not allowed to climb up on a high chair or other place and fall off. Childproof the home when the child begins to move about.

1.11 Teething

At the time when the child's teeth are coming in, keep all hard things out of his mouth, for if the child gnaws on them, the substance that is becoming the teeth may be worn away and dissolve, leaving deformed teeth. Allow the child to chew on a piece of arrowroot instead, and rub the back of the neck with warm oils after the teeth do break through the gums. A few drops of the same oil may be dropped into the ears. As soon as the baby realizes he has teeth, he may try to bite his own fingers, so give him a stick of dry licorice root to chew on. Rubbing the gums with salt and honey will take away some of the pain of teething. When most of the first teeth are in, they should be rubbed several times a week, at the base of the gums. New teeth sometimes seem to itch. Let the child chew on a dill pickle.

1.12 Inflammation of the Gums

This condition, called gingivitis, may occur while the teeth are coming in. Swelling may also occur around the juncture of the jawbone. You should press firmly against the swollen parts in the mouth, or along the outside of the jawbone, and rub the gums with a few drops of oil of chamomile added to honey.

1.13 Diarrhea

Many babies develop diarrhea during teething. Some healers say it is due to the ingestion of saline matter excreted by the gums during dentition. Whatever the cause, it interrupts normal function and, if severe, must be treated. Suggested treatments include applying a plaster of about equal parts of caraway, rose hips, anise, and celery seeds or parsley seeds to the stomach. A plaster treated with infusion of rose leaves and caraway works also. If the skin loses its elasticity and the baby becomes senseless, this is an emergency. Take the baby to a doctor or hospital.

1.14 Constipation

A suppository may be used, made from honey cooked over a low flame until it becomes thick enough to shape for insertion into the anus. Adding a little honey or rice-bran syrup to the milk also improves bowel movement.

1.15 Incessant Crying; Loss of Sleep

The causes of incessant crying are heat, cold, bugs (flies, fleas, etc.), hunger, thirst, retention of urine, and retained feces. For retained feces, the nursing mother should eat some prunes or add a tablespoon of olive oil to her diet twice a day. If sleep must be had, make a decoction of chamomile and pepper-mint, ½ teaspoon to 4 ounces of water, and allow the infant to drink an ounce or two. Or add 1 drop of oil of peppermint to 8 ounces of water and let him drink as much as he wants.

1.16   Earache
This is caused by excess moisture in the brain, or trapped gas. It may be treated by making an oil from gur, lentils, and myrrh or cedar seeds; put 1 or 2 drops into the ear.

1.17   Difficult Breathing
Rub olive oil on the base of the ears and on the tongue. You can also depress the back of the tongue to cause vomiting, which will ensure that there is no obstruction of the airway. Water may be dropped into the mouth, drop by drop, as well as a little linseed and honey to suck on. NOTE: Loss of voice in infants is due to constipation. Give cabbage juice by mouth or rectum.

1.18   Cough
Some healers advise that the baby's head should be bathed in plenty of warm water. A steam vaporizer will also work well. Put plenty of honey on the tongue, and cause the baby to vomit and expel excess mucus in the stomach. A few grains of the following may be added to the milk: gum arabic, quince seed (set 20 or so seeds in water for half an hour, and a gummy substance will form). Give ½ teaspoon of this mixture to the baby.

1.19   Severe Vomiting
Feed three grains of very finely ground cloves.

1.20   Hiccups
Feed a piece of fresh coconut dipped in honey.

1.21   Colic
When the baby writhes and cries, apply a hot water bottle to the stomach, and give peppermint water.

1.22   Skin Rash
In all kinds of skin rash of unknown origin, treat by bathing in soothing waters. You may use any of these: rose, myrtle, tamarisk, marjoram, peppermint, or almond. Also recommended is a decoction of dates and figs, mixed in water of fennel seeds. When the rash has developed fully, bathe in rose water, then rub rose oil on the affected parts.

1.23 Fevers

As explained elsewhere, fevers are not necessarily a negative sign, but they can sometimes quickly get out of hand with small babies, or even children. Cool baths can be used to keep a fever from getting too high. Apply cold cloths to the baby's head, chest, and extremeties between baths. See the following sections and index for specific diseases accompanied by fevers. If the fever gets too high or persists more than two hours, consult a physician.

Nervous Disorders

Some people call these conditions epilepsy, while others think they are a kind of epilepsy followed by burning fever. Still others feel that they are not truly epilepsy, but some disorder related to it.

The signs of this affliction are that the child abruptly falls down, senseless, and the feet become twisted, the eyes squinted, and foam appears in the mouth. When the child is restored to his senses, he weeps a great deal, will not take the breast or bottle, and is quite restless. The cause of this illness is an accumulation of wind, or air, in the head, such that the scalp becomes slightly enlarged and the spaces between the front teeth can be seen to widen. This may be due to the evaporation of milk in the child's stomach, from which excess air is carried via the bloodstream into the brain and affects the cells, causing a kind of simulated spastic hyperventilation. Sometimes a parent will miss the signs of the disease and call it a temper tantrum.

If there is no deterioration of the brain cells, the child recovers quickly. But if untreated, this affliction can indeed lead to full and more frequent seizures, sometimes ending in death. The sign of illness increasing is that the attacks come more frequently, one after the other, each time more violent than before. Regardless of the severity, the cause is the excess of air being carried to and filling the brain cavity. If the attacks come with less frequency and intensity, it is a sign that there is a decrease of the air and its assimilation.

The first prudent measure is to avoid eating foods that cause evaporation and spoil very easily—such as eggs—overeating, intake of air with breast or bottle, and emotional disturbance such as anger and fear. Standing in places where strong winds blow, and other extremes, should be avoided. Constipation also worsens the condition, as it blocks the natural flow-off and excretion of waste from digestion. If the condition worsens, the palms and soles should be massaged, and any influence that causes anxiety should be screened from the child. In extreme cases, the hands and arms should be bound to the sides to prevent self-injury. The foregoing should alleviate mild cases.

If the illness lingers on or becomes complicated (a plethora of phlegm is a sign of increase of illness), further measures should be taken such as increasing the child's water intake, rubbing the body with mild salves, and softening the abdomen by using suppositories or feeding laxatives. Good laxatives for this consist of decoctions extracted from boiled chickory, fish eggs, rose, jujube, senna pods, borage, or plum. This should be filtered and mixed with sweet almond oil. Warm the mixture and eat 1 teaspoonful with liquid.

Since the condition itself is brought on by what really is staleness of the mind, or entry into the brain of rotted matter, however minute, the best thing to refresh the mind is to obtain some milk from a nursing mother. Gently tilt back the head of the ill child and drop some of this fresh milk into his nose. Also, a piece of clean cloth can be soaked in the mother's milk and put on the top of the child's head like a scarf. Other efficacious means are to rub his body with flower oil and butter. These applications are useful in reducing tension. When phlegm is present in large amounts, it is important to keep the child warm. A most effective medicine for phlegm is to take $1/8$ teaspoon each of wild thyme, pennyroyal, and cumin. These should be ground and dissolved in mother's milk, shaped into pills, and eaten, one with each meal.

Honey suppositories are a useful remedy for constipation. Boiled gum of plum with sugar in lukewarm water, taken by mouth, also helps soften the bowels and produce movement. The vapor of aloeswood and saffron will cause sneezing, thereby loosening the muscles; the vapor of mustard soaked in vinegar will have the same effect. Any milk from a nursing mother used in the foregoing medicines should be pure, and her diet should also be free from foods producing gas and phlegm.

Coughing

The reflexive action of the lungs and throat known as coughing is often taken for granted as a natural effort of the system to expel foreign matter. However, whatever the underlying causes, coughing can be the precursive sign of more serious diseases in formation, and in every case disturbs the normal harmony of breathing. Breath is the bridge to life, and its frequent disturbance in childhood can upset the entire mental and physiological process of development.

Several conditions can produce coughing. The first cause is penetration of smoke (from fire, stoves, or cigarettes) into the throat. Remove the child from the source of the smoke, and give him a small amount of honey to alleviate the cough.

A second cause of coughing is dust. Shield the child from the dust, and oil the breast and throat with almond oil or violet oil. If the child is old enough to eat solid foods, he should be fed oily food and gargle with milk.

A third condition of which coughing is a symptom is dryness and coarseness of the lungs. The remedy is again rubbing the throat and breast with oil and wax and feeding a decoction of quince seeds with a little sugar. If the child is bilious, give black mulberry water or black cherry decoction. If the child is old enough to eat regular meals, the medicine should be given prior to meals. Sometimes an enema or laxative is helpful.

A fourth cause is flu. Children are especially susceptible to flu, which is generally known in its milder, natural form as a children's disease. The medication for coughing without running nose (or before the condition can be called flu) is a decoction of plum, violet, borage, or hyssop, to be given for three days.

Pills made from dried egg white ground with a little sugar and dissolved in mother's milk can be given at night. Give the child one or two small balls. In the morning, feed him a sweet paste of almonds and walnuts, and keep the chest warm by rubbing with lanolin to stop the coughing.

If there is constipation, give a few leaves of senna in a decoction, and rub the chest with almond oil.

To prevent phlegm from developing when the weather is cold, keep the child from breathing cold air, talking too much, and drinking cold water. Rub castoreum on the temples, palms, and soles of the feet, and in the nose. If there is a lot of phlegm, mix 1 tablespoon of honey in 1 cup of lukewarm water and feed it to the child. If that doesn't remove the congestion, take a dab of honey on the tip of the finger, add a dash of confectioner's sugar, and rub it on the end of the child's tongue to draw the congestion out of the chest.

It helps to expel the phlegm if it is ripe, which will happen automatically if the cause of the coughing is the phlegm. To assist expulsion of phlegm, mash a pinch of gum arabic or a dozen seeds of quince with 1 teaspoon sugar; mix with mother's milk, and feed to the child. Syrup of hyssop seed has a great effect as well. The best diet for this condition is vetch or a rice dish.

If the coughing is followed by phlegm, the child shouldn't eat foods that are dry and produce many calories, especially when there is fever. All efforts should be made to control the fever by lowering the temperature, which alone may cause the phlegm to disappear.

If the coughing and phlegm persist, place a steam vaporizer near the child in the morning. Because the nostrils are blocked by the cold air of dawn, the inside of the chest is warmed by this vapor, and thus the congested matter that is causing the flu is dissolved and the flu will disappear. Keep the head covered as much as possible.

If the coughing is followed by both phlegm and fever, give the following: quince seeds, violet flower, and borage. If you want to soften the stomach and help to promote digestion, dissolve $1/_8$ teaspoon senna pods in this mixture and feed to the child. If the child is under seven years, give 3 teaspoons; if older, a little more. Vinegar should not be consumed, nor should calorie-rich foods. To stop coughing, especially at night, grind equal parts of bitter almond, gum arabic, and clove.

CAUTION: Opium, although illegal in the West for general consumption, has found its way into some homes. It is very effective in stopping coughs, as well as relieving pain and promoting sleep and rest. However, when the person has coughing followed by phlegm and fever, opium will increase the temperature and dry and harden the phlegm, which may result in emphysema, typhoid fever, swelling of the lungs, or death. In January 1978, a young couple in Arizona gave a very small quantity of opium to their child to stem a cough and promote sleep. The child never awoke. As it is an illegal substance and the dangers inherent in its ignorant use are great, it is not recommended. Great care must be taken when giving any psychoactive or central-nervous-system agent to a child. In all cases, a doctor or experienced medical practitioner should be sought first to correctly diagnose the disease.

Measles, Chicken Pox, and Smallpox

Measles are characterized by small red boils the size of millet. Before the red spots can be seen, the skin swells in small bumps; the skin then wrinkles, and finally small boils develop on the surface of the skin. These boils contain a type of blood that is not mature or has not been properly assimilated into the blood composition. Usually, the boil dries to an outer scale which separates and falls off.

Smallpox is a disease characterized by boils as big as lentils, sometimes bigger, filled with rheum. Chicken pox is similar to smallpox but less intense. The appearance of measles or smallpox is preceded by fever, accompanied by pain in the back region, itching, scratchy nose, redness and tearing of the eyes, nightmares, burning sensation of the skin, and/or prickly feeling over the whole body. Some children are also affected by coughing, earache, emphysema, and hoarseness.

Fever in measles is milder or less hot than smallpox fever, and pain in the back, if present, is less severe than with smallpox. Also, measles appear suddenly, "breaking out" more or less at once, while smallpox and chicken pox appear over a three- to seven-day period. Measles are usually more dangerous to the life of a child, especially the worst type of measles.

A severe infection of smallpox is indicated by pox that are connected to one another and appear as one piece, or great numbers of pox on the chest and abdomen, or pox that ripen late or ooze blood. If the pox appear followed by fever or if the fever does not weaken immediately after the pox appear, both are signs of severity, especially the latter sign.

The signs of the mildest forms of measles, chicken pox, and smallpox are that the child is fully conscious, there is no change or coarseness in voice, and the appetite for food and water remains stable. The cause of these diseases is the boiling of the blood, due to the rawness and presence of phlegm that is in the nature of children. Congestion of the blood and other bodily systems results in this boiling of the blood (as evidenced by fever), and the skin boils are the signs of the completion of the boiling process. Rarely, pox or boils appear without the attendant fevering and boiling of the blood.

Prevention of Measles and Smallpox

Measles and smallpox have been controlled or eliminated (to some extent) by inoculation programs of public health authorities. However, some people do not have access to even rural health care (in the United States as well as many underdeveloped nations), so the following measures are recommended for diet and prevention of these afflictions, especially during the summer, when these diseases are prevalent.

In general, these foods, all of which increase biliousness and heat of the blood, should be avoided: milk, sweet peas, syrups, meat, and eggplant; honey, figs, dates, melons, and grapes should not be eaten by mother or baby. Instead, foods that keep children in a good mood should be given, such as juice of pomegranate, tamarind juice, and other *fresh* juices. Children should be kept from running and walking in direct sunlight for long periods, sitting close to fire, and any other activities that overexert or overheat their systems.

The best foods during summer months are cold and sour vegetables such as spinach, pumpkin, and purslane, and occasionally beef with vegetables and vinegar.

The best precaution against pox and measles, especially when outbreaks of these diseases occur, is to stop children from eating candies, dry foods, and other foods that cause high-caloric burning inside the body.

When either of these diseases appears, it is necessary also to purify the blood. This can be done by giving special diet and drinks. If the child is full of phlegm, it must be cleared out, and bad or difficult digestion should be avoided. Since smallpox has been eradicated in the United States by vaccines, only information on measles and chicken pox will be given.

The following recipes are given as the most frequently mentioned preventive medicines for measles and chicken pox:

3 teaspoons red rose
3 teaspoons magnesia
2 teaspoons sandalwood paste
2 teaspoons each chickory seeds, purslane seeds, pumpkin seeds, and lettuce seeds
1 teaspoon gum tragacanth
½ teaspoon camphor

Grind all together, then sieve and form pills with infusion of fleawort. Adults take 2 pills, children 1 pill. During the warmer summer months, cold showers sometimes prevent smallpox and measles or greatly lessen the severity if contracted.

Fevers of Measles or Chicken Pox

The fever accompanying measles or chicken pox is usually very hot. The child's mouth is bitter, the eyes are yellow, and the urine is rose- or red-colored. The remedy is first to reduce phlegm by mild laxatives; if the fever is mild, a pain reliever can be given, such as herbal tea. Some physicians forbid using medicines that make the blood cold or thick when there are measles *with no boils on the skin*. They reason that the boiling of the blood at this time is a process of nature to remove waste matter from the system. Medicines that thicken the blood, and thus slow the elimination process, are acting against the natural bodily function.

When boils do finally appear on the skin, cover the child's body with soft clothes and keep warm. The temperature of the room should be moderate. The boils will surface quickly. Burn sandalwood incense and make a slight vapor of camphor to strengthen the heart and mind, and stimulate the natural process of transfer of matter to the surface of the skin. The sign that the matter is thickened is that more boils appear on the chest and do not completely disappear after four days. The sign that the boils are blocked below the surface of the skin is that the skin is rough and very little sweat comes out.

The general condition of the child must be taken into account in treatment. For example, if the pulse and breathing are normal and there is no fainting or loss of consciousness, and if the temperature is normal and there is no blackness of the tongue, make the room a little warm. Do not give cold water, but rather lukewarm water, perhaps with a little anise water from time to time. This formula is useful: 4 teaspoons mother's milk, 4 teaspoons lentils, 3 teaspoons gum arabic. Mix all together and boil until half remains. Give a teaspoonful every few hours. The medicine is more efficacious if you add 2 teaspoons rose water, a few ground figs, and 2 teaspoons anise to the mixture. An alternative: boil a few figs and add a pinch of saffron. You can put a hot-water bottle under the child's blanket to vaporize and open the pores. The child's head should not be under the blanket, for if the vapor goes into his nose, it will cause itching and restlessness.

When the boils have appeared completely, the child should be given cold juices, as much as is readily accepted. Special attention should be paid to the condition of the stomach and bowels. When the boils have completely come out, protection of the eyes, nose, throat, lungs, and intestines is necessary. If boils are appearing in these areas, they will be slight and light in color.

Protection of the Eyes

Put a drop of the following mixture in each eye: sumac soaked in rose water, three times daily. Another good mixture is water of fresh coriander seeds, with seeds of sour pomegranate, and rose water in equal parts; put these drops in the child's eyes. Both medicines have the same effect. If the eyes are swollen, put a bandage over them after using the medicine to cure the swelling. If the child becomes very nervous or restless, untie and remove the bandage from time to time.

Care of the Nose

Drops of vinegar with rose water or flower oil with a little camphor should be rubbed up inside the nose. Apply cold compresses over the nose area. If the blood coming out of the nose is blackish and the child will not sleep and has severe coughing, the illness is severe and medical aid should be sought at once.

Care of the Throat

When the boils appear on the surface of the skin, or even during the preceding time of fever, it is good to give pomegranate (this should not be given to children under two years old). The child should chew the seeds and swallow the juice. Three useful gargles:

• a decoction of sumac, red clover blossoms, and lentils boiled in rose water
• iced water mixed with rose water
• black cherry juice

Care of the Lungs

When boils appear, if there is no hoarseness in the throat, take the temperature and check whether the bowels are moving fast or slow. If the temperature is high and the bowels are sluggish, give water of quince and fleawort with sugar in small doses, and put ground almond in the child's mouth. Licking this medicine can be tried if the child won't take it into the mouth. If, in spite of the temperature, the bowels remain loose, take gum arabic, almonds, pumpkin seeds, and seeds of cucumber (1 teaspoon each) and fry each one separately; then grind them together and fry in an infusion of fleawort. Let the child lick this medicine. If the temperature is not high and the bowels are not soft, give fresh butter with sugar, gradually and in small doses.

Care of the Joints

For sore joints and boils, grind sandalwood, clay, and red clover blossoms with a little camphor, add a little rose water and vinegar, and rub onto joints. If a boil appears and opens by itself, no further treatment is necessary. If it doesn't open, a doctor may have to pierce the boil to let out the rheum.

Care of the Intestines

Sometimes, although the boils of measles seem to be drying and clearing, their remnants are left under the skin and transferred to the intestines, spreading the infection there. To avoid this complication, give the child a syrup of myrtle, pills of magnesia, and quince juice, at the time the boils seem to be drying. Care of the intestines is very important at this time.

When the boils have completely appeared, cold juices should be given, and constipation and looseness of bowels regulated. Do not give any laxatives at this time. If the stomach is loosening on its own, do not give anything that will block the bowels too quickly.

Diet

Generally, children affected with measles should be given cold and dry foods, such as barley composite, which can be prepared as follows: Take one pound of barley, split the corns into halves, grind, and remove skins after one hour. Then fry the remaining split barley, put through a sieve, and add lentils and juice of sour pomegranate or green grapes.

If the child's bowels are not soft or loose and there is a feeling of coarseness in the chest and throat but no temperature elevation, give the above mixture with sugar syrup, but do not make it too sweet. Never feed sour foods if the bowels are constipated.

If the bowels are loose, the temperature is high, and the chest and throat are coarse, fry the above composition; cool and refry several times, and mix with magnesia. If there is severe diarrhea, give water of fried barley and 1 teaspoon pomegranate in equal parts.

Severe symptoms of measles indicate that the internal temperature is too high, which leads to burning of the blood and biliousness. Everything given should be cold and juicy, like the water of boiled barley. Vinegar can be added to the barley if there is no coughing. If there is coughing, give purslane, melon water, pumpkin water, and similar foods, but these should not be given with vinegar.

Section 2

The Head

General Considerations

Every physician knows that if the subject of disease is looked into deeply enough, every ailment can be said to have originated in the mind. Dr. Lewis Thomas, former president of the Memorial Sloan-Kettering Cancer Center in New York City, has suggested that despite the astounding advancements in removing most of the plagues of humanity, such as tuberculosis, smallpox, poliomyelitis, and other scourges of humanity, people are today more fearful about their health than ever before. He claims that the majority of people who go to a doctor's office have nothing organically wrong with them. The problem is rather that 75 percent of the people visit the doctor because they are fundamentally unhappy. What does this say about us and the times we live in?

Despite the tremendous research applied to all areas of human knowledge, the human mind cannot be fathomed, even in a small way. There are no medical methods known to control with consistent accuracy the focusing of the mind on negative aspects of life. No doubt, the sixty million legitimate prescriptions for Valium and the tens of millions of other drugs given to raise the threshold of anxiety are mute testimony to the complete failure of modern science—and medicine—to deal with the underlying true causes of human illness.

To the great healers of the past and present who truly understand human health, there is only one way to assure a stable mind, and that is by gaining contact with and discovering the full magnificence of one's immortal Being. It is immaterial what name or term is applied to this phenomenon. It is real and often accounts for spontaneous cures of the most baffling diseases.

There are probably as many paths to such awareness as there are people, and it is vital that people acknowledge this reality as something more important than any other aspect of their daily lives. Meditation, yoga, breathing exercises, shiatsu and other massage techniques, Rolfing, body balancing, and hundreds of alternative modalities of health building are really efforts to silence and harmonize the "outer" person so that the mind can be brought into balance. Violence, fear, worry, avarice, and sirens throughout the night can easily be called to task as causative agents for much of the disease produced by irregularity of living habits. All of the recognized prophetic religions of the world contain programs of organized study and application of the divine principles of fit conduct of human life on earth, and, as such, are worthy of the most intelligent and careful study. Mahatma Gandhi once wrote that the essence of all the religions of man could be summed up in these words: "Live and let live."

This is the vital prescription and message of our time for the relief of suffering humanity.

2.1   Headache

Headaches are often caused by eyestrain, stress, or the obnoxious noises of city life. Resting in a darkened room and drinking a cup of chamomile, valerian root, or peppermint tea often relieve a simple headache.

Headaches are also caused by unbalanced humors. Check for signs of a dominant humor. If the cause of headache is inharmony of the blood humor, cupping on the back of the head is useful. After cupping, give sour lemon. If the cause is biliousness, take an enema and add to the formula sandalwood and coriander, about 3 teaspoons each. If the cause is phlegm, use the phlegm adjustor, followed by boiled anise seeds mixed with honey, which should be rubbed on the neck and shoulders. If the cause is black bile, adjust by giving a black bile purgative and massage the neck and shoulders with sweet almond oil.

Washing of the feet and foot massage are the best method for every kind of

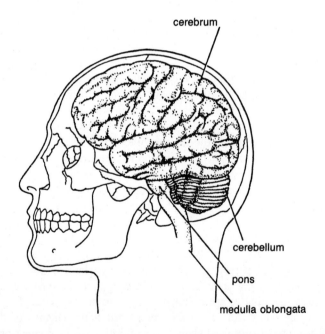

Brain and Head

headache. Do not rub the head. Although this will produce immediate relief, its long-term effect is negative. It is always better to use foot massage.

2.2 Headache Caused by Heat or Cold Intemperament without Prevalence of Phlegm

If caused by heat, give foods from the list of "cold" foods. If caused by cold, do the opposite. If the headache is linked with fever, cure the fever first. If the headache occurs on one side of the head and not the other, this formula is useful: 1 teaspoon gum arabic, ½ teaspoon cannabis sativa, ¼ teaspoon saffron. Mix these with the white of an egg or rose water. Spread this on a piece of plain paper and stick to the temple of the affected side. It is especially useful if placed on a throbbing blood vessel.

2.3 Use of Cannabis Sativa and Narcotics for Headache

It is not at all recommended to use marijuana for recreational purposes or as a regular part of one's regimen. Ill effects are quite well known in cultures that have a history of centuries of consumption by the populace. In a few cases, since it is available and legal in some areas, it is recommended in the minute doses noted, as the method of choice as opposed to using a more potent drug.

If this or other narcotic drugs are to be used in any case at all, side effects can be minimized by taking a small amount of saffron along with it (note formula in 2.2). Some also recommend bathing the head with rose water; it should be applied copiously to wet the entire head. Headache followed by nosebleed is a sign of a healing crisis.

2.4 Delirium

Delirium is swelling of the membranes of the head, either from viruses or bacteria in the brain. If the cause is imbalance of the blood humor, the person is happy or giddy. If it is due to biliousness, there is ill-temper and constant frowning. If due to phlegm humor imbalance, the person is perplexed and weak; if due to black bile, the person is manic and wild (this happens very rarely). Furthermore, if the cause is blood humor, the temperature is often quite high. The delirium caused by yellow or black bile will cause raving. In all forms, the senses are not sharp. Valerian root as a tea is helpful to calm the person. Adjust the proper humor according to the signs. Cupping the lower legs is advised as well; also a massage of the legs to absorb gas. If the cause is bacterial or viral, medical treatment is necessary.

2.5 False Delirium

Raving and talking nonsense sometimes happen without swelling of the brain membranes, as when the person is feverish. This condition is called false delirium. Treatment is treating the cause, as false delirium does not occur alone. Check the other signs and refer to appropriate section.

2.6   Stiffness

This condition comes on suddenly, and the person becomes motionless. Black bile is the cause, bringing obstruction to the lower section of the brain. The person is senseless and should be given a hot suppository or enema of 2 teaspoons lobelia in 1 quart water. If the person cannot be roused, a few drops of tincture of lobelia taken orally will usually suffice to bring him to his senses. When the senses are restored, give a black bile purgative, hot drinks and food, and rub the back of the head with a preparation of almond and ginger oils. If castoreum can be added, it is better.

2.7   Heart Failure

The signs of this are similar to stiffness, but in addition to the person being motionless and senseless, there is no breathing. The person falls down like a dead body. A complete obstruction of the brain causes this. Rubbing the feet and hands, especially the left hand, at the juncture of the thumb and palm on the beefy part, should be done with great force. Cardiac massage should be begun and an ambulance called. If it is caused by prevalence of blood, some must be let out. Otherwise, an enema and suppository should be given to take out phlegm. Vomiting is a good sign. If there is no breathing at all and no pulse, recovery is improbable. The difference between a heart failure and a fatal condition is that in simple heart failure, you can see a reflection of yourself in the person's eyes, but in a fatal condition, you cannot. In rural settings, with no help available, it is recommended that even though the person may look dead, he should not be buried for seventy hours, because cases of spontaneous recovery have been recorded. If a mirror held to the lips shows no frosting, the person has turned blue, and the stomach is swollen, death is certain.

2.8   Lethargy

This is like a very heavy, unnatural sleep. Its cause is the prevalence of moisture in the brain, brought on either by phlegm or by blood. The remedy is to adjust the humor and use an enema. Make the person smell vinegar and feed him only light, easily digested foods. Another cause of lethargy is stomach gas. Clean the stomach by making this mixture: 5 teaspoons crushed fennel seed, 5 teaspoons powdered ginger, and enough honey to make a thick paste. Take 1 teaspoon with tea at each meal. Follow with a chickory-root enema. Use coriander as a spice in as many meals as possible.

2.9   Sleeplessness

The cause of sleeplessness is prevalence of dryness in the brain. It can come from imbalance of black or yellow bile or phlegm humor. Give an enema. Don't allow vinegar vapor to be inhaled, and avoid vinegar in foods, for it will increase sleeplessness. Put common dill under the pillow before sleep. Sweet basil in rose water can be smelled, too. Valerian root tea is also very effective, as is rubbing the neck with violet oil.

2.10 Lethargy and Sleeplessness

This combination of conditions is caused by a kind of brain swelling due to biliousness and phlegm, according to most healers. The signs are lengthy sleep, tiredness, or sometimes inability to sleep at all. If it is caused by swelling of the brain, the person will be wide-eyed and talking nonsense. The remedy is to combine the formulas given in sections 2.8 and 2.9 for the single signs of lethargy and sleeplessness. If there is much phlegm, use hot herbs; if biliousness is prevalent, give cold herbs.

2.11 Nightmares

The person imagines during sleep that some heavy object has fallen on him, or someone is chasing him, or some catastrophe is occurring. Therefore, shortness of breath is felt, and often a change in the tone of the voice. Cupping on the cephalic veins and on the legs, light eating before retiring, and enemas are all recommended.

2.12 Epilepsy

The person falls down completely senseless and has seizures, causing the limbs to assume contorted shapes. There is much restlessness and a feeling of heaviness in the head, and the veins under the tongue turn a greenish hue. This occurs spontaneously from time to time; if frequent enough, it can be fatal. Sometimes, with children, it will occur seven or eight times in one day and never return. Something soft but firm, like a piece of wood wrapped with cloth, should be inserted in the mouth to prevent self-injury from choking on the tongue. When the seizure is over, give an enema. Do not give fresh fruit or goat milk, but instead allow the person to smell aloeswood incense or hang a piece of aloeswood around his neck.

2.13 Epilepsy in Children

This condition is sometimes called hydrocephalus, and even children's gas or colic when the attack is mild. Children should not be carried too much or kept excessively warm or cold. Most healers recommend that nursing mothers avoid sexual intercourse until the signs pass, as it is felt this spoils the mother's milk and affects the child's brain. If the child is constipated, give him a suppository, as it has an immediate effect.

2.14 Melancholy

This is an imbalance that prevents a person from thinking soundly and often leads to acting foolish, excessive loving, or sometimes to libertinism and great vanity. It is caused by an imbalance of the phlegm humor. Use an enema at waking and at bedtime. Eat only soft foods. Sexual intercourse has a remarkable effect in removing melancholy.

2.15   Madness

There are several kinds of madness. If it comes with anger and annoyance, it is called mania. If it comes with laughing, teasing, and annoying others, it is called "dog's disease." If it comes with frowning and being afraid of people it is called chorea. Some say madness is a kind of advanced melancholy, but it is not, for one of the factors of true madness is the burning of unnatural (corrupted) phlegm. Burning of natural phlegm causes melancholy, not madness. Adjust for phlegm humor inharmony. Pour mother's milk over the head and into the nostrils. Rub the body with violet and almond oils, and take frequent warm baths.

2.16   Vertigo and Giddiness

When someone stands up or moves abruptly and a "darkness" comes over the eyes, it is called giddiness. When the person feels everything turning around him, it is called vertigo. The remedy is to take an emetic and vomit. The cause is either in the brain or in the stomach. In either case, vomiting corrects it. Give 1 teaspoon lobelia tincture every ten minutes until the effect is achieved. Lemon juice, sandalwood tea, and pomegranate juice are helpful to avoid this condition. If there is frequent vertigo, do not let the person become cold, and give hot foods.

2.17   Forgetfulness

The cause of forgetfulness is an excess of phlegm and its effect on the brain. Hot temperature causes forgetfulness, too. Remedy: give a chickory-root enema. Small amounts of tea made of ⅓ teaspoon each of frankincense, sugar, and ginger are useful. Avoid cold water.

2.18   Paralysis

In this imbalance, half of the body becomes senseless and motionless. The cause of this is usually an excess of moisture in the phlegm humor, but sometimes imbalance in the blood humor can also be the cause. The cause of paralysis is swelling of the nerve endings. (If only one limb is affected, it is called slackness.) Do not give strong foods or herbs for four days. A light soup with cumin and cinnamon is good. After the fourth day, give the formula that ripens phlegm. Beneficial foods are pea water, clove, cinnamon, and black pepper. The phlegm will ripen from the ninth to the fourteenth day, at which time a purgative for phlegm should be given. After this, use an enema and lubricate the body with olive oil. If the temperature is high, lower it. Never give hot medicine.

It should be noted that this kind of paralysis is not the same as that caused by viral infection from poliomyelitis. The only known treatment for the latter is large doses of organic iodine, as reported by J. F. Edward, M.D., in *The Manitoba Medical Review* (vol. 34, no. 6, June-July 1954, pp. 337-339). NOTE: A young man in Arizona died from poliomyelitis in 1977, after contracting an active case from his three-month-old daughter, who had been given a vaccine for polio. While the origin of his case has not been conclusively proved, it is possible and probable that this was the cause. Since polio has been nearly eradicated in the United States through use of the vaccine, most physicians under forty years of age have never seen a case. Whenever there is total paralysis and swelling of the thyroid glands, polio may be suspected. There is an urgent need for medical assistance if this is the case.

2.19 Weakness of the Limbs

A feeling of numbness or loss of sensation in a limb can be caused by either blood or phlegm imbalance. Adjust the proper humor and fast moderately for several days.

2.20 Paralysis of the Face

This happens when a part of the face is weakened. The signs are displeasure of the senses (corrupted sense of smell and the like) and a lack of appetite. Convulsions may appear if there is a stretching of the skin of the forehead and cessation of saliva and dryness in the mouth.

If there are no convulsions, start treatment four to seven days after the signs appear in the face. Eliminate as much food and as many liquids as possible. Put the person in a dark room, with a mirror so that he can see himself. Have the person chew on a bit of nutmeg. It is said that if the paralysis of the face persists for longer than three months, it cannot be reversed.

2.21 Convulsions

There are two kinds of convulsion: moist and dry. There is excretion of phlegm in moist convulsions, and the onset is sudden. Dry convulsions come on gradually and there is excessive vomiting, sleeplessness, and depression. There may be weight loss.

The preparation for moist convulsion is the same as for ripening of phlegm. For dry convulsion, mix equal parts of violet herb and almond oil and massage the body, and have the person gargle with mother's milk.

Convulsions can also be caused by stings of scorpion and other insects, by a wound to the head or other part of the body, and by intestinal worms. Fight the poison, cure the wound, or expel the worm. In a city, any of these would be treated at a hospital emergency room facility or by a physician.

Epilepsy can also cause convulsions, as discussed in 2.12. There is another kind of convulsion that occurs just after yawning and affects primarily the lower jaw and face. In this case, rub the body with warm flower oils.

2.22 Muscular Tension

There are so many sources of tension that it would be impossible to list them all in one book. The main cause of them all is that a nerve is pulled at from both sides, due to muscle spasm affecting a part of the body. The remedy is to discover where the spasm is located and apply constant direct pressure upon the place with the thumb and first three fingers bunched together. Apply steady pressure for twenty seconds, release for five seconds, and repeat until the spasm subsides. Follow with a massage with warm rose oil, accompanied by soothing music and a hot bath for ten minutes. Valerian root tea is specific for muscular tension.

2.23 Dystaxia

Dystaxia is the trembling of a limb. If the cause is phlegm, the signs are forgetfulness and the other signs of an imbalance of phlegm humor. The remedy is to use an enema. Excessive sexual intercourse can also cause spontaneous trembling of the legs and arms. If this is the case, drinking fresh goat's milk and rubbing the body with warm rose oil and eating lightly fried eggs are recommended.

2.24 Nictitation

This is the continuous blinking of the eyes. The remedy is to warm salt and apply it as a plaster to the affected part. If it is not relieved, balance phlegm humor. Suppression of the menses can also cause this, in which case an emmenagogue is recommended (see 17.1) and also cupping on the pubis.

2.25 Heaviness

In this condition, the person feels heavy all over and the eyelids may droop. The upper lids become red. There is frequent yawning and restlessness as before a fever, but no fever appears. The condition comes and goes. The preparation for balancing the blood and yellow bile humors should be given; allow some food even if the signs return. Chickory seeds with a little sugar are useful.

2.26 Nose Itching

The sign of this is itching in the nose but no pain. Give the person cold things to eat. The cause is found in biliousness, so give a biliousness purgative. If there is excess of blood, signaled by flushed face, nosebleed, or excessive heat, adjust the blood.

2.27 Eyebrow Pain

This is often caused by excess internal heat, in which case the pain commences at sunrise, along with fever, which continues until noon. It then gradually dies down until no sign is left throughout the night, but it starts up again in the morning. Dissolve 3 grains of camphor in flower oil and drop it in the nose, but do not inhale it into the nasal passages. Apply cupping on the cephalic vein on the side of the pain.

Section 3

The Eye

General Considerations

To understand the function of the eye in terms of natural medicine, we must understand that it is the main receptacle of light in the body. It is related most closely with the lungs, as light is converted by plants into oxygen through photosynthesis, which is then breathed in by humans and other animals to sustain life. The direct rays of the sun, then, are the essence of life in that they are the pure form of oxygen.

Most often, little thought is given to how we use the eyes. First of all, we should endeavor to "see no evil," for if we accept that the mind originates much disease, looking upon harmful things is just like pouring sludge into the mind. Furthermore, at least once per day, one should rest the eyes. This is done by placing the palms of the hands tightly over the eyes, yet not so close as to cause much pressure. The object is to block out all light. Sit forward in a chair with the elbows on the knees, and rest the head in the palms of the hands. Remain in this position for twenty seconds, take the palms away for a few seconds, then repeat. Continue this for two minutes in the evening, to allow time for the eyes to regenerate their inherent strength.

As with all of the self-regulating organs, the eyes work nearly all the time without respite. The eyes are used in ways we are not aware of. For instance, in driving down the road, we pay attention to the many signs of traffic, looking out for other drivers, and so forth. But we also look at all of the many advertising signs, and things in the sky, and often over at other passengers. An advertising trade journal reported that the average person views 1,200 such advertising messages each day! The mystics of the East sometimes seclude themselves for extended periods in darkness for the purpose of training the eyes to be under better control. We should all endeavor to have as much conscious control over what we look at as possible, for the same reason.

For the purposes of natural medicine, the eye is divided into parts consisting of seven layers, three moist vacuums, and one hollow nerve, which is the receptacle for light. That portion which makes contact with the air and which can be touched is called the flesh layer and cornea. Under the cornea and flesh layer is the *original layer*, which is colored (in the normal eye, either blue or brown). In the middle of this is the "hole" that is the intake valve for light (*iris*). Behind the original layer is the *ball of moisture*. After the ball layer is the *spider layer*. After this, there is a layer called *solid moisture*, and finally the *crystalline layer*. After these layers there is the *retina*, then the *choroid coat*, and finally the *sclerotic*

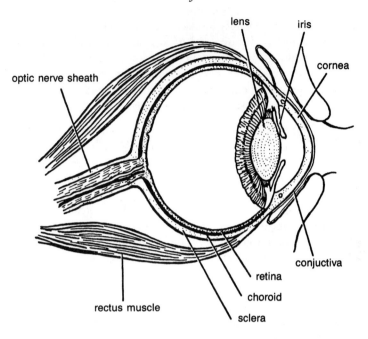

The Eye

coat. These approximate the usual anatomical terms for the eye used in Western medicine, but we will use the terminology above in this section.

Iridology

There has appeared in the past century a science of diagnosing states of health by looking at the eye, called iridology. A comprehensive study manual for iridology is Bernard Jensen's *Science and Practice of Iridology*, published by Dr. Jensen (D.C.), Route 1, Box 52, Escondido, CA 92025. Some medical doctors and many alternative health practitioners use this tool as a guide for looking inside the body without using surgery. It cannot determine *what* is wrong but in most cases can tell *where* the problem is located and how far the condition has progressed.

3.1 Swelling of the Flesh Layer

If the cause is with the blood humor, the signs are that the eye is red, heavy, and painful and much secretion is noticed. If the cause is yellow bile, the signs are much burning and pain, but little or no secretion. With phlegm humor imbalance, the signs are swelling and a great quantity of excretion. If the cause is black bile, there is no swelling and no excretion, but the eyelids cannot close

and touch each other and there is headache. If the cause is gas, there is no
heaviness and no excretion. The remedy in each case is an enema and detoxification. Never drop any medicine into the eyes without consulting a physician
first. Purgatives are advised for the appropriate humor, and an enema, followed
by bathing the eyes with mother's milk. Meat should be avoided, as should any
boil-producing foods that are known to the person.

3.2   Appearance of Bloody Spot in Conjunctiva

Consult an eye specialist.

3.3   Pterygium

This is an inflammation of the wing or side of the bone of the nose, in line
with the eye. Make a poultice of sea salt and apply to the affected place several
times a day. Burn frankincense and allow the smoke to reach the eyes. Avoid
phlegm-producing foods. A physician should be consulted as soon as possible.

3.4   White Spot in the Black Part

A white dot appearing in the black part, or diaphragm, of the eye should be
treated by washing with sea water (an infusion of nigari is an acceptable substitute). Using this procedure several times should remove the spot. If it remains,
the brain needs to be cleared by taking a chickory-root enema for that purpose.

3.5   Swelling and Redness of Veins

If the eyes are red and swollen and there is copious tearing, and even the
eyelids are wet, it is called wet pannus. If there is no wetness, it is called dry
pannus. In both cases, relieve by enema. If there is only very slight redness of
the veins, use the "golden suppository" composed of 3 parts tumeric, and one-
half part each of aloe vera juice and rainwater, in a cacao base. Take a tub bath
before and after application to the eyes. If there is swelling accompanying the
redness, do not eat hot foods or herbs—use cold ones. Cupping may be done
on the forehead and cephalic veins.

3.6   Conjunctivitis

The difference between swelling and conjunctivitis is that the nature of swelling affects the whole eye (due to excess fluid and the like), whereas conjunctivitis affects the parts of the eye or skin. Conjunctivitis can be caused by gas,
in which case the inflammation comes on suddenly. First a burning is felt on
the corner of the eye, like the burning one feels when bitten by a mosquito or
fly. If the cause is phlegm, the onset is more gradual and there is little or no
pain. The remedy is to use a phlegm purgative. If the cause is gas, nothing is
necessary, as it will disappear by itself after three or four days.

3.7   Itching of Conjunctivitis

Itching accompanies conjunctivitis when the eyelids become red and sore. Salty and hot foods should be avoided. In addition to a phlegm purgative, if indicated, the eyelids should be rubbed very lightly with olive oil and the face and eyes washed every hour or so with warm water.

3.8   Hard Boil (Sty) in the Corner of the Eye

Such knobby boils sometimes appear in the corner of the eye. Their removal can be assisted by using a phlegm purgative. As it softens, apply rose water as a wash.

3.9   Excessive Tearing

Excretion of tears is a normal bodily function, to remove foreign objects as well as an expression of human emotion of sadness or exalted joy. It is also the means to expel various superfluities that accumulate internally. What is spoken of here is tearing when none of the above causes is present. It is usually caused by overheating of the body, which can be corrected by rubbing with collyrium. If the cause is coldness, use lobelia infusion as an eyewash. It is sometimes also caused by weakness of the eye muscles. In this case, use exercises to strengthen the muscles. If there is unexplained tearing which stops after a few moments, it means that superfluities are trying to escape. Use a purgative and expose the eyes to vapors of fresh onion.

3.10   Burning of the Eyes

A burning sensation in the eyes is also caused by excess heat of a part or organ of the body. Use a purgative. Pound fresh chickory, add safflower oil to it, and use as an ointment on the eyes.

3.11   Foreign Object in the Eye

If there is something in the eye, never rub it; it may be forced into the eye and damage it. The best procedure is to wash the eye with warm water and pour mother's milk in as an eyewash. If the object that has fallen into the eye can be seen, use a piece of cotton twirled into a point to capture it. If it is an insect stuck in the eye, remove in the same way. If there is glass or metal or any object that cannot be identified in the eye, go to a doctor for removal with instruments appropriate for this purpose. After the object is removed, pour in mother's milk and add some white of egg to help soothe any damage.

3.12   Injuries to the Eye by Force

When the eye is hit and becomes swollen and red, the remedy is to boil fresh fruits like apricot, plum, or tamarind together for fifteen minutes, leave overnight, then filter in the morning and give to the injured person. Cup behind the head on the side of the injured eye. Afterward use a purgative, and put an ointment made of whole shirred egg and rose oil on the eye. This should remove the pain. If bruising is present, put egg yolk with coriander on the eye to speed recovery. Following any injury to the eye, an examination should be made to make certain that undetected damage has not occurred.

3.13   Ulcer of the Eye

An ulcer may appear on any layer of the eye. The least dangerous place is in the conjunctiva. Conjunctival and corneal ulcers can be seen. Other ulcers occurring in the deeper layers cannot be seen, but cause severe pain. In time they may grow through the various layers and appear on the surface layer. Cupping should be applied on the cephalic vein at the beginning of each week. If there is pain, a few drops of mother's milk will soothe. The ulcer must "ripen" to heal. Wash it with rose water to hasten the ripening, and afterward mix mother's milk with honey and apply as a salve. Then use a suppository of frankincense.

3.14   Heaviness of Eyelid

This can be caused by gas, which is known by a feeling of sand in the eyes after waking up. Wash with juice of fenugreek. If this doesn't work, do not rub the eyes too much as they may be injured. If there is no relief, apply the phlegm purgative for conjunctivitis as given in section 3.6.

3.15   Nyctalopia (Night Blindness)

The inability to see after sunset is often caused by prolonged exposure to a strong bright light. Apply honey with water of anise seed to the eyes. If it is severe, use a purgative and cupping.

3.16   Hemeralopia (Day Blindness)

The cause of day blindness is uncertain. Effective diet includes leg of lamb, beef brains, and unleavened bread. Massage the scalp with mother's milk and wash the eyes with cold water.

3.17   Eye Ache

A person feels a kind of beating deep in the eye that may extend outward toward the temples, and there is a slight prickling sensation. The pain is intermittent. Massage or apply cupping between the eye and the ear to stop this sensation.

3.18   Bulging Eyes

Projection of the eyes without swelling can be relieved by taking an enema, using a purgative, cupping, and applying honey over the eye as a salve. The diet should be restricted to smaller quantities of food until the eyes return to normal.

3.19 Projection of Cornea

This is caused by imbalance of both the phlegm and bile systems, so adjust for these both. Wash the eyes with warm water.

3.20 Ulcers of the Cornea

Since the cornea has four layers, ulcers may sometimes appear in any of them, sometimes in all. The remedy is to use purgatives and follow with the frankincense suppository.

3.21 Double Vision or Diplopia

If a person is born with this affliction, it usually cannot be cured. If it develops in childhood or later on, the causes may be epilepsy, sleeping on one side of the head, or extreme fright by loud noises. For children, it is recommended to hang down some bright red object on alternating sides of the head. (For a baby in a crib, suspend the object from the sides. For older children, have them sit in a chair for 5 minutes several times a day, with the object at the edge of their field of vision.) In the case of the elderly, the cause is excess dryness. Dryness is always a sign of hot ailments, and the remedy is to consume a fruit diet and mother's milk. If the cause is slackness of the muscles of the eyeball, exercises must be done to strengthen them.

3.22 Dilation of the Eyes

Dilation is widening of the pupil, whether of the hollow nerve itself or the pupil. Another condition, called spreading, is the scattering of light in various parts of the eye, which is definitely a trouble of the nerve, not the pupil. When there is a widening of the hollow nerve, the pupil will usually widen, giving the impression of a dilated pupil. This is difficult to remedy, but mere widening of the pupil aperture can be cured, depending on the cause. A blow to the head should be treated the same as any injury to the eye. Excess phlegm can also cause dilation, in which case, use a chickory-root enema. If it is due to excess wetness in the eyeball, which happens mostly with boys, or swelling of the flesh layer, use a purgative. If the cause is dryness of the eye, the eye muscles must be strengthened the same as for poor vision.

3.23 Constriction of the Pupil

If the pupil contracts for no functional reason, the cause must be determined; it can be from excess wetness or dryness or a defect of the eyeball. Wetness and dryness can both be observed. A defect of the eyeball is apparent when there is an actual reduction in its size. The remedy for wetness and dryness is to massage the scalp with mother's milk and drop olive oil into each nostril (3 drops each side). If there is an excess of wetness, a purgative should be taken.

3.24 Imaginary Visions

This means the imagination of forms and figures, insects, and such. There are three stages to this problem. The first stage is prior to tears coming from the eyes. The second is appearance of stomach gas and wetness of the eye. The third stage is sharpness of the sense of vision. The clue to the onset of this condition is the appearance of more and more tearing in the eyes each day. When the imaginary visions become excessive, the stage of stomach gas has arrived. The clue that corruption of the layers and wetness of the eye has occurred is that the iris takes on different colors. The appearance of the third stage is accompanied by loss of health of vision and mind. This is not, in fact, a disease, as the vision actually becomes sharper as the stages progress. The person may actually "see" particles of gas ascending from his stomach and being scattered in the air. Because the person sees things that are not supposed to be there, he becomes totally confused. Sheep's brain and leg of lamb are recommended, along with detoxification of the system.

3.25 Glaucoma

This is a kind of wetness that enters from above in the head, suddenly or gradually, and stops in the pupil of the eye, and over time completely obscures vision. When the wetness thickens in the eye, it completely fills the hole for vision, and blindness occurs. If the wetness is thin, there may be some vision for color or form. The sign that it is glaucoma is that the pupil actually changes and vision is corrupted.

The only remedy mentioned by Hakims for glaucoma involves cauterization, and since there are few practitioners of this, it would be difficult to locate a physician competent to perform such surgical procedure.

It should be known that there are several kinds of glaucoma, called cloudy, blue, glassy, green, white, yellow and red, gold, black, and scattered lightly. None of these is recoverable with natural medicine, except the white kind.

Western medicine has, to my knowledge, no cure for glaucoma, although there are drugs which can arrest its development if the condition is discovered and treated soon enough. My judgement is that Western medicine would be the treatment of choice in glaucoma. Wetness and overheating of the eyes occurs more in black, brown, and dark eyes, thus glaucoma appears more frequently in persons with dark eyes.

3.26 Change in Eye Color

According to the science of iridology, there are only two true eye colors at birth, blue and brown. The eye contains delicate and sensitive nerves that pick up changes occurring in the body and reflect these in the eye. Drugs taken but not eliminated can cause a golden-brownish discoloration. The eye must be checked under magnification to see what the normal eye color actually is.

3.27   Poor Vision

The cause may be excess of blood or phlegm. For excess of blood, balance the blood humor, use cupping, and take a purgative. Use rose water as an eyewash. For phlegm, use a phlegm purgative and apply kohl (antimony sulfate) to the lower rims of the eyelids. Poor vision can also result from lack of natural heat, a usual condition of declining age. There is no cure for this circumstance, but kohl may be used on the eyelids. Eyestrain and certain diseases may affect vision. Consult an eye specialist.

3.28   Loss of Sight after Extended Darkness

If the cause is sudden emergence from a dark place, cover the eyes with a blue veil and avoid looking at sunshine until the eyes regain their ability to function normally.

3.29   Weak Day Sight

A few people are born with ultrasensitive eyes and cannot look at light. They usually cannot be cured of this condition and must adjust to it by wearing sunglasses. Rubbing the eyes with smoke from ignited oil of violets is recommended to strengthen the eyelids and eye.

3.30   Snow Blindness

This is caused by looking for too long a time at sun reflected upon snow. The remedy is to hang black purslane from the person's neck and have him cast down his eyes at it. In addition, the room where he stays should have dark or very subdued light, dark carpets, and so forth. Pour mother's milk in the person's eyes. It is also very effective to put pounded bitter almond or apricot kernels on the eyelids as a poultice.

3.31   Feeling of Sand in the Eyes upon Waking

Though this feeling will go away on its own, the eyes should be cleaned with warm water, followed by a shower or warm bath. See also 3.14.

3.32   Slackness of Eyelids

Clean the eyelids with warm water, then apply juice of aloe vera as a salve. If the problem persists, the only remedy is corrective plastic surgery.

3.33   Eyelids Sticking Together

This occurs sometimes when there is excessive excretion from the eyes, as during allergy seasons. Pull the eyelids apart carefully, using warm water to help dissolve the mucus. If they have stuck to the eyeball, use great care in pulling the eyelids away and separating them. After that, take a ½ teaspoon cumin and ½ teaspoon of salt in ½ cup of water; soak a ball of cotton in this solution and apply to the eyelids for ten minutes. At night, rub rose oil on the lids.

3.34   Excess Skin Flap Growing on Eyelid

When small bits of skin appear spontaneously, the eyelids may actually thicken. It causes the eyes to be wet all the time from the excess weight bearing upon the eyeball surface. Use purgatives and dress the eye as in 3.33. If this does no good, go on a detoxification diet.

3.35   Growth of Extra Eyelashes

There is no particular danger from the growth of excess eyelashes. They can be plucked out. To help keep them from turning in and irritating the eye, make the lashes straight and firm with honey to keep them from pricking the eye. A physician can probably cauterize the roots of a few excess hairs to stop them from growing back as a last resort.

3.36   Shedding of Eyelashes

The cause is usually food putrefying in the stomach. Use a stomach purgative to take out excess phlegm, which is sure to be present. A fruit diet is recommended until the shedding stops. The cause may also be a lack of nutrients reaching the area, in which case foods rich in niacin along with rigorous exercise should be the program.

3.37   Whitening of Eyelashes

Use a purgative, and afterward take leaves of wild tulips, bruise them in olive oil, and apply to lashes.

3.38   Mange of Eyelids

Only diet will help here. Use a purgative first, then employ detoxification diet, emphasizing foods of a cold nature.

3.39   Excessive Perspiration of Eyelids

The pores of the eyelid need to be opened. Make them soft with olive oil, then use rose water eyewash.

3.40   Hardening of the Eyelids

This is caused by excess bile, which causes difficulty in opening and closing the lids. Use the biliousness purgative and keep the eyelids soft with olive oil.

3.41 Swelling of the Eye

Swellings of the eye that are not due to any of the foregoing may respond to a fruit-juice diet. Along with this, soak a few leaves of sumac in ½ pint of rose water and use as eye drops during the day. At night, prepare a salve of purslane and chickory with rose oil. Cupping and purgatives are also useful.

3.42 Ulcers of Eyelids

Boil the skin of a large pomegranate along with the inner skins from about two dozen pistachio nuts, and add to ¼ cup lentils that have been soaked in vinegar for several hours. Make a salve of this and apply to the eye until the ulcer subsides. Then put yolk of egg with a grain of saffron on the ulcer.

3.43 Swelling of Eyelids

The eyelids alone will swell when there is weakness of the intestine. The cause is almost invariably excess of phlegm, so use a phlegm purgative, follow with the detoxification diet, and use colonic irrigation if needed.

3.44 Boil on the Eyelid

Balance the yellow bile humor. Apply Bentonite (a diatomaceous earth preparation sold in most health food stores) to the affected area. Cupping and purgatives are also recommended.

3.45 Dandruff of the Eyelids

Use a phlegm humor balancer. If it is chronic, scratch the area with a piece of hardened gur until it is slightly raw, then apply collyrium.

3.46 Ulcer in the Inner Corner of Eye

For these ulcers, called sties, use cupping, then treat the body with a purgative. Then, clean the ulcerated part with a piece of clean cotton and take away all pus. Keep it clean, and it will go away by itself. If the tear duct is infected and blocked, clean the eye as above, then use rose water wash, followed by a few drops of mother's milk to which a grain of finely ground saffron has been added. Put this on the ulcer to open it.

3.47 Itching of Eyelids or Duct without Boils

Use a systemic purgative, and afterward apply ½ teaspoon of pounded chickory with rose oil to the site of irritation.

Section 4

The Ear

General Considerations

The sense of hearing is above all the other senses, as sound is connected with memory, intellect, knowledge, and the higher faculties. For example, music is heard by the ears and affects the sense of hearing in a way that can produce an aesthetic sensation or even religious feelings. The trained mystics of the East work in practical ways with sound. The long sound of the vowel *a* (as in *father*) is often intoned in all of the esoteric schools to stimulate the heart center. The vibratory level of the sound *ah* has the ability to move the heart and mind in ways that other senses cannot perceive. All of the prophetic books have first been recited as poetry, and the faculty of hearing is necessary to respond to this. According to the science of breath, the vibratory level of the letter *a* radiates a *feeling* of sympathy, power, and magnetism. Likewise, the vowel sound of a long *e* (as in *see*) gives a clear sound and feeling, like diving deep into the recesses of one's own soul. Physiologically, the *a* vibrates in the heart; the *e* vibrates up the nasal septum and stimulates the root of the pineal body, an organ of uncertain function.

Figure 3 gives the basic anatomy of the ear. Generally speaking, little goes wrong with the ear, but when something does disturb the delicate inner mechanisms, the cure is difficult. For minor ailments use only enemas and do not put anything into the ear. (Anything that *is* put into the ear should always be warm and never cold.)

4.1 Earache

Earache due to swelling or ulcer is explained in 4.2 and 4.3. Other causes are from hot or cold temperament, which should be balanced with a purgative. Water retained in the ear after swimming or bathing can cause earache. Remove the water by jumping on one foot, on the side of the ache. A small piece of sterile sponge or cotton can be made into a wick and gently inserted into the ear opening to absorb the water. If there still remains water in the ear, take a piece of anise wood 20 cm long and bind a piece of cotton to one end, soak it with oil, and ignite it with a match. Insert the end without the cotton a small distance into the ear, and the water will be completely absorbed.

If there is a worm or insect in the ear, try blowing smoke into the ear, which will probably cause it to come out. If this doesn't work, you probably will have to go to a doctor and have the ear irrigated to remove the foreign object. If a doctor is unavailable, try boiling peach leaves, or bruise the juice out of the leaves when fresh, and use this fluid (or the juice of aloe vera or vinegar) to kill the insect, which can then be removed with a cotton swab.

4.2 Swelling of the Ear

After first using a purgative, examine the ear to determine whether the swelling is coming from the inside or the outside. If it is swollen inside, there is severe pain, weakness of hearing sense, and often fever. Rub a composition of equal parts of sandalwood, magnesia and camphor, and coriander water inside and outside the ear, and pour a few drops of mother's milk into the ear to stop the pain. If this has no effect, drop linseed water into the ear to ripen the infection.

If the swelling is on the outside of the ear, there is obvious enlargement but usually no severe pain and no fever. If there is severe pain, soak hot cloths and apply as a compress. After two days, put this poultice on the ear: four large cabbage leaves boiled in pure butter. Keep this on the swollen part for twelve hours and repeat if necessary. Warm salt in a cotton sock is also effective.

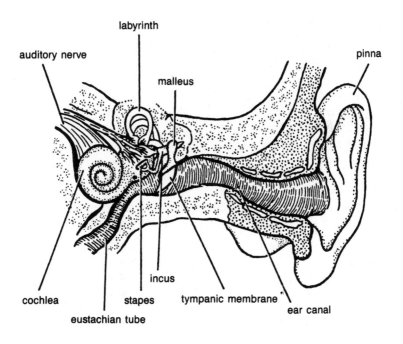

Basic Parts of the Ear

4.3 Ulcer of the Ear

The signs are swelling and excretion of rheum. The remedy is to soak a wick with honey to clean the infection. Then mix together honey, dragon's-blood, and frankincense in equal parts and add a few drops of rose oil; apply to the ear with a cotton swab.

4.4 Weakness of Hearing

Weakness of hearing, deafness, or lack of an orifice should all be treated with purgatives. The cause can be hereditary or due to old age. These cannot be helped by herbs, so the person with them is advised to consult a hearing specialist to see if a mechanical hearing aid will help.

4.5 Entrance of Stones and Similar Objects into the Ear

Drop 3 drops of olive oil into the ear and have the person sniff black pepper to cause sneezing. When the person is about to sneeze, block the nose and mouth completely, and force the ear to expel the object. If this is not effective, seek medical help.

4.6 Ringing in the Ear (Tinnitus)

This trouble has psychic origins and often comes upon people who are overly intellectual and very anxious. Detoxification of the system should be accomplished first, along with relaxation techniques. It is helpful for the person to take up pastimes unrelated to his intellectual pursuits. There is no certain herbal cure. It has been determined that those who suffer from a constant ringing in the ears continue to "hear" the sound even if the auditory nerve is severed. This gives some credence to the view that there are signals that are constantly going on but are normally beyond the range of our hearing. Many people have temporary ringing or buzzing of some kind in their ears. It is not understood by medicine why this occurs, but in the view of natural medicine, it is a signal and tone from another, higher dimension that needs to be heard. It can also be a temporary reaction to a blow or a very loud noise. Include leg of lamb in the diet.

4.7 Bleeding of the Ear

The cause can be from a befouled stomach or from injury. In the former case use a stomachic, and in the latter case apply first aid. If the bleeding will not stop, boil ¼ ounce gallnut in 4 ounces vinegar and put a few drops in the ear, which should stop the flow of blood. If there is spontaneous bleeding from the ear from no apparent cause, it may be that the body is eliminating toxic blood or excess blood pressure in the brain. This condition will regulate itself. If the bleeding is due to the bite of a snake, consult the section on snakebite (see

21.27). Any blood coming from the ear should be examined by a physician promptly.

4.8 Cracks in the Ear

This mostly happens with children. Apply cupping between the shoulder blades and under the ear on the side of the injury. Wash the ear with mother's milk and apply a pomade made with juice of aloe vera, false acacia, henna, and sweet almond oil.

4.9 Itching of the Ear

Boil ¼ ounce wormwood in 3 ounces vinegar; add 10 drops bitter almond oil to it and put a few drops in the ear.

4.10 Injuries Caused by Extremely Loud Noise

Strengthen the brain with a diet rich in greens, keep sweet scents about all the time, and burn rose incense.

Section 5

The Nose

General Considerations

According to natural medicine, the nose has two outlets, one going to the brain and the other to the throat and then on to the lungs. In yoga and other mystical disciplines, there are practices that involve breathing through alternate nostrils in order to balance both the brain and the lungs.

Relatively few ailments, apart from injuries, affect the nose. The hairs that grow in the nose gather minute particles and keep them from entering the head or lungs. The sense of smell is necessary for proper appetite and to perceive certain danger signals in the environment. Afflictions of the nose are often accompanied by troubles in another part of the head or face—thus specialists treat the group of "eye, ear, nose, and throat" diseases.

5.1 Corruption of the Sense of Smell

There are three kinds: (1) that a person perceives all scents as the same; (2) that different smells are perceived from the same scent; and (3) that some scents are perceived but others are not. In the last case, sometimes only sweet smells are noticed, or only sour scents. The remedy is to detoxify the brain by diet. If the person smells everything as foul odor, drop a few drops of musk oil into the nose. If only sweet smells are perceived, use castoreum.

A New York physician published information about ten years ago that the complete corruption of the sense of smell is due to a zinc deficiency: he used massive doses of zinc to cure several drastic cases![1]

5.2 Hemorrhoids of the Nose

An extra piece of flesh growing in the nose can be relieved by cupping the back of the head and using a purgative. A salve of myrrh is recommended as a nasal suppository. If this does not bring relief, surgical removal of the skin piece is necessary if there is obstruction of breathing.

5.3 Boils in the Nose

Use a purgative. If the boil is hard, soften with wax and oil.

5.4 Ulcers of the Nose

If the ulcer is wet and draining, apply cupping to the sides of the nose, then

---

[1] Arthur Berton Roueche, "Annals of Medicine (Disorders of Taste)," *New Yorker*, September 12, 1977, pp. 97-117.

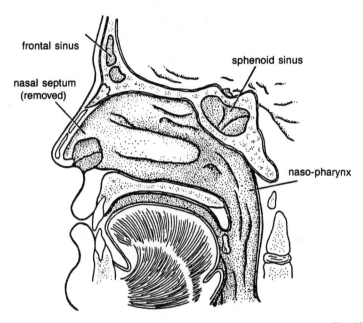

The Nose

use a purgative. Afterward, rub with rose oil. If the ulcer is dry, rub it with wax and oil.

5.5 Nosebleed

There are many causes of nosebleed, some of which are discussed in other sections as a sign of another ailment. Check these sections in the index, especially if there are other signs present such as fever, vomiting, diarrhea, and the like.

A nosebleed can be controlled by binding the arms, thighs, and ears tightly and cupping the back of the head. If blood is coming out of the right nostril only, also apply cupping to the area of the liver. Apply cupping over the spleen if there is blood coming out of the left nostril only. The blood should be thickened after bleeding, which can be done with a diet of rice and lemon juice. In some mental diseases, blood must escape from the head, and does so through this mechanism. If the bleeding does not stop on its own, consult a physician.

5.6 Foul Odor Coming from the Nose

The cause may be a boil or ulcer, which must be treated. If the bad odor is from phlegm, it may mean that the brain is infected. It may also be from gas rising from a foul stomach. In either case, purge the brain or stomach. Gargle afterward with oxymel and mustard seeds soaked in water for an hour, then strained. Dropping sweet-smelling oils in the nose is also recommended.

5.7   Bruising of the Nose

If there is an injury followed by blood and rheum, immediately try to put the nose back in its correct placement, as it may have been broken, and this will prevent a wrong mending that could obstruct breathing. Then make a paste of equal parts aloe vera juice, false acacia, and myrrh oil on a clean sheet of paper and paste this over the nose.

5.8   Excessive Sneezing

The usual cause of this is thought to be allergy. Sensitivity to substances can often be minimized by eliminating intake of all sugar, including the sugars of fruit, along with a general detoxification program. For intermittent irritation that causes frequent sneezing, drop rose oil into the nose and rub the same oil over the hands, feet, eyelids, and ears, and on the palate in the mouth. Mild sneezing is a sign of healthy reflexes; anything in excess is a bad sign.

5.9   Dryness of the Nose

The nose can become overly dry in the heat of summer or cold of winter. Eat warming or cooling foods and beverages. A few drops of mother's milk or olive oil will soothe and moisten the membranes.

5.10   Itching of the Nose

The nose often gets itchy in the colder months. Adjust the temperament for cold weather with a hot diet. If it seems to be the start of flu, mix ¼ teaspoon cayenne pepper and 1 teaspoon ginger root, and boil in 2 cups water for 8 minutes. Strain and sip the mixture, drinking ¼ cup every half hour.

Section 6
The Mouth

6.1 Swelling of the Tongue

The remedy is to use a purgative and gargle with oxymel. If the swelling is not gone in three days, use syrup of lettuce seeds, chickory, and purslane in equal parts as a gargle. If this still does not help, first wash the tongue with linseed water, then use a gargle composed of feverfew herb, melilot, violet, and fresh seeds of senna in equal parts, and add to 1 pint pure water. In case of phlegmatic condition, mix some honey in with the formula; in the case of biliousness, mix some cooked figs in with it and add 2 drops of violet oil and $^1/_8$ teaspoon senna pods. If the swelling becomes chronic, chewing on chickory and fresh coriander is recommended.

6.2 Heaviness of the Tongue

In this condition, the person has difficulty pronouncing words. If it is severe, the person cannot pronounce words at all. The cause is languor of the brain, which needs purging and a detoxification regimen. If the cause is not languor

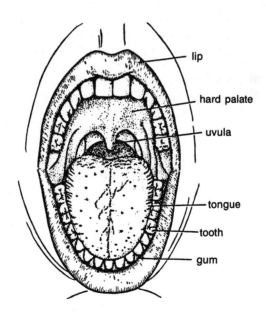

The Mouth

the brain but humoral imbalance, use the remedy for paralysis as found in 2.20. Cupping under the chin is sometimes helpful.

6.3 Enlargement of the Tongue

When the tongue becomes so large that it protrudes from the mouth, imbalance of the blood or phlegm humor is the cause. In the case of blood imbalance, balance the humor and rub sour pomegranate on the tongue. If it is a phlegm imbalance, adjust for phlegm and rub salt and vinegar on the tongue.

6.4 Slackness of the Tongue

The remedy is the same as for enlargement; see 6.3.

6.5 Split of the Tongue

If a taut, dry feeling exists in the brain, give the person plenty of fluids with a drop of voilet oil in each glass. Rub cucumber foam (obtained from rubbing two pieces of cucumber together) on the tongue. If the cause is stomach gas, it means that the digestion is off and a stomachic tea is needed. After cleansing the stomach, keep a few capers in the mouth.

6.6 Dryness of the Tongue

Lack of salivation is caused by excessive internal heat. Keep water of quince seeds, white water lily, and a little sugar handy, and sip frequently. If phlegm also appears on the coating of the tongue and there is further drying, rub oxymel on a piece of willow wood and put it in the mouth.

6.7 Burning Sensation on the Tongue

If this is due to eating a scalding substance, use a purgative and eat very cold substances such as ice chips.

6.8 Itching of the Tongue

After using a purgative, gargle first with warm water, then with milk, then with sugar water, then with vinegar, then with rose oil. Put honey on the tongue to soothe.

6.9 Growths under the Tongue

When something hard, like a gland, appears under the tongue, the cause is watery phlegm or blood. It must be surgically removed by a physician. Purge the phlegm humor.

6.10 Corruption of the Sense of Taste

This is a feeling of a bad taste in the mouth. The cause is prevalence of phlegm. Purge the phlegm, use cupping, and gargle with oxymel.

6.11 False Taste

False taste means that the person cannot taste at all. It sometimes happens that the general sense of temperature is also corrupted, and the tongue cannot distinguish between hot and cold. The cause is prevalence of moisture in the nerves of the tongue. Purge the brain; then, if signs of heat are present, cook ½ teaspoon mustard seeds with ½ teaspoon pellitory root in 2 cups of water. Cool and gargle. For signs of cold, boil 2 teaspoons rose petals and ½ teaspoon myrrh in 1 cup water. Mix in 1 teaspoon oxymel, and use as a gargle.

6.12 Lesions of Skin of Tongue

Use a purgative and then boil equal parts of rose leaves, pomegranate flowers, and myrtle in 2 cups vinegar, and gargle.

6.13 Boils of the Mouth

Use a purgative and follow with a gargle made of vinegar in which coriander has been boiled for ten minutes. Cool and gargle.

6.14 Other Mouth Sores

First use a general purgative. Then determine the basic imbalance of humor. If it is due to blood or black bile humor imbalance, gargle with a preparation of magnesia, pomegranate flower, and camphor. If the sore has a foul odor, gargle with vinegar and salt to remove the wetness and secretions. If the cause is phlegm, boil celadine and ½ teaspoon pellitory root in 1 cup vinegar. Add 1 teaspoon honey, and gargle. If the cause is bile, chew henna leaves or boil coriander with gallnut and pomegranate skins in vinegar and gargle.

6.15 Excessive Salivation

This can occur during sleep or at time of waking up. The cause may be excessive heat or moisture in the stomach. Purge the stomach by rubbing fresh chickory with a little salt and drinking it in water. If the cause is cold, use frankincense with mastic.

6.16 Bad Breath

If the cause is poor hygiene of the mouth parts, clean them with a teaspoon of salt in a glass of water. Gargle rosewater or sesame water in the morning. Try to brush the teeth and clean the mouth three or four times a day.

6.17 Swelling of the Palate

The cause may be blood or phlegm humor. If the cause is blood, the appearance of the swelling is red and there is soreness. If the cause is phlegm, the appearance is white and there is no pain. Use proper purgative and gargle with the formula given in 6.14.

6.18   Whiteness of the Lips

Remove phlegm with detoxification regimen; afterward eat thick foods (breads, meat broths, and the like) and drop diluted jasmine oil into the nose.

6.19   Cracks, Separation, and Dryness of Skin of Lips

Check the sections on mouth ailments to see if there are accompanying signs. Keep the lips covered with a pomade made of powdered tragacanth gum, cooking starch, and powdered gallnut. Mix a little olive oil with it for consistency. Every pomade put on the lips should be covered with the skin that is inside an egg.

6.20   Trembling of the Lips

If the cause is excessive blood entering the veins of the lips, cupping on the cephalic vein is recommended. Fasting should be commenced. If there is a great deal of stomach gas at the same time as the trembling, apply the remedy in 2.23. If the cause is in the brain, it can be a sign of the beginning of epilepsy or paralysis. Consult 2.12 and 2.18. Begin detoxification diet.

6.21   Shrinking of Lips

Stomach convulsions can cause this. Use a purgative and massage the body with warm oils.

6.22   Hemorrhoids of the Lips

The appearance of a projected piece of the lower lip from inside the mouth should be treated by purging the blood humor and black bile humor, followed by the pomade given in 6.19.

6.23   Swelling of the Lips

Purge the phlegm humor and use pomade.

6.24   Boils on the Lips

Use a purgative and see 6.13 and 5.3.

6.25   Ulcers of the Lips

Apply pomades (see 6.19) and correct humor according to the signs.

6.26   Toothache

If the cause is eating excessively hot foods, swirl ice water in the mouth. If the cause is cold food, do the opposite.

Another cause is ill-temperament brought on by overheating of the body. In this case, gargle with vinegar and rose water. In the case of a cold temperament and lowered body temperature, gargle with water in which cooked basmati rice has been soaked, and use an enema.

Putrefying food in the stomach also causes toothache. Cleanse the stomach and use more coriander in cooking. If the cause is gas from improper digestion, gargle with cooked anise seed and cumin (about ½ teaspoon of each mixed together in a pint of water).

A toothache can usually be stopped quickly by putting one tablet of betaine hydrochloride on the offending tooth. If there are frequent toothaches, a visit to the dentist is in order, as well as a review of one's dietary patterns.

6.27 Dull Feeling of Teeth

Where there is a general ill-temperament along with the dullness, the cause is from excessive eating of very hard and sour foods. The remedy is chewing leaves of purslane, seeds included if possible. Eating warm lamb kabob or fresh warm bread is recommended. In the case of cold intemperament, the preparation is apricot kernels mixed with the core of nutmeg, chewed well. If the cause is in the stomach, sour belching and sour taste in the mouth are the signs. Remedy: Purge the phlegm and black bile humors and see a dentist regularly.

6.28 Decay, Cavities, and Worn Teeth

Purge the brain, using gallnut and pellitory in equal parts as a tea, and see a dentist.

6.29 Accumulation of Tartar at Base of Teeth

The cause is the same as for facial paralysis. Consult 2.20. The teeth should be cleaned regularly by a dentist.

6.30 Discoloration of Teeth

Yellowness of teeth is a sign of biliousness. Blackness is a sign of canker. For yellowness, clean teeth by rubbing with lentil flower and vinegar. For blackness, rub rose oil with powdered root of caper on the teeth. With excessive whiteness of teeth, rub with mastic.

6.31 Loose Teeth

In children and the elderly, loose teeth are a natural condition, and nothing should be done. In others, the causes are prevalence of moisture in the system, hot blood, and decay of gums. Cupping on the cephalic vein and the chin is recommended. A dentist is recommended for treatment to try to save the teeth. If one is not near a dentist and the tooth has to be removed, pound fresh fig leaves to make a syrup of green figs and put on the tooth for three days. The tooth should come out quite easily. Afterward, consume many oranges and other citrus fruits.

6.32 Spaces between the Teeth

This occurs as normal variation of growth in some children. For cosmetic reasons, some people want such spaces to be corrected by orthodontic appliances, which can be quite expensive. If it happens in adults, the cause may be prevalence of blood, so use a blood humor purgative. If there is pain with the widening, it is prevalence of blood. If prevalence of phlegm is the cause, there is no pain. Give a phlegm humor balancer.

There is some normal stretching due to the wear of teeth as aging proceeds. This can be adjusted somewhat with special devices, for which a dentist must be consulted.

6.33 Itching of Teeth

In this condition, one cannot help gnashing the teeth. Take a purgative and avoid hot, salty, and sour foods. Gargle with vinegar, taking care not to swallow any sourness.

6.34 Gnashing of Teeth While Sleeping

Give a purgative for the brain, and massage the neck with oil before sleeping.

NOTE: To help children grow teeth easily rub butter, honey, and gum arabic on the gums. Rub the roots of the gums with oil of aloeswood to help stop gnashing.

6.35 Swelling of Gums

Use brain purgative and gargle with formula given in 6.28.

6.36 Bleeding Gums

The cause is usually poor nutrition or hygiene. Correct these factors, and help the gums back to health by rubbing with powdered lentil, magnesia, and gallnut in equal parts. Cold gargles are also helpful. A teaspoon of liquid chlorophyll as a mouthwash helps supply healing nutrients.

6.37 Ulcers of the Gums

If the gums are infected, it is called ulcer of the gum. After forty days, it is called unsound ulcer. Follow the advice given in 6.31 and balance the phlegm humor.

6.38 Diminishing and Receding of Gums

In children, receding of gums helps stimulate tooth growth. In other cases, use this formula: soak equal parts (about 1 teaspoon each) of red rose petals, pomegranate flower, oak leaves, sumac leaves, pellitory, and carob bean in water for several hours. Mash soaked substances together and apply the pulp to the gums. Consume oranges and other citrus fruits in season.

6.39 Swelling of the Uvula

Use a purgative and gargle. In case of presence of bloody discharge and biliousness, gargle with a preparation of equal parts of vinegar and rose water. In case of phlegm with the swelling, mix oxymel with mustard seed. In case of canker, use $1/_8$ teaspoon powdered senna pods in fresh cow's milk.

6.40 Slackness of Uvula

If blood humor is the cause, apply cupping, and gargle with vinegar and rose water and rub the throat with red flowers, sandalwood, pomegranate flower, and camphor. If it is caused by inharmony of phlegm humor, gargle with honey water and use a purgative. For children, soak pieces of hard gallnut in vinegar and apply to top of the child's head.

6.41 Diphtheria

This is a bacterially caused acute inflammation of the throat, which should be treated by a doctor, or at least tested to determine if this is the specific ailment. According to natural medicine, the remedy is to take a purgative and afterward gargle with sumac water and other humorally cold things such as boiled barley water. If there is no coughing, sour things can be given. If blood humor is the cause, cupping on the lower part of the legs is recommended. After about three days, the diphtheria will begin to ripen, at which time the person should gargle with senna leaves mixed with fresh goat's milk. Gargling with diluted, warmed rose oil helps eliminate the canker in the throat. After the canker sloughs off, gargle with cow's milk and honey to clean the rheum. Afterward, feed a dish of wheat bran, almond oil, and sugar.

If the cause of diphtheria is felt to be phlegm, use enemas and gargle with radish juice and honey with a little vinegar; apply cupping to the back of the head and under the chin.

In the case of black bile imbalance, cup as for phlegm and gargle with cow's milk and senna leaves. Make a pomade of ground and sifted feverfew herb mixed with some narcissus and chicken fat for consistency, and apply to throat.

There is an intense kind of diphtheria in which the person is forced to open his mouth by spasms of the muscles, and the tongue hangs out like a dog's. The cause of this is swelling of the throat muscles, which needs to be cured by enemas and treatment according to the trouble with the muscles.

In another kind of diphtheria, the person cannot talk and everything given as food comes out through the nose. If redness appears on the neck under the throat, it is a good sign. If difficulty in swallowing occurs, cup on the second vertebra on the back of the neck. If breathing becomes impossible, a tracheotomy is necessary. Treatment by a physician is suggested from the earliest stages.

6.42 Burning Hot Boils in the Throat, Gullet, and Trachea

The sign of gullet boils is severe pain in the gullet, especially when eating sour and hot foods. The sign of throat and trachea boils is feeling severe pain when talking and chewing. Remedy for all three kinds of boils is to drink fresh fruit juices but avoid cold water. Eat soft foods only. For throat boils, gargling with the medicines mentioned in diphtheria, such as sumac water or barley water, is advised.

6.43 Swallowed Needles

Take the person to a hospital emergency room. In the absence of medical aid, grind magnetic stone, such as iron ore, and drink 1 tablespoon with water in the morning. After a half hour, give a purgative. After the needle is emitted, try to strengthen the stomach (see Section 9, General Considerations, and 9.1 and 9.2).

6.44 Fishbone Stuck in the Throat

If it is possible to see the bone and remove it with a tweezers, do so. If not, have the person take in something slippery, such as seeds of mango. Make a fist and beat the person on the back between the shoulders to cause the bone to be expelled or to cause it to fall into the stomach, where it will probably be digested. If it is stuck halfway up or down, tie a whole dried fig on a string, let the person swallow it, and then draw it back out suddenly, to withdraw the bone. Another technique, called the Heimlich maneuver, is to grasp the choking person from behind with a "bear hug" by reaching under his arms so that a fist can be made and held right in the solar plexus. Make the person bend over and, quickly and with force, pull up and backward to expel the object. If breathing is interrupted, seek emergency aid.

6.45 Narrowness of Food Passage

This can be determined if light things such as water and soup will not go down, but large hunks of food in mouthfuls are easy and painless. The remedy is to purge the phlegm humor. Also drink a tea made from anise seed, frankincense, mastic, and hyacinth, $1/8$ teaspoon of each. Apply cupping under the chin.

6.46 Slackness of the Throat

Its sign is that there is difficulty in expelling breath through the throat. The remedy is the same as for narrowness of the throat, as given above in 6.45.

6.47   Itching of the Gullet

Remedy: Take ½ teaspoon tincture of lobelia every ten minutes until vomiting occurs. Afterward, gargle with vinegar.

6.48   Vibration of Trachea

Vibration is a sign of convulsion, which often causes some hesitation and impediment to speech. The sign of vibration is often seen in the aged, whose voice may vibrate constantly. Gargling with honey and water is very useful.

6.49   Drowning

Use the techniques recommended by the Red Cross or other first aid for resuscitation. After the person has been revived, this regimen is prescribed: boil ½ teaspoon cayenne pepper with ½ teaspoon ground ginger in ½ pint vinegar, filter, and pour in the mouth to arouse the senses. Then feed a dish of pea flour and milk to assist the lungs to work better.

6.50   Choking by Hanging

If the person is still breathing, free the neck and immediately check to see if there is foam in his mouth. If there isn't, immediately give an enema and massage the feet with ground mustard seeds. When the person has come to his senses, have him gargle with violet oil and warm water. (The Hakims note that if there is foam in the mouth, there is no hope of reviving the person.)

6.51   Difficulty in Swallowing

This may be due to diphtheria or other signs mentioned in this section. If it is from bad temperament of the gullet itself, adjust the temperament according to the cause of humoral inharmony. Apply rose oil between the shoulder blades because the gullet is closer to the back than to the front.

6.52   Ulcers of the Gullet

The signs are pain in the gullet and extreme sensitivity to hot and sour foods, while oily foods alone can be eaten with no pain. Remedy: Take a small piece of white wax, put a few drops of rose oil on it, and eat little by little. After this, drink honey water mixed with milk and sugar for two or three days, until the ulcer is gone.

6.53   Coarseness (Hoarseness) of Voice

The cause can be either catarrh or bad temperament. For catarrh, give syrup of marshmallow herb and gargle to stop the catarrh. Bad temperament needs a humor adjustment, according to the signs. The coarseness of the voice can be filtered by eating beans, dates, figs, almonds, sugar cane, honey water, or large raisins; each will smooth the voice.

Section 7

The Chest and Lungs

General Considerations

We can live without food for several weeks and without water for days, but without breath, life ceases after a few minutes. The lungs are the largest organ in the body, and we tend to think in terms of functions of the lungs rather than of the entire process of breathing.

According to natural medical philosophers, breath is not the lungs as such or the air moved by them but a divine emanation of potentiality, carrying the essence of every human faculty at its beginning and making it manifest in the various physical organs as it circulates through the body.

It is assumed that God created the original breath of Creation out of the finer particles of the fire humor and created the hollow left side of the heart to serve as the storehouse and seat of manufacture of the breath in the body. The tissues and bones and all other parts of the body are also produced from the four humors; the breath is thus related to manifest matter.

From the heart, the breath passes throughout the body, pausing long enough at each part to convey the specific properties: the sense of sight to the moist crystalline lens of the eye, the sense of hearing from union with the auditory nerve, and so forth. While there is much to be said in relation to the theory of modern medicine that the mind originates all vegetative faculties, the only view of natural medicine is that the breath carries the divine vital essence of the faculty of an organ. It is interesting to note that the word *human* comes from two Sanskrit words, *hu* (divine) and *manas* (mind).

If an organ is missing, there then remains on the breath a vital potential that cannot be used up and so becomes superfluous, resulting in persistent ill-health, which seems to have no cure. Whenever an organ is surgically removed, the channels of breath are destroyed due to the severance of the nerve fibers and often of important ganglia. The circulating "divine mind" of breath, coming to an absent organ, is turned back upon itself, and there is a great sense of distress which nothing can relieve.

The breath thus relates very closely to temperament and emotional character. For example, moist intemperament occurs when the breath lingers overlong in any one of the phases of earth, air, or fire. An imbalance in the fire element would be characterized by a personality that is hot, impetuous, prone to anger, physically strong, courageous in danger, strong in desires, and so forth. The whole range of human emotional types can be worked out on this same scale of the breath in relation to the elements.

Inherent in the view of natural medicine is the idea that willpower should dominate the breath. Since breathing is a function of the autonomic nervous system, we do not need to apply intelligence to continue breathing, although this should be done as a regular part of health maintenance.

A balanced breathing pattern is necessary for stable emotions and intelligent living. This is obvious when one takes the trouble to catch oneself in the midst of anger. The breath is always out of rhythm in anger, fear, or any extreme emotional state. Application of willpower to the intake and expulsion of breath can open a whole new dimension of living. Mystics, yogis, and other Eastern people use exactly this principle to gain control over the lower kinds of appetitive actions—anger, fear, perverse desires, and so on.

In the inhalation phase of the breath, the innate heat or vital force is built up, and on expulsion it is dispersed. Simultaneous with the expulsion of breath is the appearance of the phenomenon known as the aura or atmosphere (a sensation resembling a gentle current of air, sometimes perceived as a color, rising from the limbs or body to the head).

There are in every community teachers of yoga and others who teach conscious control of the breath as a means to regulated health. Great profit can be had in this discipline.

The expelled breath is that which separates the superfluous matters from healthy matter. Thus, one who has poor breath also has poor internal health. Disease can also be explained from this doctrine, in that the cycle of the breath is not in harmony with the process of formation of the humors of the body. Presence of the signs of disease indicates an abnormal humoral state, either an unbalanced innate heat or a conflict between innate heat and the heat of foreign substances (such as bacterial decomposition).

Any change in rhythm of the breath will in itself cause loss of natural immunity to bacterial agents. Since there must be an outflow of superfluous matter, any holding back of isolated microorganisms in the tissues will allow them time to develop into active colonies. This leads to structural organic changes in the body, called symptoms of disease.

A rational explanation for certain "miraculous" cures can be found in cases where long-standing blockages of the circulation of the breath have been removed, either suddenly or gradually. Restoration of the normal flow is often enough to allow the body to rid itself of the accumulated superfluities and resultant symptoms.

It should be remembered that smoking, air pollution, and poor posture can all contribute to disease by disturbing the regulated flow of the breath.

7.1 Asthma

Asthma is a chronic affliction of the throat and chest, recurrent and difficult to cure. The sooner it is treated, the better. The signs are expulsion of phlegm when coughing, hoarseness in the chest, wheezing, difficulty in breathing, and rasp in the lungs—all signs that the cause is phlegm.

The remedy is first to eliminate all foods that produce mucus, such as milk, eggs, cheese, fruits, and all sugars of any kind. Foods high in iodine must be eaten, such as kelp, which also help replace minerals stripped out with the phlegm (consult the chapter on detoxification). Use purgatives. If vomiting is provoked, there is no harm. Coffee or chickory-root enemas should be employed whenever there is danger of an attack that could interrupt or stop breathing. They can be given every ten or fifteen minutes for up to two hours, if necessary, to keep the elimination of phlegm continuous.

Syrup of hyssop with warm water three times a day is recommended after a bout with asthma. White turkey meat with plenty of spices is also recommended. When the phlegm seems to be building up, take garlic with honey to soothe the throat if it is raw from coughing.

Dr. Edward Shook's preparation or remedy for asthma attacks and all afflictions of the lungs is one of the finest herbal remedies I have used. It is prepared as follows:

2 ounces powdered slippery elm bark
1 ounce cut horehound
1 ounce cut garden thyme
1 ounce cut red clover tops
1 ounce yerba santa
1 ounce lobelia inflata
1 dram capsicum (cayenne pepper)

Put all the above into 2 quarts distilled water. Stir well and let stand for two hours. Cover tightly and simmer for thirty minutes. Strain, pressing out all liquid. Return to saucepan and reduce to 1 pint. Add 24 ounces blackstrap molasses and 8 ounces glycerin. Bring to a boil and simmer five minutes very slowly. Cool and bottle. For spasmodic asthmas, the dose is 1 tablespoon every hour until relief is obtained. After this, take 1 tablespoon three or four times a day. For children, 1 teaspoon according to age; ages four and up, half the adult dose.

If there is pain, give about ¼ teaspoon of half-pounded linseed with honey, which should relieve the pain immediately. Rub the chest with linseed oil and beeswax.

There are several causes of asthma, according to the Hakims. One is called *heart gas*, which is evidenced by these signs: thirst, hard beating of the pulse, and labored breathing, coming in hard gasps. For this, apply cupping on the cephalic vein of the left arm, give laxatives in beverages, and rub the sides.

Another cause given is *internal heat affecting the lungs*. The signs are hard beating of the pulse and thirst, but the breathing is not as labored. Remedy:

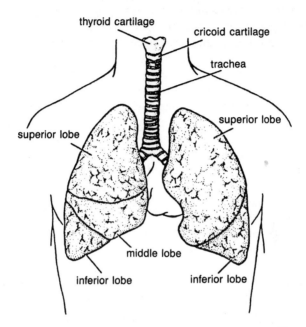

thyroid cartilage

cricoid cartilage

trachea

superior lobe

superior lobe

middle lobe

inferior lobe

inferior lobe

Chest and Lungs

Adjust with cold drinks and a cucumber pomade on the chest. Another cause is *slackness of the chest muscles,* which is evidenced by soft beating of the pulse and soft breathing. The muscles must be strengthened. Rub oil of narcissus on the chest and balance the humor as for paralysis in 2.20. Gargling with milk and cinnamon with honey added is also recommended.

If the cause of asthma is *excess dryness in the tissues,* the voice is changed to a somewhat higher pitch, and there may be thirst and a tendency to desire to drink liquor. Remedy: Give fruit juices and take sitting baths in water made from violet, cucumber, chamomile, and marshmallow. Drink plenty of fresh milk.

If the cause is *cold nature of the lungs* (known from lack of thirst and soft pulse) give the person hot-natured foods. If the cause is *inflammation of the lungs,* a sense of lightness of the body, and coughing without phlegm are the signs. In this case, as with all others, use a coffee enema and adjust the proper humor. Put a pomade made of common dill and fennel seed on the chest.

Fullness of the stomach can also cause asthma. This can be corrected by enemas, fasting, and improving the digestion.

Other causes are *swelling of the lungs, diaphragm, or liver,* which are discussed later.

7.2   Coughing
The signs and kinds of coughing remedies are as follows.

Blood humor The signs are hard beating of the pulse, hot temperament of the breath, and redness of the face. All these are due to hot temperament of the liver. Drink cold-natured drinks, and apply cupping.

Descending of superfluities from the brain There is a tendency to sleep all the time, along with coughing. Gargle with cooked marijuana seeds and keep a bit of gum arabic in the mouth. A variation of this problem is that the substance coming down from the brain goes into the lungs and is thickened there. The signs are expulsion of phlegm while coughing, heaviness of the chest, runny nose, and congestion. This is treated with a drink of equal parts cooked fig, milk, and hyssop. Keep some cayenne pepper with sugar and rose conserve in the mouth.

Moisture of lungs and chest A great deal of phlegm comes out when coughing, and the voice is hoarse. This happens mostly with the elderly and those who have moist temperament. Use the treatment given for asthma in 7.1.

Roughness of lungs from smoke or dust or loud shouting Remove the person from the cause. Moisten the lungs with syrups of (equal parts) barley and marshmallow; mix in a glass of water with ½ teaspoon each of sugar and almond oil added. Also, rub the navel with olive oil and the anus with butter.

Boils or ulcer of the lungs The signs are fast beating of the pulse and a burning sensation on urination. Cold drinks make the person feel better. The remedy is to cup the chest and use purgatives.

Fullness of the stomach Use an enema and limit intake of food.

Black bile If corrupted bile has reached the lungs, a blackish or dark-greenish substance comes out when coughing. Give boiled wheat bran with sugar or honey, then purge the black bile humor. Eat chicken or mutton stew.

Water or fluid entering the larynx The coughing will not stop unless the substance is thrown out. No treatment is advised. If there is so much congestion that it becomes difficult to breathe or swallow, the throat and chest should be rubbed with oil and an emetic is advised to clear the larynx and trachea so that function can be restored.

Cough powder This is a good remedy for cough to relieve general irritation of the throat and lungs. Use $1/_8$ teaspoon, all powdered fine, of each of the following:

skunk cabbage
horehound
African cayenne
bayberry bark
valerian root
gentian

Mix with 3 ounces molasses, and take 1 teaspoon with hot tea.

7.3 Blood Coming from the Mouth

The source of the blood must be determined. Blood can be coming from the parts of the mouth, from the head, or from the inner organs. What comes from the mouth parts is ejected with saliva. If it is coming from the head, it seems to come from the palate, and there may be light-headedness. If it is coming from the larynx and trachea, the blood is emitted when clearing the throat and comes out a little at a time. There is no coughing. Blood coming from the trachea is foamy, and there is coughing and pain.

There is also foamy blood if it is from the lungs, but there is coughing with or without pain. Blood coming from the chest is small in amount and is ejected with severe coughing. If the blood is coming from the stomach, spleen, or liver, it comes out by vomiting.

Remedies of each of these sources of bleeding are:

Parts of mouth:
Gargle with cooked astringent things such as pomegranate flowers, gallnut, and myrtle.

Head:
Cup on the cephalic vein and gargle with cooked astringent things such as pomegranate flowers, gallnut, and myrtle.

Larynx and trachea:
The above medicine, held in the mouth but not swallowed, should stop bleeding.

Lungs:
Apply cupping on the saphena vein and legs, and adjust the temperament. If further measures are needed, put astringents on the chest, but only if the lungs are not swollen.

Chest:
Take the medicine as above and rub the chest. Chest ulcers often heal easily, due to the large supply of fresh oxygen in that part.

Stomach and other parts: Consult appropriate section for specific body part.

In every case of bleeding, chewing purslane leaves or drinking a little syrup of purslane is recommended. If pressure of blood is felt in the lungs but there is no coughing, gargle with vinegar and rose water and drink a few ounces, too. If there is coughing, mix ash of fig wood with water and sip this occasionally. Consult a physician as soon as possible.

7.4   Rheum Coming from the Mouth

This may be caused by the discharges of pneumonia, pleurisy, or tuberculosis (these are discussed in their own sections). If rheum is coming from the mouth parts or the larynx or throat, the cause may be diphtheria or other swellings. If rheum is coming from the chest, the remedy is to soften the phlegm. Make a pomade of beeswax, oil of chamomile, and a little hen's fat and apply to chest. Never use astringents or cold foods. A drink made of cooked hyssop, fig, and licorice root is useful to open all swellings of the diaphragm and chest.

Substances from the chest entering the lungs are expelled via the trachea. There is no need to force it out.

7.5   Pleurisy

Pleurisy is an inflammation of the membrane lining the chest and surrounding the lungs. It is caused by imbalance of heat, whether of the blood, bile, or phlegm. The signs are high fever, severe asthma, heaviness of the chest, redness of the face and cheeks, and thirst. Apply cupping on the chest, then use a laxative or enema.

If the pain and swelling are on the left side, the left cheek will be red, there will be a feeling of heaviness in the left side, and the person will prefer to lie on his left side. If the swelling is in the right lung, the opposite signs will be noticed; also in this case there will be some saliva running out of the mouth. If only one side is affected, the cupping should be done on that side.

After cupping on the appropriate side, put on a pomade made of ½ teaspoon each of violet flowers, linseed, chamomile, milk, barley flour, and common dill. Boil them all in water, with a little sesame oil mixed in, and apply lukewarm to the chest.

In chest afflictions, astringent medicines such as fennel or even cold water should never be given. To lower a fever, give nonastringent substances like cucumber juice, watermelon, and pumpkin juice. A fairly sweet mixture of vinegar and honey may also be given. If there is difficulty in breathing, give an enema and laxatives, and pour lukewarm water on the chest and sides to relieve pain.

7.6   Notes on Swelling

It should be known that swelling has three resolutions: (1) It ripens and comes out, (2) it jells, or (3) it becomes hard.

The sign of ripening is the gradual day-by-day diminishing of signs.

The sign of jelling, or turning to pus, is a worsening of the signs, especially as it begins to ripen. The fever and pain then go away, but heaviness is still felt in the chest. Then severe asthma and dry coughing, heaviness, and pain reappear. This kind of swelling, when ripened, will open and try to find its way out. Usually, blood alone or blood with a little unripened substance will first come out, followed by expulsion of the ripened phlegm. Pus usually "opens out" by means of reflexive actions, such as vomiting, severe anger, or a sudden movement. If, after ripening, it does not come out, it must be assisted.

If the swelling is hardening into phlegm, the signs are excess saliva, heaviness in the stomach, asthma, and absence of signs of heat. Make a pomade of mother's milk and soft wax and apply to the chest. If there is phlegm, the temperament must be adjusted for phlegm. When there is hardened phlegm, sometimes it beads into small stones, and then the coughing stops. Pleurisy sometimes results in tuberculosis.

7.7 Tuberculosis

This is a lung ulcer. While it can be detected by chest x-rays, the active stage is known by the signs of hectic fever, and phlegm matter emitted in coughing. The matter ejected is some form of moisture. A natural test for tuberculosis is that the substance coughed up will sink in water and has a very foul odor when burned. While there is no immediate cure, the use of fresh air, sunshine, exercise, heat, light, rest, and similar aspects of nature cure are recommended. Avicenna said that a person affected with tuberculosis could live for twenty years, with proper care. Galen said that he cured every tuberculosis patient whose treatment had been initiated from practically the first day of signs.

If there is pain, apply cupping to the chest and give a soup of cooked barley with honey. Everything useful for hectic fever is useful in this case. Avicenna recommended giving rose conserve for tuberculosis, except to pregnant women.

7.8 Swelling of the Diaphragm or Internal Pleura

There are many names for vague symptoms of upper stomach pain; some call this pleurisy. True pleurisy, as described above, is a swelling of the pleura, or the membranes of the respiratory organs. Impure pleurisy, which is what is described here, is swelling of the muscles between the ribs, or the swelling of the membranes covering the back muscles. Diaphragmitis is a swelling of the membrane surrounding the stomach and the liver. There are other forms of swelling that affect the membrane between the digestive organs and respiratory organs, but there is no differentiation of these forms in treatment. In these cases of swelling, put a flower oil on the chest, or between the shoulders if the signs are coming from there. The difference between pneumonia and these swellings is that in pneumonia the pulse is erratic or "wavy" and there is severe asthma. In diaphragmitis, the person may become irrational.

Sometimes swelling of the liver is quite similar to pleurisy. The difference is that with swelling of the liver, the person's skin usually has a yellow color and there is no coughing; there is heaviness and pain in the liver, and the urine is very dense and concentrated in color.

Each of the above swellings will become ripened and should be treated before they turn into rheum. Give cabbage water, barley water with sugar, lots of butter and honey. Lying down on the affected side is helpful.

There is false pleurisy that can be mistaken for swelling. In this case, gas is imprisoned between the membranes around the sides and the person feels pain. Because the gas cannot escape, it appears almost like actual swelling of the membranes. The test for false pleurisy is that with simple gas, there is a lightness to the chest or other part, and also an absence of fever.

7.9   Rheum in the Chest

When swelling of the lungs ripens and the phlegm matter gathers and becomes thickened in the area around the lungs, it cannot be excreted by the lungs or in the urine. This is difficult to cure. Since the substance is not eliminated, hectic fever comes. To soften the substance and help eliminate it, give roots of fig, hyssop, plum, licorice, black raisins (in equal parts, ground together), and mix with almond oil and sugar to form little pills. Diuretics will also help. The substance may penetrate to the bladder or kidneys in an attempt to come out, and if this occurs, give any remedy that cleans the bladder and bowels.

7.10   Chest Pressure

The causes are exposure to extremely cold weather, cold wind, excess consumption of ice water, and smoking marijuana. The sign is lack of ability to expand and contract chest. Put warm rose oil or olive oil on the chest and drink warm milk with honey.

The Heart

General Considerations

Heart disease is the leading cause of death among adults in America. There is a great deal of information and research about the causes of heart problems, much of which is focused upon diet and exercise. It is beyond the scope of this book to review all of the available literature on the subject of heart disease, but a few directions for keeping the heart healthy are in order.

Good exercise habits, are vital, for if the heart is not strong it may lead to stagnation of all inherent functions of the body. It is possible that "heart attacks" are nothing more (or less) than the atrophy of its capacity to generate the vital force of life itself. In the view of natural medicine, therefore, exercise is necessary not only to strengthen the heart but also for the health of all the bodily systems.

Obviously, one must map out a reasonable program of physical fitness in keeping with age, general level of health, season, and so forth. Dr. Sheldon Deal of Tucson, a prominent natural physician in the Southwest, said that if one performed a simple set of exercises, it could be virtually *guaranteed* that one would never die of a circulatory congestion. Here are his recommendations for keeping off the page of coronary statistics:

1. Begin with a thorough physical checkup to make sure there are no present medical problems.

2. Run in place, lifting the feet lightly, for one minute every other day for a week.

3. For the second week, extend the time to two minutes.

4. For each successive week, increase the time you run in place by one minute per week. After four weeks, run every day and increase the time until you are running five minutes every day.

5. After reaching five minutes, you can increase the tempo of the running and lift the legs higher, to promote more vigorous stimulation of the circulatory system.

Although it may not be possible to guarantee that someone won't die from heart attacks, this simple regimen, done each day, will certainly ensure that the all-important circulatory and respiratory systems are getting ample exercise.

Common sense dictates that smoking be eliminated and a healthy diet adopted, low in salt, meat, and animal fats. It is impossible to provide a single diet in this book for all people, because every person's needs and general state of health are different, but it is important to become conscious of what you eat, to begin to study and learn about the composition of foods and how the food affects the body. Many people advocate a salt-free diet, but the chlorides in salt are the only readily available source of manufacturing ingredients for hydrochloric acid in the stomach. This may explain why people use salt to excess: the body craves it to produce more hydrochloric acid to assist digestion of excessive amounts of food. Remembering the principle of natural medicine, "Fasting is the best medicine," it can safely be recommended for the average American that at least *less* food be consumed daily.

Avicenna's View of Heart Disease

In Tibb, the heart is considered the most important organ. Avicenna subscribed to and repeated the Prophetic Tradition of Muhammad (peace be upon him) in this regard: "There is one organ in the body, which, if it is well, the whole body is well; and if it is ill, the whole body is ill. And this organ is the heart."

In the *Canon*, Avicenna assesses the condition and state of the heart by eight means: (1) pulse, (2) respiration patterns, (3) form or shape of the chest, (4) hair growth on chest, (5) general feel of the body, (6) other palpable conditions, (7) general strength or weakness, and (8) thoughts and hallucinations.

Among the diseases of the heart Avicenna lists intemperament, inflammation, embolism of cardiac arteries, functional diseases, and discontinuity.

Amazingly, my teacher Hakim Sherif denied ever having seen or heard of anyone suffering a heart attack. In fact, he never did understand precisely what I tried to convey when I explained that the person's heart stopped and he or she fell down dead. "Human beings do not die in that way," he answered with disdain.

To Avicenna, the heart possessed a greater function than being simply a muscular pump. He believed that the heart served as the repository of divine potentialities and was greatly affected by emotions such as pleasure, sorrow, joy, grief, revenge, anxiety, and exhilaration.

The first purpose in treatment of any cardiovascular disease was to "purify the blood, which refines the pneuma or vital force." To accomplish this purification, many substances were used, especially finely ground amber stone, lapis lazuli, and shaved gold and silver.

General treatment was both symptomatic and tonic. Avicenna advised single and compound herbs, smelling salts, teas, foods, change in climate, pastes over the heart, and perfumes.

For Avicenna, the breath was the link between the manifest and unmanifest realms, between God and humans, and he believed that the "vital power of the heart is attracted to aromas. In cardiac drugs great consideration is given to aromas, because the heart is the seat of the production of the vital force of the body." In fact, Avicenna was so convinced of the value of essential oils in heart conditions that he once remarked, "All aromatic oils are cardiac drugs." One very important difference between the oils used by Avicenna and contemporary "perfumes" is that the use of alcohol, even in minute quantities, was forbidden, because it is believed the alcohol destroys the "essence" or vital force of the floral oil. Of the sixty-three cardiac drugs mentioned by Avicenna, forty, more than half, were aromatic oils. Attars—non-alcoholic, distilled essential oils—of lavender, rose, cinnamon, frankincense, water lily, mint, aloeswood, and basil were among those often prescribed in heart conditions.

Purgatives were extremely valuable for cleansing the body of toxins, especially in the area of the heart, but Avicenna urged caution in their use "because they can remove beneficial elements as well as detrimental." A tea made from senna pods ranked highest in Avicenna's formulary of purgatives.

Intemperament caused by coldness was treated by its opposite, the heating herbs—musk, amber, saffron, aloeswood, and cardamom. Cooling drugs included camphor, sandalwood, rose, and coriander.

For palpitations of the heart, Avicenna advised extracts of fragrant fruits—apple, quince, guava—especially after meals. Many of the cardiac oils are advised to be added to the diet, such as clove, saffron, coriander, mint, cucumber, and lettuce.

8.1 Heart Palpitation

When palpitation becomes severe, it will be followed by fainting. There are three causes of palpitation: (1) the heart itself, (2) the stomach, brain, intestine, womb, lungs, or diaphragm, or (3) the total system, including the heart.

If the whole body is affected, the specific parts must be located and corrected. Check the index for sections which have palpitation as a sign of a specific ailment. If only the heart is affected, use a purgative and enemas. Sometimes a person who has the "dry heaves" or excessive vomiting will have heart palpitation. Give spearmint tea as a stimulant, and energetic high-calorie foods.

Another cause for palpitation is living in an excessively warm climate. If one's temperament cannot take excessive heat, a change in climate is recommended.

8.2 Fainting

If the causes of palpitation are not removed, fainting will result. When the cause of fainting is not corrected, it can lead to death. There are three kinds of fainting: (1) the soul is weakening, (2) the soul is congested, and (3) the soul lacks generative force. The causes of weakening of the soul are vomiting, extremes of happiness, overindulgences, and physical pain. The causes of congestion of the soul are excess of fullness (especially of drinks), sadness, great and sudden fear, or shock. The cause of lack of generative force is a bad temperament, or poor food, which cannot increase the potentiality of the soul. The

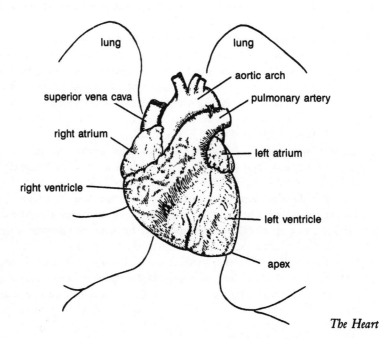

lung

lung

aortic arch

superior vena cava

pulmonary artery

right atrium

left atrium

right ventricle

left ventricle

apex

The Heart

long-term remedy in each case is to remove the cause and strengthen the soul and temperament by meditation, breathing practices, and religious contemplation. If the cause of fainting is excess of heat, give cold foods and energetic drinks like sandalwood tea after the patient is aroused. If the cause is cold, allow the person to smell hot vapors, such as musk. Adjust the temperament, in the case of heat, by pouring rose water and cold water on the chest. However, never pour cold substances on the chest if the cause of fainting is from stomach foulness. In this case, make a tea from ½ ounce powdered ginger and ½ ounce crushed fennel seed, mixed with honey for consistency. Give ½ teaspoon before each meal to balance digestion. Once the stomach is cleansed, eat stewed chicken and meat broth, and rub the chest with cabbage oil.

One of these substances may be substituted for the hot ones given above: musk, saffron, ambergris, aloeswood, mint, cardamom, amber, camphor, marshmallow, apple, and coriander.

If there is great perspiration when the person faints, it is because the pores are opening to allow toxic matters to escape. Excessive perspiration can be stopped to avoid dehydration by grinding leaves of myrtle, soaking in water, and rubbing this on the body.

In all cases of fainting except excess of perspiration, vomiting is recommended immediately after fainting. This can be effected by successive teaspoon doses of tincture of lobelia, every 10 minutes until the result is achieved. Usually 1 teaspoon is sufficient.

Strangulation of the womb can cause fainting (see 17.26).

A person who faints may have a slightly yellow color to the skin and a weak pulse. In a serious case of fainting, the person cannot open the eyes but will understand you if you call his name. If the person cannot understand or hear you, that is apoplexy, not simple fainting, and needs immediate medical help.

8.3 Swelling of the Heart

When the soul becomes weak because of long illness and this weakness reaches the heart, it causes swelling. It is said that this swelling is mostly of a cold nature, because if it were of a hot nature, it would cause death immediately. Of course, cold-nature swelling that reaches the heart can also be fatal, but if it reaches only to the outer surface or skin of the heart, it can be cured. If it is not cured, the person loses weight day by day until he dies. The sign is a feeling of heaviness in the chest close to the cardia. The person looks as though he may faint. There is heart pressure, the face is very yellow, and the eyes become excited. The remedy is to put a poultice of chamomile, white clover, and wheat bran on the chest and cardiac area. Give foods to strengthen the heart, such as beef heart, brewer's yeast, bone marrow, dairy products, egg yolk, green leafy vegetables, peas, beans, nuts, lemons, and oranges.

8.4 Odd Sensations in the Heart

The person may feel as if "smoke" inside the chest were coming from the heart or other strange feelings. This can cause fainting and confusion. Give foods to moisten the temperament and use a purgative to purge the black bile humor.

8.5 Heart Pressure

When pressure is felt, there may be fainting and saliva running out of the mouth, followed by hiccups. Give a coffee enema to take pressure off the liver, give a black bile purgative, and use relaxation techniques of massage and soothing calmative drinks such as chamomile, valerian root, catnip, hops, and the like.

8.6 Heart Attack

The person feels senseless for a short time, but immediately comes back to his senses. There may be convulsions because of the pain, and thus perspiration. Obviously emergency medical aid should be summoned immediately. If there is none available, a coffee enema can relieve pressure on the internal organs; first aid for resuscitation should also be given if necessary. If the attack is not fatal and you are away from any medical aid at all, purge the black bile humor and try to rebuild the heart with a strengthening diet as in 8.3, but eliminate the eggs and dairy products.

8.7   Sensation of the Heart Coming out of the Chest

This is caused by toxic matter in the blood and befouled black bile humor. Give bile humor purgative, rose water, willow water, and syrup of sandalwood. Apply cupping.

8.8   Feeling the Heart is Being Pulled Downward

This feeling is caused by phlegm reaching the area of the liver and surrounding it. The person may feel slight pain and appear to be ready to faint. Use a phlegm purgative.

8.9   Feeling of Fluid in Heart Area

The person feels that his heart is moving in water in a convulsive movement. The Hakims say this is a kind of palpitation caused by excess moisture imprisoned under the tissues of the heart. Make a salve of red rose blossoms, saffron, and hyacinth, mix with mint, and apply to chest. Fortunately or unfortunately, the best way to assimilate heart moisture is by feeling anger!

Sometimes the above-mentioned moisture becomes dried, yet remains inside because of unbalanced heat. The sign of this is that the heart doesn't expand, breathing becomes difficult, the strength dissipates, and anger appears. The remedy is to use laxatives and moistening pomades on the chest.

Section 9

The Stomach

General Considerations

According to natural medicine, most illness originates in disordered digestion. It has been explained in earlier chapters that if the stomach is overburdened or is not functioning efficiently, there will eventually be damage to other organs of the body. Where the damage occurs depends on each individual's inherited constitution and other factors.

One of the first problems with digestion, usually due to excess food consumption over a long period of time, is insufficient hydrochloric-acid production, often due to lack of salt.

9.1 Bad Temperament of the Stomach

In a person with hot temperament, the softness of low-calorie foods causes the stomach to become foul. Hard food and food of high caloric value is the answer. Sometimes there is thirst caused by salty phlegm. This can be relieved by drinking warm water; cold water will not quench the thirst. However, if the cause is bile or excess internal heat, cold water will suffice.

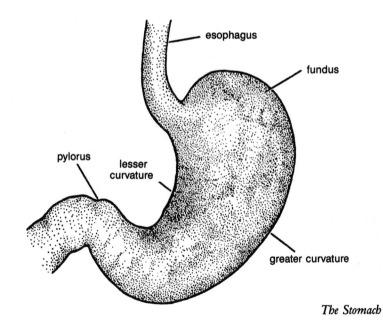

The Stomach

9.2   Stomachache

If the cause of pain is gas, there is much belching and hiccupping and the stomach is distended from the gas. When partially digested food reaches to the bottom of the stomach, pain is felt in the area of the spleen. Remedy. Apply a hot pack to the stomach and drink peppermint tea, with a few drops of rose oil added. Chewing pennyroyal is useful to cause belching and expel gas. If the gas is quite dense, use the phlegm purgative. An immediate effect is gained by applying cupping to the stomach. Honey and vinegar or anise-seed tea may also be used to relieve the pain of gaseousness.

Another cause of stomachache is prevalence of dense gas in the empty bowel. Another cause is that bile has poured into the stomach from the liver because the stomach has been empty for a long time. Another cause is that impure bile spills onto the cardia of the spleen. In the case of gas, use a purgative. For black bile, purge the black bile humor and use a purgative, followed by cupping on the brachial artery of the right arm.

9.3   Weakness of Digestion

The sign of bad digestion is that the food comes out in the stools in an almost unchanged condition, or sometimes by vomiting or diarrhea. The food does not remain in the stomach more than a few hours. Ground fennel seed, with ginger, mixed in honey is the specific remedy for all cases of poor digestion.

9.4   Cholera

This disease causes corrupted substances to come to the stomach from various parts of the body and be emitted by vomiting or diarrhea. If the cholera is very severe, there is no vomiting, and all the substance is eliminated by diarrhea. The accompanying signs of fainting, lowered pulse, and occasional convulsions are not as dangerous as they seem. They can be reversed easily, especially in children. But if cholera becomes chronic, it is dangerous, and is the leading cause of death among infants in underdeveloped nations. The remedy is to remove the corrupted substance completely. While it may seem illogical, one should try to increase the diarrhea or vomiting, as the body realizes that there is a toxic substance and is trying to eliminate it by the quickest route possible. Use laxatives and provoke vomiting by giving tincture of lobelia in ½ teaspoon doses. If the person feels faint, give lemons to chew on. Restrict the diet to simple foods, ensure ample rest, keeping the patient in bed, because nothing works better than rest and fasting. Uncomplicated cholera is self-limiting, with recovery evident by the third to sixth day. Vaccines are available for cholera protection. All cases should be attended by a doctor.

9.5   Deficient and Invalid Appetite

There are many causes. First, it can be bad temperament, whether excessively hot or cold, which affects the cardia. Second is the collection of phlegm in the stomach. Third is the body being filled with raw phlegm, which interferes with the normal appetitive signals of the body to the stomach. Fourth is density of skin pores and roughness of skin, which stop absorption. Fifth is that the liver is weak and obstruction occurs, either in the liver itself or in the mesentery. Sixth is that obstruction occurs in the valve between the spleen and the cardia. Seventh is that the nerve sensors in the cardia are impaired. (NOTE: When the parts of the body need food, they "ask" the veins. The veins carry this message to the liver, which conveys this request to the mesentery, which alerts the stomach via a very sensitive nerve network in the cardia. At this time, bile is secreted from the spleen into the stomach, causing what we call hunger. If any part of this process is blocked, delayed, or altered, the sense of hunger is corrupted or fails.)

The remedies are as follows: *foul substances in the stomach:* purge; for *density of pores:* open by bathing and loofa scrubbing; for *liver weakness:* reinforce liver (see section 10.2, on the liver); for *obstruction of spleen:* purge spleen (see 11.4); and for *nerve failure in cardia:* reinforce the brain (see 2.2).

Sometimes anemia or quitting an addiction can slacken hunger. If there is deficient appetite over an extended period—a month or longer—the stomach is the seat of the anemia. Cure it by using foods and herbs that increase appetite, such as oxymel, lemon juice, spearmint, vinegar, onion, salty fish, and pomegranate.

9.6 Corrupted Appetite

Corrupted or inordinate appetite includes the desire for such things as mud or the tendency of the pregnant woman to crave a peculiar food, such as pickles. I once treated a woman who desired to eat cotton and paper. Ultimately, the cause is accumulation of corrupted phlegm in the stomach. Use a purgative, except in the case of pregnant women, who should take nothing, as these cravings will pass after three months without treatment.

9.7 Excessive Appetite

The person cannot satisfy his hunger and wants to eat "like a dog." If the cause is a cold-natured temperament, the signs are insufficient thirst and intense gas. The remedy is to warm up the cardia by eating fresh, hot bread and rubbing a salve made of nutmeg and valerian on the stomach. If there is phlegm in the stomach, purge the stomach. If the cause is bile spilling on the cardia from the spleen, the signs are great hunger along with burning sensation on the cardia. The burning will not go away unless food is eaten. Purge the black bile humor and apply cupping over the spleen. If the cause is phlegm coming down from the brain into the stomach, the sign is that the food turns sour in the stomach, followed by much belching. Purge the brain.

9.8 Loss of Appetite

The person wants no food, not even one mouthful, even though the body needs nourishment. The signs are emaciation and loss of vitality. When this ailment lingers, it causes fainting. For fainting, consult the proper section. If the person is very weak, enemas are not advised. Instead, reinforce the stomach (see 9.2, 9.3).

9.9 Impatient Hunger

The person acts as though he won't be able to refrain from eating and seems always to be hunting for something to eat. Reinforce the cardia by feeding apple juice and pomegranate juice (not too sour).

9.10 Severe Thirst

There are two kinds: true thirst and false thirst. True thirst is that which is experienced to offset heat. Signs of the effect of heat and dryness are apparent, and the person benefits from cold water. This is normal desire. False thirst occurs when salty phlegm and burning canker collect in the stomach and the temperament needs water to wash these away. The signs are that the body is not relieved by cold water, and the taste in the mouth is changed. In this case, breathing cold air and inhaling cold-natured substances are useful. If there are signs that the person has cold-natured substances in the stomach, he should vomit after drinking warm water with honey and vinegar. Afterward, feed anise water, chicken, and pea water. Eating garlic and honey is also effective.

In the case of salty phlegm caused by excess internal heat, allow only anise water or a little sweet almond oil. If the cause is swelling of the liver or fever, consult the sections on those problems.

9.11 Swelling of the Stomach

If the cause is cold-natured substances in the stomach, the person is slightly feverish. If it is from hot-natured substances, there is high fever and pain. In hot nature, cup the stomach but do not give strong laxatives, and induce vomiting. If there is constipation, give purging cassia, tamarind, and red clover tea. An external pomade made of sandalwood and scallions is recommended. After three days of this, change the pomade to one composed of barley flower, marshmallow, and rose water.

For cold-natured corruption, make the pomade of sweet flag root and cooked hyssop. If the cause is black bile humor, give willow oil mixed with senna pod decoction for three days.

9.12 Corruption of Stomach Juices into Rheum

If the cause is swelling of the liver, the remedy calls for ripening the rheum with a pomade made of bitter almond, willow oil, and bruised thyme. Have the person drink plenty of warm water to assist ripening. If the rheum ripens by itself, it is fine. After three days of ripening, clean it out with milk and honey water. After cleaning, drink tea of pomegranate blossoms, ammoniac, and dragon's-blood herb.

9.13 Ulcers and Boils of the Stomach

The sign is severe pain immediately after eating sour or hot foods. The location of the pain reveals whether the ulcer is in the cardia or lower part of the stomach. Apply the remedies found in 9.11 according to the signs, or give buttermilk with a little magnesia, red clover blossoms, and sour grape seeds.

In the case of boils, use the remedy for swelling of the stomach, but never forget to use an enema. For a laxative, use senna pods with syrup of chickory. If the stomach seems loose, give magnesia with barley bran.

9.14 Stomach Gas

The cause is bad cold temperament or corruption of the food in the stomach, or collection of phlegm in the stomach. See 9.1 and 9.3 for weak digestion and bad temperament. Fennel seed boiled in rose water is very useful.

9.15 Belching, Yawning, and Gasping

These are caused by excess gas. Use a purgative and correct digestion. Relief of gas can be had from ground anise in rose water or honey.

9.16 Vomiting and Nausea

Expelling matter forcibly via the mouth is called vomiting. If you have the desire to vomit and can't, it is called nausea. Use the purgative for the phlegm humor. To cause vomiting, use 1 teaspoon of tincture of lobelia every ten minutes until the effect is secured; or, for a less violent emetic, drink ¼ glass lukewarm water with 1 tablespoon honey and 5 tablespoons vinegar.

To stop vomiting caused by biliousness, give a mixture of 1 teaspoon each dates, tamarind, purslane, magnesia, and barley bran.

To stop vomiting from phlegm imbalance and to reinforce the stomach, take 1 teaspoon each aloeswood, ground clove, pennyroyal, and mastic, and add to 10 teaspoons of rose preserve. Pound and sift together, and give 1 teaspoon of the compound with 10 teaspoons of rose water.

A pomade recommended for vomiting caused by black bile humor imbalance is watercress, melilot, moss, myrtle leaves, and white clover, in equal parts, plus a little honey for texture, placed on the spleen.

Cupping close to the navel and between the shoulders and vigorous massage also have a good effect to stop vomiting.

9.17 Vomiting Blood

There are two sources: one is that a vein from the gullet or stomach is pierced or broken. It is known by a recent injury to the gullet or stomach. If there is pain between the shoulders, it is a sign that there is an ulcer in the gullet or stomach. Binding the arms and cupping the legs are recommended, as is eating large seeded raisins to help congest the vein openings.

The other source of vomited blood is an internal injury or other calamity to the liver, spleen, or head, whereby blood is poured into the stomach and thrown off. Emergency medical aid must be sought as soon as possible.

If there is a crushing chest injury and emergency medical aid is not available, this remedy is given: acacia, ammonia salt, aloe vera juice, and myrrh in equal parts, mixed with myrtle water; place over the affected organ.

9.18   Clotting of Blood

When blood spills into the stomach from an internal source and is not expelled due to lack of internal heat, it forms a clot. The signs that this has happened are that cold sweat and fainting appear and the person trembles. Boil ½ ounce each dill weed and pennyroyal, along with ½ ounce honey and the same amount of vinegar. Strain and drink hot.

9.19   Milk in the Stomach

It often happens that milk is coagulated in a nursing baby's stomach due to the illness of the mother. Adjust the mother's food during illness and give relaxing teas, such as peppermint, to both mother and baby. During the mother's illness, never feed the baby fully.

9.20   Hiccups

Mild hiccups after eating will pass without drastic treatment. If they persist for several hours, the cause must be determined and treated accordingly. If the cause is overeating, it happens immediately after the meal; remove the food with an emetic and correct the digestion.

If the vomiting continues after the food is expelled, take a decoction of pennyroyal.

If the cause is gas, which is common with babies, the hiccups occur after eating gas-producing foods. The remedy for gas is given in 9.14.

Hiccups can also be caused by excess of phlegm. If this is the cause, induce vomiting with honey and vinegar or lobelia, and adjust the digestion with fresh fruit juices and milk. Drinking warm water and 1 tablespoon of plain almond oil or butter with meals will have the same effect.

Another cause of hiccups is that moisture of phlegm has adhered to the surface of the stomach lining. The signs of this are watery mouth, sour belching, and incomplete digestion. The remedy is to use an enema.

If the cause of hiccups is bad cold nature of temperament, the signs are sleepiness, cold hands, and low pulse and are corrected by eating hot-natured foods.

If the cause is due to swelling of the liver or stomach, consult 9.11 and 10.7.

Making a person sneeze is quite effective in relieving hiccups. Sniff some black pepper. Other remedies include drinking a tea of pennyroyal with juice of pomegranate and lots of ice-cold water. Cooked cinnamon and mastic are also mentioned as effective, as is holding the breath for as long as possible.

9.21 Vomiting after Food Is Digested

The cause of this is usually that there are lesions in the intestine—when the intestine is unable to assimilate food, it must be gotten rid of (ejected) by vomiting. The remedy is given in 13.2.

9.22 Upset Stomach

Right after eating, the person feels a kind of "fearful churning" of the stomach, similar to the sensation when confronting a dangerous situation. Use a phlegm purgative and drink peppermint tea.

9.23 Convulsion of the Stomach

There is a throbbing movement in the cardia. Use a phlegm humor purgative. The cause may also be worms, which must be removed. Presence of parasites can be detected by laboratory tests.

9.24 Heartache

Severe pain is felt in the cardia. The hands become cold and clammy, and the person may faint. Consult 9.2.

9.25 Heartburn or Stomach Burn

If the cause of the burning sensation is from eating unleavened bread or green fruit or imprisonment of raw moisture in the stomach, eating moist foods will correct it. Remedy: Reinforce the digestion (see 9.2).

The cause may also be from black bile humor imbalance. If so, cup on the right or left arm, then give dates, jams, and honey. Drink fennel tea with ¼ teaspoon ground ginger added.

9.26 Slackness of the Stomach

There are two kinds: one is in the nature of the stomach. Its signs are poor digestion and projection of the chest. The other type of slackness relates to the parts that connect to the stomach. Apply what was given in the sections on slackness (2.19) and paralysis (2.18) and feed soft foods. Allow the person to inhale the fragrance of sweet flowers, and use astringent herbs.

9.27 Slackness of the Stomach Tissues

This is a degeneration of tissue that involves all parts of the stomach, and is the worst stomach affliction. The signs are false or incomplete digestion, despite eating very soft foods, and constipation. Rub the stomach with amber oil and mastic. Feed only fowl. It will take a long time and wise guidance from a physician to relieve this affliction.

9.28 Hardness of the Stomach

This hard swelling occurs mostly in the area of the cardia and can be felt, so no other signs are necessary. If the swelling is severe enough, it can even be seen. The cause is usually hot temperament. Apply cupping on the veins of the arms and make a salve of white wax, bitter almond, balsam, chicken fat, and everything that will absorb phlegm. Especially recommended is iodine, available in pure kelp and sea food or as organic iodine from a physician.

It sometimes occurs that due to hardness of the spleen, coarseness is felt in parts of the stomach. See also 11.1.

9.29 Hardness of the Stomach Muscles

Such hardness happens in the lengthwise striations of the muscle fibers. The remedy is the same as for bad, hot intemperament of the stomach (9.1).

9.30 Stomach Corruption

This can be caused from bad temperament and is treated in 9.1. The cause can also be an ulcer or boil, discussed in 9.13. Another cause is catarrh, called brain "diarrhea," and is signaled by continuous diarrhea. The person usually falls asleep for a twelve- or fourteen-hour period, and the signs do not reappear for a long time. The remedy is given in Section 2.

In this latter case, never try to stop the diarrhea. The remedy is in correcting the diet and improving digestion. If the cause is weakness of the liver, the sign is gradually increasing weakness. Remedy: Reinforce the liver and stomach, and take some mastic with a diet plentiful in fresh green vegetables.

9.31 Smallness of the Stomach

The stomach can naturally become smaller due to decreased intake of food over a period of time. If this is the case, ingesting large amounts of food at one sitting can be harmful, even if the food is soft, for the stomach is not accustomed to the quantity. The stomach may also be shriveled because of convulsion or swelling, as discussed in 9.11 and 9.23.

9.32 Stomach Flu

The sign of the heat of flu is the softness of the feces. The sign of flu from cold intemperament is thickness of the matter coming out of the nose. The remedy is to adjust the temperament and endure the symptoms. Eat soft foods, and keep the body warm and the head covered. Avoid lying flat on the back and eating sour things, milk, or meat.

Section 10
The Liver

General Considerations

The liver is a compound tubular gland located in the upper right part of the abdominal cavity immediately below the diaphragm. It is the largest gland of the body, weighing about 1,500 grams.

The main functions of the liver are the secretion of bile, the formation of blood, metabolic functions, detoxification, and a thermal function. Two of these functions—the regulation of blood volume and the production of heat—make this the most important organ from the view of natural medicine. (While the liver produces bile, this substance is stored in the gallbladder.) Some researchers believe that the liver can accomplish reoxidations and metabolic regenerations.

The functions of the liver are so vitally important for the body that they can be compared to the activity of chlorophyll in plants. Indeed, the liver is so crucial biologically that it can be called the balance of the wheel of life. Dr. Max Gerson, a pioneer of nontoxic cancer therapy, concluded that the possi-

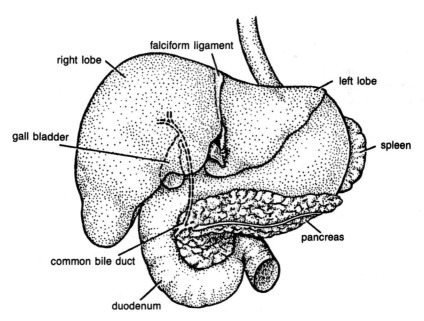

The Liver, Spleen, and Gallbladder

bility of recovery from cancer depends directly on the degree of damage to liver function. The liver can remain damaged for a long time because the deterioration of the liver cannot be detected before its great functional reserves have been consumed. The liver has great capacity to regenerate. Therefore, a partial destruction may be restored if deterioration is not extensive and rapid. The great difficulty is to determine when pathological destruction of the liver actually begins. For this purpose, the science of iridology is useful in evaluating the degree of liver degeneration.

In view of the unanimous agreement among all medical systems, new and old, on the supreme place the liver holds in human health, it is easy to see why all concern should be exercised to avoid any activities or substances that interfere with correct liver function.

One of the main conditions that affects the liver is cirrhosis, as it is called by Western medicine. It is well known that excessive consumption of alcohol in any form may lead to cirrhosis; it is also well worth considering the potential benefits to health and longevity of eliminating the consumption of alcoholic beverages. Excessive drinking (which can be the daily two or three martinis of the "social" drinker) often carries other patterns of living with it, such as lack of exercise, anxiety from high-stress vocations, large consumption of meat and fats, and high coronary-disease risks, among others.

10.1   Bad Temperament of the Liver

All the Hakims I consulted were in agreement that chickory is the best remedy for bad temperament of the liver. Senna pods are also recommended if the cause is any kind of substance obstructing the liver. When there is constipation, give laxatives and cold-natured substances such as pomegranate juice, oxymel, barley water, cold buttermilk, and sandalwood syrup. To these can be added honey and vinegar and barberry water. If the stomach is soft and queasy, drink astringent teas such as yellow dock or bayberry and magnesia with quince or apple conserve.

If imbalance of the blood humor is the cause of liver intemperament and there is no obstruction of the liver, cup the veins on the arms. If the cause is biliousness, putting cold-natured compresses over the liver will reduce the overheating. Cucumber works well.

If the person has diarrhea, fry 1 teaspoon each of purslane seeds, sweet basil seeds, and gum arabic together for ten minutes in a little oil, soak in rose water, and take 1 teaspoon several times a day.

To purge the black bile humor affecting the liver, moistening medicines are required. Apply a salve of cooked rose leaves and give a tea made from equal parts of rose hips, cowslip, mint, and anise. Be careful not to use this preparation for more than two days, for too much moisture can lead to dropsy.

10.2   Weakness of the Liver

The signs of weakness of the liver are a foul odor of the urine as it is emitted, and the color of the urine, which is like the water one would have from washing fresh meat. The appetite is lessened, and there may be general weakness. The person may complain of pain on the right side just below the last rib, especially after eating. The face color may be of a greenish tint, or sometimes yellowish. Give coffee or chickory-root enemas, and apply the remedy from 10.1 according to the signs.

10.3   Obstruction of the Liver

The tissues of the liver, or the blood vessels supplying the liver, are obstructed with phlegm. The signs of this are a lessened production of blood in the body, yellow face, diarrhea, and a feeling of heaviness in the liver. If the obstruction is in the convex portion of the liver, more heaviness is felt, and reduced amounts of thin urine are excreted. If the obstruction is in the concave part, much thick, moist fecal matter are passed. The difference between obstruction and swelling of the liver is that in swelling there is fever and pain, whereas in obstruction there is seldom pain and more heaviness is felt.

Remedy: First use enemas. Also, if the obstruction is in the convex part of the liver, give diuretics; if in the concave portion, use laxatives. Watch the diet carefully. If the obstruction is caused by eating astringent foods, it may be removed by eating such things as milk, sugar, almond oil, chicken soup, and pomegranates.

Obstruction may also be caused by narrowness of the blood vessels of the liver; this is usually apparent from childhood. The remedy is to drink diuretics and avoid eating hot and energetic foods.

10.4   Gas of the Liver

The first sign is that pain is felt under the right rib. No heaviness is felt in the liver, and there is no fever. After digestion of food, the gas increases. Eat millet, take warm baths at noon, and keep warm packs over the place where pain is felt. Give laxatives and diuretics, and follow the remedy for gas in the stomach (see 9.1, 9.3, and 9.14). Detoxification is recommended.

10.5   Liver Ache

The causes are bad temperament, gas, or swelling, discussed above.

10.6   Liver Pain after Drinking Cold Water

For some reason, this most often occurs before noon and after getting out of a warm bath. The remedy is to soak ½ ounce purslane in warm water and apply it as a poultice to the liver. A pomade of hyacinth and mastic applied over the liver is also recommended. This pain soon goes away, but has to be treated if it recurs, as it can lead to dropsy.

10.7   Swelling of the Liver

If the cause is imbalance of the blood or yellow bile humor, the signs are fever, thirst, heaviness of the stomach, pain in the area of the liver, vomiting, fainting, coldness in the extremeties, asthma, and retention of urine (or some combination of these signs). The remedy in cases of blood humor imbalance is to apply cupping on the right arm, followed by chickory water and pomegranate juice mixed with a little vinegar and honey. If there is any constipation, give laxatives, and always remember chickory enemas.

If the cause is inharmony of the yellow bile humor, apply the same remedy as for blood humor, but follow with a pomade made of barley flour, sandalwood, rose water, chickory, and vinegar (in equal parts).

If the cause is phlegm humor inharmony, the signs are an extreme heavy feeling, a salty taste of phlegm in the mouth, and a very slight pain in the liver, but no fever. Laxatives are advised.

A feeling of hardness is a sign that black bile humor is affected and must be adjusted. After the canker has been softened, milk with a little sugar can be given to good effect if there is no high temperature.

If the liver is swelling due to a blow to the body or a fall, apply this pomade: grind and sift 3 teaspoons powdered dried peas with the skins removed (soaking for fifteen minutes in water will assist easy removal) and 2 teaspoons of beeswax. Mix these with oil of violet to make into a pomade. Apply over liver.

10.8   Large, Round Swelling of Liver

Apply what was recommended for bad temperament (10.1), and follow with the remedy for swelling of the stomach (9.11). If the swelling is inclined downward toward the intestines, give a light purgative. If it is inclined toward the kidneys, give a diuretic. If the swelling tends toward the interior of the body, it is a warning sign of dropsy.

If the cause of swelling is relieved by these measures, the signs will go away, even though no rheum of phlegm passes in the urine or feces. It is difficult to determine whether the corrupted substance may have been dumped into the interior of the body.

10.9   Boils on Surface of Liver

The sign of boils is the appearance of red marks on the skin over the area of the liver, which proves there is hot, burning intemperament of the liver. The remedy is the same as prescribed for hot intemperament of the liver (10.1).

10.10   Palpitation of the Liver

The liver palpitates in convulsive movements, and there is a feeling as if someone were blowing on the liver. This condition goes away soon. Its cause is a slight obstruction of the liver, which can often relieve itself. Massage the feet and cup on the right hand.

10.11 Liver Stones

The signs of stones forming in the liver are vomiting after eating and pain felt in the liver. Swelling can be felt by touch and sometimes can be seen. There is a peculiar "sandy" quality to blood that is drawn and examined. Consult the remedy in 14.9 for kidney stones.

10.12 Shrinking of Liver

The causes and signs are the same as for smallness of the stomach. Purge the liver with laxatives and diuretics.

10.13 Diarrhea of the Liver

There are five forms of this ailment. (1) If it is caused by rupture during swelling of the liver, consult the remedy in 9.11 on swollen stomach. (2) If the urine is of a watery pink color, caused by chronic degeneration of the liver, the remedy is the same as for liver weakness (10.2). Eating raisins is good. (3) Third is the type caused by blood. This is called *zusentar* in Persian, a derivative from the Greek word that means "stomach ulcer." Its cause is an excess fullness of blood manufactured by the liver, without any internal broken blood vessels. (If the cause is from an internal injury, a fall, or the like, blood comes out continuously from the rectum. Any case of internal bleeding needs the immediate attention of a physician. It is not good to stop the flow of blood, as it may back up and inflate the kidneys.) Use enemas to assist elimination if no medical help is available. It is advisable to constipate the system to stem excessive flow of blood; syrup of purslane and mother's milk are recommended, 1 teaspoon of each. (4) In the type caused by biliousness, the sign is red pocklike marks over the liver area, indicating excessive heating of the liver and thus overproduction of bile. Apply the remedy for bad temperament of the liver (10.1). (5) Finally, there is the serum form of this ailment. This is caused by very hot blood humor and phlegm in the liver. Removing bile with a laxative is necessary. Afterward, apply a pomade made of sandalwood and rose water on the heart and liver. Cup on the right hand.

10.14 Dropsy

There are three kinds: (1) the bowel is projected because there are impacted substances in it; (2) the bowel and other parts of the body are distended due to water accumulating in the layers of the bowel (it can also be due to gas distention, in which case the bowel sounds like a drum when you tap on it); and (3) heat of the liver. In the third case, apply the remedy found in 10.1.

For dropsy, laxatives and diuretics are recommended, along with methods to open up external elimination such as steam baths, dry heat, and hot pomades. Avoid anything of a hot nature in foods, and also avoid an extreme of coldness. Drink only pure water to which anise or chickory has been added. It should be sipped plentifully during the day and at each meal. Reduce the amount of food eaten to one-sixth the amount normally eaten. The most useful single food is pomegranate; eat as much as you like. Meat-eaters should concentrate on white meat of chicken, lamb, and green vegetables such as peas. Cereals and grains should be avoided as much as possible. If they are demanded, give only rice. In dropsy types 1 and 2, use enemas and keep up with diuretics, changing the herbs from time to time since the body will gradually become immune to its efforts. If you consume herbs in capsules, grind them very fine first so that they will take immediate effect.

To induce perspiration, lie in a bath or other suitable place. Rub salt mixed with a little oil over the body, then cover it with soft sand. If the sand is cold, add more, as much as can be tolerated, as this takes the swelling away. Usually only a part of the body is treated in this way (rather than the whole body). If sand is not available, sitting with the back exposed to the sun for fifteen to thirty minutes, or bathing in warm fresh springs or mineral baths will have the same effect. The best treatment is bathing in the sea. If there is no sea water, put sun-evaporated sea salt in distilled water for three or four days and expose it to the sun. This will make an acceptable substitute for sea water. Some health food stores sell a product called Nigari, which has the therapeutic properties of sea water.

For the second kind of dropsy mentioned, distension due to accumulated water, boil 100 parts of water with 1 part of very old grape vinegar. Boil until reduced to one-third, cool, and drink. If there is coughing, do not give sour things. A pomade is also recommended for this form of dropsy, as follows: 3 teaspoons gur, 3 teaspoons lily of the valley root, 7 teaspoons beet seeds, 60 teaspoons barley flour. Grind and mix with anise water or chickory water and apply to belly.

When dropsy is chronic, as indicated by the "drum" sound on tapping, the hardness of the liver will increase, even though the person feels better. There is no problem except the swelling of the belly. This is the time to use softening pomades. When the hardness is softened, make this mixture and apply to the belly to absorb the substance: Pound together feverfew herb, melilot, seeds of wild rue, castoreum, white rose (each $1/_6$ ounce), and mix with rue water to make a pomade.

Section 11

The Spleen and Gallbladder

11.1 Jaundice

The main disease of the spleen is jaundice. It occurs in two main forms, characterized by either yellow skin (imbalance of the yellow bile humor) or brownish-black skin (black bile humor). The black form originates in the spleen itself, while the yellow type is generally caused by malfunction of the liver and gallbladder. Yellow jaundice will be discussed first.

11.2 Yellow Jaundice

1. The severe form of yellow jaundice occurs *as a complication of other illness.* The nature of the body is to expel toxic matters, so if the skin is yellow, it is a good sign that there is no failure of organ function. Bathe in warm water, and drink honey and vinegar or chickory syrup; the color will go away by itself.

2. Another form of yellow jaundice is caused by *bad temperament of the liver.* This must be treated according to 10.1.

3. *Hot temperament of the gallbladder* also causes the sign of yellowing skin. The sign that this is the problem is that it comes on suddenly, and the urine is white in color, changing a few days later to dark yellow and finally to a dark, almost brown color. There is no sign of bad temperament of the liver or obstruction. The person has a good appetite. Give honey and vinegar with chickory syrup.

4. Yellow jaundice caused by *swelling of the gallbladder* is evidenced by fever, vomiting, roughness of the tongue, and nausea. Apply the remedy given in 10.7.

5. Yellow skin is also a sign of *extreme high temperature* of the whole body. The signs are feeling the heat of the skin by touch and constipation of the bowels. If the cause is from simple excess heat, give cold foods and herbs; if it is from a corrupt substance in the body, use purgatives and general adjustment of the diet.

6. Another cause of yellowing is *obstruction of the pores,* from traveling without protection for long periods of time under a hot sun and from dust covering the skin. Open the pores by washing with cooked violet flowers, chamomile, melilot, marshmallow, and bran in equal parts.

7. Yellow jaundice is also caused by a *poisonous insect sting* or from eating *poisonous drugs or foods.* The skin is activated as an organ of elimination in such an emergency. First remove the effect. Then see sections on insect bites and poisoning (21.27). Seek emergency first aid for any accidental poisoning or serious insect or animal bite.

8. *Weakness of the gallbladder* can cause yellow jaundice. The gallbladder becomes weak and cannot absorb bile from the liver, finally resulting in jaundice. The signs are vomiting, constipation, and yellow feces. See 10.2 for the remedy.

9. *Obstruction of the vessel connection between the gallbladder and the liver* also causes jaundice. The feces gradually lighten in color until they are almost white. See next paragraph and the remedy given in 10.2.

10. *Obstruction between the gallbladder and intestine* will also cause the feces to become white suddenly, along with great constipation. The remedy is an enema to remove the obstruction. In both cases of obstruction dissolve ½ teaspoon powdered senna pods and 1 teaspoon cabbage seeds in 1 cup water; mix with 6 or 8 ground apricot kernels, and take 1 teaspoon twice a day.

11. *Fleshy growth over organ valves.* Additional tissue sometimes grows over an outlet for no known reason. Sometimes it is present from birth. There is no natural cure; sometimes the impairment can be corrected by surgery.

12. Jaundice is also caused by a kind of *phlegm colic*, due to very watery phlegm blocking the mouth of the vein going to the stomach. This is the place that bile enters the stomach. The remedy is to remove the colic.

If you want to remove the yellowness from the eyes during jaundice, inhale some stale vinegar in a warm bath and put a few drops of rose water, vinegar, and sour pomegranate juice in the eyes.

11.3   Black Jaundice

1. The bad temperament of the *spleen causes lymph fluid to be thrown off.* This is very severe and spleen diseases follow. The remedy is to assist nature in its elimination, as was mentioned in 10.13(4). Also massage with oil of feverfew herb.

2. *Obstruction of outlet between spleen and cardia;* or

3. *Obstruction of outlet between the liver and spleen* are both recognized by these signs: the jaundice appears slowly, the liver is heavy, and the appetite gradually diminishes. Open the obstruction by taking laxatives.

4. *Burning of blood humor* due to excess heat in liver. Consult 10.1.

5. *Weakness of the spleen* is seen in the signs of loss of appetite and the whites of the eyes becoming swollen. The signs of weakness of self-regulating faculty of the spleen are excretion of black bile by vomiting and diarrhea.

6. Caused by bad and *excessive cold temperament of the liver.* The remedy is given in 10.1.

If jaundice is both yellow and black, apply cupping on the veins of both arms every three days. Soften the stomach by drinking teas for purging yellow or black bile. Correct the temperament of the liver and the spleen. Foods recommended to strengthen the spleen are lemon juice, citrus, green pepper, and buckwheat.

11.4 Bad Temperament of the Spleen

If the cause is heat, the signs are burning of the spleen and redness or blackness of urine and feces. If the cause is cold, there is stomach grumbling and lack of hunger. If there is dryness, the spleen is hard, the blood is thick, and the body is generally weak. If due to moisture imbalance in the spleen, there is heaviness in the area of the spleen and the body color is ashen.

If the cause is heat, this remedy is useful: water of wormwood with ½ teaspoon each of honey and vinegar. For softening the hardness of the spleen, give honey in senna-pod tea. Give cold foods as well.

In case of cold intemperament of the spleen, give celery water with honey and vinegar, or mix two parts grape juice with one part water and reduce to half by boiling; add a teaspoon of rose water and give in the mornings.

For dryness, violet syrup is recommended.

If the cause is corrupt substances in the spleen, laxatives are advised.

For dryness, make pills from ¼ teaspoon each of red clover blossoms, hyssop, hyacinth, and barberry herb, and take two several times a day.

11.5 Swelling of the Spleen

If the cause is heat, there is fever. If the cause is phlegm, there is convulsion of the spleen. In black bile or canker, the spleen is hard.

For heat, make a pomade of barley flour and water of valerian.

For phlegm, make a pomade of rose oil and hyssop:

1. Mix with one part vinegar
2. Or mix pennyroyal and wild rue with a little vinegar
3. Or boil an ounce of bran in vinegar, add a few drops of ammoniac
and make a pomade of it.

The Hakims also recommend eating only from wooden bowls for forty days. For those suffering from a hardened spleen, cupping on the veins of the left arm is recommended.

11.6 Detoxifying the Spleen

Swelling of the spleen usually goes away by itself or becomes hard; it rarely ripens and becomes rheum. If it does become rheum, the rheum enters the stomach and is thrown off by vomiting or diarrhea. The remedy is given in 10.8. Adjust the temperament by giving diuretics.

If hardness remains after detoxifying, use the pomade in 11.5 for swelling of canker, and generally avoid using astringents. When hard swelling becomes chronic, it requires surgery.

11.7 Weakness of the Spleen

If the weakness is due to absorption of spleen fluids, there is no appetite.

If it is from lack of self-control, there is diarrhea and vomiting. If it is from bad digestion, there is good appetite and diarrhea. To reinforce the spleen, make this pomade and apply to the spleen: hyacinth, caraway, tamarisk, red clover blossoms in equal parts; grind and mix with wild rue water and vinegar and apply.

11.8 Obstructions of the Spleen

This is caused by weakness of the digestion. Remedy: Reinforce the spleen. Make a fomentation of wheat bran and salt, and add to a pomade made of gur, pennyroyal, and wild rue in equal parts. Oxymel is very useful. Apply cupping over the spleen.

11.9 Spleen Stones

The sign is a sandy granulation coming out with the urine and prickling sensation of the spleen. Eat lots of figs and apply the measures given in section 14.9.

Section 12

The Intestines

General Considerations

The small intestine has three digestive juices: pancreatic juice, intestinal juices, and bile. The first two help complete digestion by the effect of various enzymes on the food. Bile, while not a digestive juice, serves an important function by emulsifying fats and aiding in excretion of waste products.

By the time food reaches the large intestine, the digestible materials have been acted upon by the enzymes and are nearing the stage of elimination as end products. The main functions of the large intestine, then, are absorption of water and elimination of waste products.

The consistency of semifluid chyme when it leaves the stomach through the ileocecal valve remains about the same through the rest of digestion. Feces leaving the rectum are semisolid, indicating that the large intestine absorbs a very considerable amount of water.

The fluid secreted by the intestines is thick and full of mucus. Foreign substances, including drugs, are eliminated by the intestines.

Large numbers of bacteria are usually consumed with the food eaten. Most of these are destroyed by the sterilizing and digestive action of the acids in the stomach, but some pass through unaffected and appear in the large intestines.

The principal changes brought about by bacteria in the intestines are fermentations. Carbohydrates are decomposed, with alcohol and acid products as a result. Proteins are also acted upon, giving rise to putrefactive products that include amines, volatile acids, and several gases (H_2S, H_2, CO_2, and CH_4). These are primarily responsible for the characteristic odor of feces.

Some of the amines are toxic, but usually have no effect upon the body, for even if absorbed into the body, they are rendered harmless by the detoxifying action of the liver. If intestinal putrefaction is excessive, if the mucus is hard and thick, or if the liver is weak and unable to perform its detoxifying action well, toxic products of digestion may enter the general circulation of the bloodstream and produce toxic effects.

12.1 Food Passing Quickly through the Intestines

The cause may be boils in the *inner* surface of the intestines, the symptoms of which are heat in the abdomen, a feeling of pain when the food reaches the intestines, and emission of bile with the stools. The remedy is to purge the yellow bile humor and use cold drinks and enemas for relief.

If the cause is boils on the *outer* surface of the intestines, itching is felt in the intestine and pain is felt in the area of the navel and the sides of the body. Food comes out undigested. Remedy: Apply a pomade of cold-natured herbs under the navel, and use enemas.

If the cause is moisture covering the inner surface of the intestine, moisture coming out with undigested food in the stools is the sign. Remedy: Vomiting with emetics, and senna-pod tea.

The intestine can become befouled with accumulated toxins that cause bad temperament of the intestine. Signs of moisture appear (sweating, tears), but no moisture is excreted with the stools. Use enemas, and very light-acting herbs, and rub rose oil on the abdomen.

If the cause is phlegm, the passing of mucus is noticed and the person may desire to eat fruits before meals. Use enemas and increase the intake of iodine by eating kelp, watercress, and lots of greens and dates. Eliminate sugars, fruits, and bread. This herbal medicine is useful: 2 teaspoons yellow dates, and 4 teaspoons each of ground myrtle, sumac, and parsley. Pound and add honey water to make a syrup. Take 1 teaspoon with meals.

If weakness is felt in the intestine because of paralysis or slackness of the peristaltic action, consult the section on paralysis (2.20).

12.2   Diarrhea Caused by Bleeding in the Intestine

There are two forms: one is from internal scratches of the intestine; the other is that the nerves of the intestine are engorged with blood, and the ending of one or more of the nerves is raw and bleeding. One of the causes of *intestinal scratches* is eating refined salt and sugars. When these are processed, the extreme heat causes the molecular structure to change so that they cannot be completely liquefied. The resultant crystals are like minute glass particles that scratch and damage the interior of the intestines. It can also be caused by bile irritation over a long period, and the sign is diarrhea. The treatment at the beginning of the signs is to drink plenty of grape juice (if you can make your own from green grapes, it is better). Pomegranate juice and sour, astringent things such as sauerkraut and strawberries are good. If there is constipation, plantain enemas are recommended.

If the cause is phlegm, diarrhea with phlegm occurs, along with flu and catarrh of the bowels. Use an emetic, and then make an infusion from fresh basil seeds, along with black dates fried in safflower oil, and take three pills formed from this mixture twice a day.

If the cause of intestinal scratches is black bile, the sign is continuous gripe and the appearance of hardened mucus mixed with blood in the feces. After purging the black bile humor, reinforce the spleen (see 11.4) and give laxatives.

If the cause is excess of dryness in the intestine, the sign is constipation. Give moistening foods like quince, and take syrup of violet with almond oil. Use enemas. When the intestine is clear of digested foods, give astringent medicine, but never give astringents before cleaning out the colon.

If the irritation of the intestine is due to taking too many laxatives, stop them and drink plenty of buttermilk.

The second cause of diarrhea is *irritation of the nerve endings in the intestines.* Its sign is slight emission of blood with diarrhea of the stools, but there are no signs of diarrhea of the liver and no hemorrhoids. There is usually no pain. It is opposite to the signs for the other type of irritation, which has severe pain and considerable blood excreted.

Apply cupping on the arms, then take 2 drops amber oil to stop the bleeding. Apply cupping on the bowels, below the navel, alternating right to left side. Keep up the cupping for four hours to stop the diarrhea.

12.3   Phlegm Coming from Intestines

The cause is irritation of the intestinal walls or a bursting of a ballooned part of the colon. Use this herbal preparation: In 8 ounces water, boil 1 teaspoon each of pomegranate skin, sumac, myrtle, and cooked white rice; add 1 teaspoon of limestone, and use as an enema.

12.4   Gripe

Generally a little moisture comes out with the stools; it may be mixed with a little blood. There is pain. There may be an obstruction of the bowels the body wants to expel, but it cannot do it by itself. The sign is that when the person eats melon seeds and other dried seeds, they won't pass out through the bowels. Soften the intestines with warm drinks and enemas, and consult a physician. Never give astringents; this is sometimes fatal.

Phlegm, yellow, and black bile can also cause gripe. These remedies were given in 12.2.

Using enemas and suppositories is more helpful in intestinal ailments than drinking teas, as the enemas are able to go directly to the afflicted area.

If the gripe is caused by intense heat accumulating in the lower part of the intestine, the sign is feeling heavy palpitation; sometimes a fever arises, and there is difficulty in urinating. Apply cupping just under the waist, above the pubic bone, and go on a moderate fast.

If the cause is an excess of cold temperament reaching to the rectum, the remedy is applying warm fomentations to the lower abdomen, rubbing aloeswood oil on the anus, and sitting on a "hot seat" (made by heating bricks and covering with a towel folded over several times—a hot-water bottle works as well). If the anus and intestines are painful and sore on sitting down, it is enough just to rub with beeswax and egg yolk with rose oil added.

12.5   Intestinal Pain from Gripe, Swelling, and Colic

If there is pain in the intestine without any of the causes mentioned in 12.4, the cause must be determined by a doctor. If the pain is felt after drinking laxative medicines, drinking warm water in large mouthfuls and rubbing the abdomen with rose oil are sufficient.

12.6   Gas and Grumbling of Intestines

If the cause is eating gas-producing foods or overeating, the remedy is to alter the diet and eating habits. Eat rose preserves and add 1 or 2 teaspoons rosewater to tea several times a day. If the cause is coldness and weakness of the intestines, the sounds of grumbling in the intestines are there in spite of good foods in proper amounts. Remedy: Reduce the amount of food eaten at one sitting, and add cayenne pepper as a condiment to foods.

12.7   About Colic

This is a severe pain felt in the intestine, accompanied by constipation or very small hard stools passed with great difficulty. If the cause is an excess of thick phlegm in the system, the signs are constipation and the tendency to desire sour and salty things. Soften the intestines with enemas and suppositories, and afterward give a laxative to cleanse the colon completely. Adding rice-bran syrup to the diet can help alleviate constipation, especially in children.

After the constipation is removed, do not consume food for twenty-four hours. The best food after this day-long fast is pea soup containing a little chicken meat. Partridge and young lamb are also good. Don't drink much water; instead, drink 6 ounces of rose water, anise water, or honey water. Eating fresh wheat bread is also helpful.

Stomach-gas colic is caused by melancholy feelings, and the signs are that the pain happens very suddenly, even though there is no gas in the intestines or stomach. In another form, there is a great deal of sour belching but no pain. The black bile humor must be purged and a good body massage performed with oil. If there is swelling in the intestine, rub with rose oil and drink warm water.

12.8   Constipation without Pain

Remedy: Syrup of violet with almond oil, in equal parts of 2 tablespoons, to move bowels.

12.9   Intestinal Worms

There are four kinds of worms that infest the stomach or intestines. One is long; another is wide like pumpkin seeds; another is round; and another is very small, like vinegar worms. The signs of worms are that the lips are drying during the day and wet at night, and sometimes the person wakes with a little pool of saliva on the pillow. You may be able to see worms in the stool, but not always.

If the temperament is hot, which it is likely to be, never give hot medicine.

The following mixture is said to kill the worms: Make an infusion of the skin of sour pomegranate and the roots, about an ounce of each, and drink a wineglassful twice a day. If the person cannot drink the liquid, use it as an enema. The best medicine for small worms is to make a suppository of henna and wax. Insert into the rectum, but leave a little part of the suppository exposed. After a day or less, take the suppository out; some of the small worms will be embedded in it. Olive oil is also good for any kind of worms; drink a tablespoon or rub it on the anus. Ajwain added to foods is good as well.

Colonic irrigation is also quite successful in washing worm infestations out of the intestines. The addition of oxygen to the irrigation is recommended, since the worms dwell in the intestines where there is little oxygen. This should be done only by a physician.

The Anus

13.1 About Hemorrhoids

Hemorrhoids are extra skin flaps filled with swollen blood vessels, appearing along the edges of the anus. One kind is called treelike because it has many roots. Another kind is called date stone and causes corruption of the blood humor. Sometimes hemorrhoids are caused by an imbalance of the yellow bile humor. Generally burning and pain are the signs of biliousness and blood causes; pain and a prickling itch are the signs of thickened blood humor. Apply cupping on the inside of the buttocks, soften the stomach, and correct the blood humor. If there is bleeding, rub some amber oil on the anus.

If hemorrhoids are painful but there is no bleeding, make a fomentation of marshmallow and common dill, apply for half an hour at a time, and rub the anus area with peach oil. Then make a suppository of onion decoction, and use it also for enemas, to purify and cleanse the area of toxins. Hemorrhoids can usually be soothed simply by applying a flower oil. Surgical removal is sometimes recommended, but the hemorrhoids do grow back in some cases.

13.2 Flatulency

Flatulency means a thick gaseousness produced in the intestines, and it is painful. The gas sometimes goes down and is emitted as farting; other times it recedes back into the bowels or is trapped for a time in bowel pockets. There may be slight bleeding, diarrhea, and also grumbling of the lower bowels. Use the black bile purgative, and take gas-relieving remedies (see 13.6). Massage, taking warm baths, and cupping the veins of the arm is recommended.

13.3 Anus Ulcer

This has its beginning as a lesion on the interior surface, toward the intestines. There is bile being secreted consistently. First press the ulcer to take out the bile, then use a suppository (soak it in gum arabic decoction first). If the ulcer is in the intestine proper and gas and feces are emitted via the ulcer, it is a dangerous condition that needs expert medical attention.

13.4 Swelling of the Anus

Because of intemperament of heat, the anus is inflamed and painful. Apply cupping between the buttocks. Apply white of egg mixed with arnicated oil. If it is very painful, grind some marijuana seeds and add to the mixture. Vomiting is said to have a great beneficial effect.

13.5   Cracks in the Anus

This pertains to cracks of the lips of the anus on the outer, exposed surface. Avoid drinking very cold water or sour things. Try to keep the bowels soft and moving easily. Give syrup of violet, almond oil, and decoction of quince seeds and plenty of laxative foods.

13.6   Slackness of the Sphincter Muscle

The sign is the unintentional expulsion of gas. Remedy: Purge the bowels with enemas.

13.7   Protrusion of the Anus

If the cause is swelling, treat by cooking 1 teaspoon marshmallow and the same amount of violet; mix in olive oil and apply to the anus while pushing the protruded part back into the rectum. If the cause is slackness of the sphincter, the sign is that the anus protrusion goes in and out quite easily. Rub oil on the anus and make a powder of pomegranate flower and apply to the anus.

13.8   Itching of the Anus

The cause may be small worms, which are treated by oxygen colonic irrigation by a physician. If the cause is phlegm, use a phlegm purgative and apply cupping on the coccyx. Rub the anus with 1 ounce vinegar mixed with ½ dram rose oil to relieve itching. Essential oil of wormwood is effective in 3-drop doses. Consumption of pumpkin seeds is said to remove worms. Ajwain, as a tea and added to foods as a spice, is also effective.

The Kidneys

General Considerations

The kidneys are paired organs, each located next to the spine along the back wall of the abdomen at about the level of the last thoracic vertebrae. The unit of the kidney composition and function is the *nephron*, about one million to each kidney.

The nephrons maintain the constancy of the blood by filtering the reabsorbing substances that are present in excess quantity and ejecting them as urine.

The secretion of urine is accomplished by direct nerve impulses on the blood vessels leading to the kidneys, by other nerve impulses acting on endocrine glands, and through the effects of pituitary and adrenal hormones.

14.1 Bad Temperament of the Kidneys

The sign is difficult or incomplete urination or other signs of hot or cold intemperament. The remedy is to inhale vapor of camphor; its essence travels to the kidneys. Do not inhale too much of this essence, as it can lead to loss of sex drive.

14.2 Emaciation of the Kidneys

The signs are white or colorless urine and pain, weakness of the body, loss of virility, backache, and headache. Remedy: Reinforce the kidneys by diet consisting of large amounts of pure water, kidney meats, parsley, leafy green vegetables, wheat germ, and fresh green peas. Avoid coffee, alcohol, and other stimulants.

14.3 Weakness of the Kidneys

Its signs are backache, especially when bowing, bending down, or turning from side to side; weakness of virility; and lessened tendency to urinate. Cure by diet as in 14.2 and the detoxification regimen. If the cause is bad temperament, adjust it.

The Hakims say that excessive sexual intercourse will cause weakness of the kidneys, by causing the outlet of the kidneys to widen or slacken. Reinforce the kidneys by diet.

14.4 Gas of Kidney

Its sign is pain in the kidney area, but no intestinal flatulency and no heaviness. The pain diminishes as the time for eating approaches. Remedy: Make a

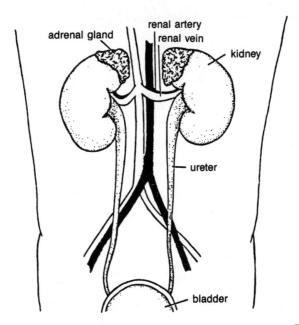

The Kidneys

pomade of equal parts common dill, cumin, wild rue, and feverfew, and apply externally to the kidneys. Drink honey water with vinegar and eat foods that remove gas (see 13.6).

14.5 Kidney Ache

Its cause is gas, swelling, weakness, kidney stones, or ulcer of the kidney. Remove the cause, consulting the appropriate sections, and afterward give this medicine: 1 teaspoon each of common dill, feverfew, and marshmallow, made into a decoction with 2 cups water; take 1 teaspoon three times a day.

14.6 Swelling of the Kidneys

The signs of this are the same as for swelling of the liver (10.7). Sometimes pain is felt in the waist. If swelling is in the right kidney, the pain is felt a little above the kidneys, close to the liver. If swelling is in the left kidney, it is felt somewhat lower, because the right kidney is a little higher than the left one. If swelling is in the ducts of the kidneys, there is difficulty in passing urine. If the swelling is in the lower part of the kidney, in the intestinal area, the pain is entirely internal and creates colic. If the swelling is chronic, go on a detoxification program, and correct the diet by including more fresh greens and cutting back on fruits. No sugar should be eaten.

14.7 Ulcers of the Kidneys

The sign is passing of phlegm, blood, and small bits of tissue with the urine, and there is pain in the kidneys. Purge the phlegm humor, but do not give strong purgatives (mild ones are all right). After adjusting the phlegm humor, diuretics are advised.

14.8 Dry Scabbing of the Kidneys

The symptom of this is itching in the area of the kidneys, and its remedy is to use a purgative. Use an emetic two times a week, and give syrup of violet. Drop 2 or 3 drops of sandalwood oil with sweet almond oil into the urethra outlet.

14.9 Kidney Stones

If the system is congested with toxins, this ailment may recur. Detoxification is recommended. The signs of a condition leading to kidney stones are heaviness of the stomach, extended abdomen, yellowness or redness of the urine, passing of small stones, and excruciating pain. The symptoms are most often severe. Adjust the digestion and avoid all stimulating foods and spices, eating very little. Refraining from sexual intercourse, sleeping on a plain cotton mattress, frequent mild baths, and drinking lots of cold water during meals and upon waking are all recommended to help prevent stone formation. Usually the pain is so severe during an attack of kidney stones that narcotics are administered. Consult a physician.

The Urinary Bladder

General Considerations

The urinary bladder is an oval-shaped muscular sac located in the front part of the pelvic cavity, just behind the pubic area.

The bladder is a storage place for urine, which is received from the ureters, which open into the bladder on the lower back side of the bladder. The urine is discharged periodically through the urethra.

The ureters enter the bladder at an oblique angle, and there is a mucous membrane at each opening that acts as a valve.

The urethra is the duct that carries the urine from the bladder to outside the body. In men, it also carries the semen. In women, its function is solely excretory.

Urine consists of 95 percent water and 5 percent solids. The principal organic constituent of urine is urea (23 percent); the two chlorides, sodium chloride (9 percent) and potassium chloride (2.5 percent), make up the main inorganic substances.

Under normal conditions, urine has the following characteristics:

1. *Color:* amber, due to urochrome, a pigment of unknown origin. Drugs, illness, or certain foods may alter the color.

2. *Transparency:* Normal urine is clear and transparent. It will become cloudy after standing for a while, due to bacterial action. Bacterial infection of the urogenital tract can produce similar cloudy urine.

3. *pH:* Urine is usually acid, with a pH around 6.0. This acidity is mainly due to the presence of sodium acid phosphate. The pH varies considerably with diet, with vegetable and fruit diets lowering the acidity and resulting in alkaline urine. Acidity increases in certain diseases (such as diabetes), and varies throughout the day as elimination of wastes and toxins occurs.

The Hakims make use of many observable characteristics of urine (see Chapter 8) to determine imbalances.

15.1 Swelling of the Bladder

If the cause is hot intemperament, there is severe pain in the pubic area, with gas, hot fever, and difficulty in urinating. The remedy calls for cupping on the leg veins and weak diuretics. Do not use pomades. If the heat is causing putrefaction and accumulated matter, try to ripen the matter and purge it.

If the cause is from cold nature intemperament, the signs are hard swelling of the bladder and the signs of black bile and phlegm humor imbalance.

For phlegm imbalance, the remedy consists of vomiting, enemas, sitz baths, drinking diuretics, honey water, and decoction of senna leaves. In black bile humor imbalance, apply pomades made of laxative herbs (cucumber seeds, cassia, dates, anise, and the like, mixed with almond oil). Do not give too many diuretic herbs, as they may cause too rapid detoxification, which can be known from a high alkaline pH of the urine.

15.2   Ulcers of the Bladder

The signs are small amounts of tissue passed with the urine, burning, and difficulty in urinating. The remedy is the same as for kidney ulcers (14.7). If there is also rheum coming out, mix 1 tablespoon of distilled water with ½ teaspoon of honey. Apply the remedy via the urethral outlet with a sterile eyedropper, so the herbs go directly to work. Women can apply herbs by douche injection.

15.3   Dry Scab of the Bladder

The signs are itching in the area of the bladder, pain, burning on urination, and blood secreted with the urine. The treatment should be designed more to adjust than to purge, because the adjustment has an immediate effect. This is the opposite of the treatment of kidney scab, in which purging is better and preferred. Put a few drops of this infusion into the urethra: equal parts of the mucilage of seeds of quince, mother's milk, and almond oil. It is always useful to use an enema in problems with the urinary bladder. The best foods are barley, oily soups, wheat germ, whole grains, green leafy vegetables, beans, and nuts. Avoid salt, coffee, and acid-forming foods as well as fruits.

15.4   Clotting of Blood in Bladder

When incomplete elimination of blood occurs, there may be clotting in the bladder itself. The signs that this has happened are fainting and both sides of the body becoming cold. There may be general trembling of the body, especially after a blow or other injury. Strong diuretics should be given, along with cooked black-eyed peas and wild rue tea. Oxymel is also very good. The diet can be amended to include chicken soup with black-eyed peas and cinnamon. Bleeding from the urethra after a wound requires medical treatment as soon as possible.

15.5   Ache of the Bladder

The cause can be either swelling, ulcer, or dry scab of the bladder. These were all discussed in earlier sections. There are two other causes to be explained:

1. *Ache caused by bad temperament.* If the temperament is too hot, the person feels thirsty and there is a burning sensation on urination. The remedy is to adjust the diet with cold-natured foods and to use pomades of cold herbs. If the cause is cold nature intemperament, the sign is whiteness or colorlessness of the urine. The remedy involves keeping the person warm under blankets,

pouring warm water over the urinary bladder, and improving the diet.

2. *Ache due to effort of bladder to repulse effete matter.* The sign is the appearance of putrid matter with the urine. Drink plenty of water to help the elimination process.

15.6 Displacement of the Bladder

The cause may be congenital or due to a fall, severe beating, or blows to the back. An internal surgeon should be consulted for congenital defects as soon as they are suspected. Otherwise, give sweet basil and sweetmeats. If the displacement lingers, imprisonment of urine may occur. Consult a physician.

15.7 Flatulency of the Bladder

The sign is the physical appearance of distension of the bladder over the pubic bone. If there is heaviness of the bladder with the area of distension moving from one place to another, the cause is only trapped air. But if there is heaviness without transference of the distention, the cause is moisture being mixed with the trapped air.

Remedy: Give a decoction of peppermint roots with 1 teaspoon of castor oil added to it for a few days. Then give 2 ounces of castor oil every few hours, and rub the bladder area with saffron oil. If there is trouble urinating, dry and pulverize the skin of a yellow melon and give 1 teaspoon of it every few hours. If there is moisture mixed with the trapped air, emetics are recommended. Marijuana tea and figs are recommended, singly or together.

15.8 Bladder Stones

The sign of presence of stones in the bladder is that immediately after emptying the bladder, the person desires to urinate again. In men, there may be a sudden erection without stimulation, which may remain for some time, but there is no pain in the bladder unless it is blocked by a stone. It is rather common that stones are formed in the bladder or pass down from the kidneys into the bladder for expulsion. A sharp pain in the area of the kidneys and back of the thighs, which then passes, is a sign that a stone is descending from the kidneys into the bladder. The remedy was given in 14.9. Surgical removal of stones may be necessary, so consult a physician if the signs persist and are severe.

If the stone is stopped in the outlet of the bladder and there is much pain and inability to urinate, a recommended first aid measure is to have the person lie on his back, lift the legs, pour warm water on the pubic bone, and apply vigorous massage from the chest down to the pubic bone. This may dislodge the stone and allow it to pass out.

15.9 Burning on Urination

If caused by dry scab of the kidney or bladder, consult 14.8 and 15.3. It may also be caused by an ulcer in the outlet of the penis, which is discussed later. The cause may also be due to liver heat or prevalence of biliousness, which signs are discussed in Chapter 6. Apply what was given in 10.1. If adjustment is not sufficient, use enemas and drop 3 or 4 drops of this mixture into the urethra: 1 ounce mother's milk, 1 drop rose oil, and ½ ounce almond oil. Males should soak the penis in alkaline water; females should bathe the urethra opening with same. Make alkaline water by soaking three figs in a pint of water and straining. Burning on urination may be a sign of venereal disease. If it persists or is accompanied by discharge of pus or blood, consult a physician.

15.10   Retention of Urine

Causes for which remedies have already been mentioned are swelling of kidney (14.6), swelling of urinary bladder (15.1), urinary or kidney stones (14.9, 15.8), rheum in the bladder (15.1), or gas of the bladder (15.7, 20.19). Retention of urine may also be caused by ulcers or boils in the bladder (see 15.2).

Retention may also be caused by internal growths on the bladder outlet or congenital smallness or other change in the outlet. The sign of congenital defects is that there are no other signs of disease; the only remedy is surgical correction.

Slackness of the muscles of the bladder is another case; this is the problem if urine is forced out when one presses on the bladder from above the pubic bone. Treat this by giving warm drinks and teas; consult the section on paralysis (2.20) for oils to rub on the bladder area.

If the cause is obstruction of the vessel between the bladder and urethra by phlegm, the sign is a sensation of heaviness in the area of the pubis. Give strong diuretics and have the person sit in warm water. If the cause is weakness of the expulsive power of the bladder, the sign is that the person can delay going to the bathroom for several hours, but when he does go, the urine will not come out. Have him sit in warm water and press the bladder to expel the urine. To revive the expulsive power of the bladder, apply oil of aloeswood on the pubis. If this doesn't work, the urine will have to be extracted with a catheter, which requires the assistance of a medical doctor.

Another cause of inability to urinate is constipation and dryness occuring in the bladder outlet, due to severe heat. The signs are heat patches over the pubis, an improved sense of well-being after drinking fluids, and inability to expel small amounts of urine (i.e., the person can only urinate after a long period). The remedy is to give moistening and cold drinks.

If the cause is weakness of the urinary urge, the remedy is dropping several drops of saffron oil into the urethra, applying sweet-smelling pomades, drinking lots of water, and taking moderate doses of castor oil.

15.11   Frequent Expulsion of Urine; Diabetes

If the cause is slackness of the bladder muscles, hot intemperament, or swelling of an adjacent part, the remedies are given in 15.10. Involuntary urination may also come from taking too many diuretics, consuming too much melon, or improper metabolism of sugar. Remove the cause. Frequent urination may signify diabetes.

This condition can also be caused by misalignment of the lumbar vertebrae after a fall or a blow to the back or urinary bladder. This needs correction by a physician. If the blow has caused improper alignment of the vertebrae toward the inside (anterior), apply cupping to the vertebrae affected. If it is toward the outside (posterior), you can probably notice the specific vertebrae out of alignment by having the person remove his clothes and bend from the waist. Have the person see a chiropractor, osteopath, naprapath, or similar practitioner. However, many masseurs can correct this as well. Cupping on the back is very effective.

If the expulsion of urine is the result of nerve damage, there is no herbal cure. Consult a physician.

15.12   Bedwetting

Although some adults are afflicted with urinating in bed, it is mainly a problem with children. (Consult 15.10 about slackness of the bladder muscles.) Do not give any food or water for two hours before bedtime. If the child begins to urinate during sleep, try to wake him up and take him to the bathroom. This medicine is advised: ¼ teaspoon each cumin, mastic, and myrtle, mixed with 2 or 3 ounces honey. Give in teaspoon doses morning and evening.

15.13   Urine Mixed with Blood

If there is no pain or mucus, this condition may be due to irritation of the nerves of the kidney. If the blood is coming in small amounts regularly, this is probably the cause. While any bleeding needs attention by a physician, you can apply first aid if necessary to stop the bleeding by cupping over the bladder, pouring cold water over the pubis, and giving a medicine of jujube syrup with coriander.

If weakness of the kidneys is causing bleeding, the urine looks white and thick; if it is caused in the liver, the urine is reddish and thin. In either case, the kidneys and liver must be reinforced.

The Male Reproductive System

In the following sections, these descriptions of tissue are given: the skin of the abdomen is called the *hypochondria*; the layer under it is called the *peritoneum*; and the fatty layer under the peritoneum which is touching the intestines is called the *omentum*.

16.1 Weakness of Virility

Completeness of the sex drive depends upon the health of the male organs. A lack of virility appears in two syndromes; one is that the libido and drive for sexual intercourse are weak, the other is that an erection is difficult to achieve and maintain.

Weakness of sex drive The first cause is eating too little food. Since the body depends on food to sustain life, the spirit, humors, and blood that are the substances of sexual energy diminish. The signs of this condition are general weakness, loss of energy, and feeling hungry much of the time. The remedy is to consume more nutritious food and stimulating herbs such as spearmint, and to remove anxiety and worry so that life may be enjoyed. Listening to music is recommended.

A second sign of weakened sex drive is that there is reduced semen production in spite of proper nutrition. The sign is emission of very small amounts of semen during intercourse. The cause of this is bad temperament in the semen-producing organs. Correct with heating foods and spices.

There is a difference between insufficient semen production and low sperm count—they can occur quite independently of each other. Also, low sperm count can be caused by excessive exposure to radiation and certain chemicals, not uncommon hazards for American workers.

A third sign of weakened sex drive is that even though semen is produced in sufficient quantity, it is not emitted during ejaculation. If this is the case, there is emission of only clear fluid, and the semen is retained or it comes out very thick and with difficulty. Also, the penis is semiflaccid during sexual foreplay, but becomes erect during intercourse. The remedy is to eat humorally hot foods and drink teas made from hot herbs.

Fourth, abstention from intercourse for an extended period will cause the sex drive to become weak. The mind must convey to the body a willingness to perform sex. Pellitory root rubbed in cottonseed oil applied to the pubis and penis is recommended.

Fifth, loss of sex drive can be due to feelings of inferiority or an imagination that the male is incapable of performing sex adequately. The man gradually loses all interest, even though he may be young and healthy and may be producing plenty of semen. This must be treated by personal guidance and counseling.

The sex drive may also become weak due to related weakness of the heart, kidney, liver, or brain. Consult the section on these organs for removal of these conditions.

16.2 Slackness of Penis

The first cause is from weakness of the sex drive or abstinence from sex for a long period. In the case of abstinence from sex, washing the penis with warm water before intercourse is helpful, as is massaging the penis with oil of musk.

The cause may be due to lack of production of the humors in the lower part of the body, and is caused by imbalance of heat, cold, or moisture.

The nerves governing the erective faculty may become blunted due to congestion of phlegm or exposure to extreme coldness, for which the signs are the thinness of the seminal fluid and that it "leaks" when there is no sexual stimulation. Seek the remedy in the section on paralysis (2.20). Using an enema

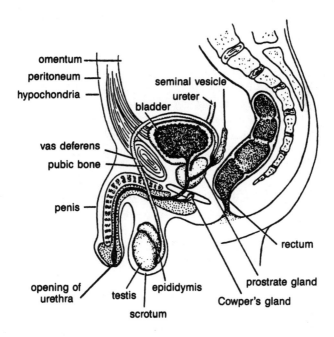

The Male Reproductive Organs

and suppositories for increasing heat and removing phlegm congestion are useful. (The Hakims say that the one whose penis does not shrink when placed in cold water cannot be cured.) Some of the remedies to stimulate full erection are washing the penis with an infusion of celery seeds and rubbing with oil of purslane. Oil of lily of the valley or bathing in celery water is said to have the same effect.

16.3   Premature Ejaculation

One of the causes is lack of self-control. The signs of this are whiteness and thinness of the semen; the remedy is purging the system with medicine for cold intemperament and taking an emetic.

Another cause is prevalence of semen and blood, which is shown by very hard and strong erections and engorgement of the glans with blood. One remedy is to increase frequency of intercourse and to eat less food, making the diet consist of more sour things and foods that decrease production of blood. If the semen is expelled with excessive force, there is burning on ejaculation and the semen is thin and yellow. Decoction of lettuce seeds and other cold-natured medicines are recommended. Hasty discharge may also be caused by weakness of the sex organs, which need to be strengthened according to 16.1.

16.4   Excessive Sex Drive

The man seems tied to his emotions and can't seem to get sex off his mind. The first cause is prevalence of semen and blood, which is known by flushed cheeks, rash on the chest, and similar signs of heat. Using laxatives and eating sour foods may help to decrease the urge. If the semen is expelled with great force, drinking honey with ice water is helpful.

There may be adequate semen but general weakness and insufficiency of blood, whose signs are excess discharge of thin and white semen and much flatulence. Remedy: Give wild rue seed and khalonji, each ¼ teaspoon, with 10 drops of oil of almond added, 1 teaspoon with tea twice a day.

Another cause of excessive sex drive is due to strength of the semen-producing organs but weakness of other important organs of the body, such as strong sperm production but weakness of the heart. The remedy is to stem the sexual energy by wholesome exercise, building up the other systems of the body.

The sex drive may be increased along with appearance of boils, ulceration, or itching of the penis outlet. The sign is primarily excessive lust and intercourse. If the boils turn into ulcers, there will be pain. The remedy is to use the purgative for the urinary bladder, given in 14.7 and 15.2.

If excessive sex drive is due to prevalence of the production of gas in the body, the sign is intense erection, for which cold-natured herbs should be given as tea several times per day. If black bile humoral inharmony signs are present, use cupping and give a black bile purgative as well.

16.5   Corrupted Semen

There are two kinds: (1) a moist substance comes out, although it is emitted not from the seminal vesicles but from another duct above the seminal vessel; (2) a sticky moisture is expelled with the urine.

The cause of either of these may be prevalence of semen or slackness of the veins serving the seminal or semen-producing organs. The remedy is given in 16.3. A second cause of corrupted semen is convulsion of the muscle of the seminal vein, which is known from expulsion of semen at the first period of erection, or successive erection and loss of erection of the penis. The remedy is rubbing rose or another mild oil on the penis and testicles, and curing the convulsion.

Corrupted semen is also caused by weakness of the kidneys, or can be due to a condition following rapid weight loss. The sign is that after intercourse, a white, thick substance similar to semen comes out with the urine. Apply what was said about weakness of the kidney in 14.3.

If semen is spontaneously emitted when a man hears others talking about sex or when he himself is thinking about engaging in sex, he should try to develop more self-control.

16.6   Excretion of Blood with Semen

The cause is weakness of the kidneys and testicles. Soak the testicles in a bowl of mastic with some olive oil added, and strengthen the kidneys (see 14.2).

16.7   Constant Erection of the Penis

If the cause is prevalence of blood, adjust the blood humor, use a blood purgative, and eat cold foods and herbal teas. If the temperament is cold and dry, procure emesis and give medicine to remove flatulency. Afterward, rub oil of wild rue on the pubis, genitals, and back.

16.8   Defecation during Ejaculation

The cause is excess moisture and weakness of the sexual organs and bowel muscles. Reinforce the bowel and abdominal muscles with exercise such as situps, and use this suppository: equal parts of pomegranate flowers, and gum arabic (or mastic). Rub the anus with oil of hyacinth. Immediately before intercourse, the stomach should be empty.

16.9   Feeling of Itch in Intestine

This comes with the urge to have intercourse with a woman, and can be caused by foul substances eaten (remedy: purgative) or prevalence of improper temperament (remedy: eat sour foods).

16.10   Swelling of the Testicles

If the cause is in the blood humor, the sign is heaviness, swelling, and heat of the testicles. If the cause is biliousness, the sign is very intense heat of the testicles. Apply cupping on the back and legs, and afterward use rose oil. (Consult the sections on general swellings.)

If the cause is imbalance of the phlegm humor, the testicles look pale and white. The remedy for phlegm imbalance is first to cause vomiting, then to give cooked anise seeds, licorice root tea, rose preserve, and the purgative for phelgm. Use a salve of equal parts of green beans and peas (dried, pounded, and sifted) and honey.

If the cause is black bile humor, the testicles are swollen and hard. Give the purgative for black bile.

If the cause is flatulency, the testicles seem full and inflated. The remedy is to apply a cloth soaked with decoction made from gas-reducing herbs such as peppermint, catnip, or chamomile. If that doesn't work, try vomiting and using diuretics. Vomiting is most recommended for conditions affecting the lower parts of the body.

NOTE: If the origin of the swelling is in the skin of the testicles, the symptoms can be felt mildly. If the cause is in the testicles themselves, the symptoms are more severe, and there is often feverishness and thirst.

16.11   Enlarged Testicles

The cause may be fatty tissue, not swelling. Make a salve of hemlock bark, apple, and infusion of coriander, and add a little vinegar to it. This can be used as an application to the testicles, or to the breasts if they are swollen. Fasting is required.

16.12   Convulsion of the Penis

The sign is shrinking or twisting up of the penis. The remedy is using a purgative, purifying the blood humor, and afterward using a purgative again. Correct the diet.

16.13   Aching Testicles

The cause may be swelling (16.10). It may also be due to accumulated gas from sexual excitement that is not gratified for an extended period. Fomentations and lubrication with olive or rose oil are usually sufficient, along with keeping a little warmer than usual. If the cause is injury to the testicles from a blow, apply a salve made of equal parts violet, marshmallow, pumpkin, and water lily (white or yellow).

16.14   Shrinking of Testicles

The cause is exposure to cold. Take a warm bath to restore elasticity of skin.

16.15   Ascended Testicles

The testicles sometimes ascend into the hypochondria, the soft part just under the cartilage of the pubic bone, and cannot be seen. When this happens, there is difficulty in urinating. If they ascend only slightly (as at time of ejaculation), it is not harmful nor painful, but if they remain up for a long time, it is harmful. The remedy is to sit in a warm bath, rub warm olive oil on the testicles and let it be absorbed. Cupping can be applied to the testicles if bathing does not cause descension.

NOTE: Sometimes the penis recedes back into the body cavity. The same measures can be applied.

16.16   Drooping Testicles

The veins of the testicles become elongated so that the testicles hang down farther than they should. The remedy is in the section on veins of the leg (18.5). If the skin of the testicles becomes hardened, apply the remedy in 16.10.

16.17   Slackness of Testicle Skin

Use a remedy composed of gallnut, myrtle, rose, and pomegranate flower. Make a salve or a weak decoction and bathe the testicles in it.

16.18   Ulcers of Penis and Testicles and Genital Area

One kind of ulceration is fresh, appearing suddenly. Use a purgative and detoxify. Another kind develops slowly and lingers. This remedy is recommended: ½ teaspoon dragon's-blood, ½ teaspoon myrrh, and 2 teaspoons juice of aloe vera. Make a salve, mix with a few drops of rose oil, and apply.

NOTE: The sign of a penis ulcer in the urethra is burning on urination and pain. The remedy for this is given in 15.2.

16.19   Swelling of the Penis

See the remedy in 16.10.

16.20   Hard Boils Appearing on the Penis

Mix ½ ounce fennel seed in 2 ounces vinegar, add a little vegetable oil, and apply to boils.

16.21   Itching of Testicles and Penis

Apply cupping on the thigh and knee. Take warm baths. Massage with vinegar and rose oil, with some egg white mixed in.

16.22   Obstruction of the Urethra

If the cause is boils, the urine is expelled with great difficulty, and burning is felt. Rub decoction of purslane and melon seeds mixed with violet oil and almond oil on the penis several times per day. When the boil opens and begins to drain, place a few drops of mother's milk and violet oil into the opening.

If the urethra is sticking together from secretions from the boil, the urine comes out with difficulty but without pain. Drink a mixture made from equal parts of waters of chamomile, melilot, and sweet marjoram. A little of this can be poured through a fine strainer and dropped into the opening of the penis.

16.23   Twisting of the Penis

This is caused either by swelling of the muscle of the penis or convulsion of the nerves in the penis. Rubbing the penis with warm oils and taking a warm bath during which the penis can be straightened are recommended.

16.24   Separation of the Peritoneum

Separation of the peritoneum occurs on the inner side of the thigh, toward the testicles. When there is a separation of this tissue, adjacent parts of the omentum or intestines (and sometimes fluids) come down into the testicles. This condition is called *cornia* in Tibb medicine, and hydrocele in Western medicine. It has four forms:

1. Water descends little by little, with gurgling, grumbling and other sounds. Sometimes it is accompanied by spastic pains like colic. The remedy is to rub the area slowly and massage the intestine. Pouring warm water on it also helps, as does sitting in warm baths. Then, put a poultice on the testicles, also covering the inner part of the groin and pubic area. The poultice is made as follows: pound equal parts of pine buds, resin (or gum), mastic, pomegranate flowers, dragon's-blood, aloe gum, and juniper berries. Mix in enough olive oil to give consistency (water will do as well), and spread on a cloth. Bind in place for three days and keep the person lying on his back. After three days, he can get up and move around carefully. Add much cumin seed to the food.

2. Gas moving around in the groin, with severe grumbling. Eat no gas-producing foods and make a binding of clean cloth that holds the area firmly in place.

3. The testicles become full of fluid and heavy. The remedy is to remove the water or liquid by applying what was said about dropsy in 10.14.

4. Thickness, hardness, and stretching of the testicles. This is different from simple swelling of the testicles in that the latter is caused by a corrupted substance. Purge the black bile humor and apply what was said in 16.10.

16.25 Hernia of the Abdomen Hypochondria (and Hernia of the Groin)

It sometimes occurs that the peritoneum tissue is torn close to the area of the navel, or higher, even though the hypochondria itself is sound. Thus, what is situated below the peritoneum is distended and lifts up the hypochondria. Sometimes it happens that in the area of the groin, a break appears in the peritoneum, also causing hernia. The only procedure that can be recommended by natural medicine is to apply heavy binding. Surgery may be necessary to repair the tears in the wall of the peritoneum. Consult a medical doctor for advice and examination.

NOTE: At the beginning of hernia, acupuncture on the toes of both feet and on the five fingers of the opposite hand is said to be helpful.

16.26 Changes in the Navel

Infrequently, due to improper cutting of the umbilical cord at birth, various changes occur in the navel scar. If it becomes protruded, it can be repaired while the infant is still a few weeks old. When it becomes healed and scar tissue forms, it is more difficult to repair.

Changes at times other than infancy may indicate herniation of the peritoneum wall, discussed in the preceding section.

Other changes can be caused by excess phlegm moisture gathering in the area of the navel (as in dropsy), gathering of excess flatulence, growth of excess flesh in the navel, or blood accumulating under the navel due to a rupture of a blood vessel.

The sign of a hernia is the turning inward of the fleshy part of the navel, with or without intestinal sounds. The sign of accumulated moisture of phlegm is heaviness in the navel area, and the sign of flatulence is extreme softness of the navel.

The remedy for flatulence is mentioned in 10.14. Extraneous growth of flesh must be treated by a physician, as must signs of broken blood vessels. An emergency salve of wax and rose oil can be applied until a doctor can treat it.

16.27 Acquired Immune Deficiency Syndrome (AIDS)

Medical research as of the date of publication of this book is inconclusive as to the specific cause of this sexually transmitted disease. While one or more viruses have been identified as causative agents, additional viruses or other factors that contribute to AIDS may ultimately be discovered. The greater proportion of those who contract the disease are homosexual males and intravenous drug users.

According to the original Tibb texts, anal intercourse is totally forbidden. The extremely toxic microbial life present in human feces makes it utterly vital to avoid anal intercourse with men or women.

Whenever the immune system is compromised, all efforts must be aimed at restoring the metabolic efficiency of the entire human organism. The first course in this process would be to undergo radical detoxification, which must be administered and supervised by a naturopathic physician.

In such a program of detoxification, the black bile humor must be purged constantly (see directions for adjusting the humors at front of Formulary). In addition, a wide range of nutritional supplements may be advised to assist the body in elimination. Organic iodine (Lugol's Solution) administered orally in 5-drop doses, twice daily, may prove especially beneficial. Once the toxic matters are thoroughly repulsed, a long-term program of rebuilding vital organs must be undertaken.

The Female Reproductive System

17.1 Suppressed Menses

A mild diuretic is recommended, as follows: take 2 teaspoons of half-pounded anise, boil in a cup of water for five minutes. Filter, and add ½ teaspoon each of powdered cucumber seeds and melon seeds. Sweeten with honey and drink.

The specific emmenagogue to open the menstrual flow is composed of ⅛ teaspoon each of senna pods and fennel seeds, and 2 teaspoons juniper berries. Take ¼ to ⅛ teaspoon every morning, followed by a cup of anise tea. This will open the menstrual flow if the cause is not due to high temperature and insufficient blood.

A medicine to open the menstrual flow or suppressed semen is composed of 2 teaspoons each fennel seeds, wild rue, wormwood, and celery seeds, 5 figs, rose hips, and honey, combined to make ½ cup. Boil together for five minutes and consume in tablespoon doses twice a day for three days. Stop for three days, then repeat dose for three more days.

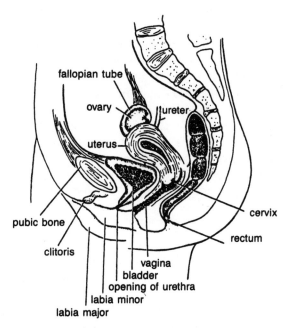

The Female Reproductive Organs

17.2   Excessive Menstrual Flow

The prevalence of menstrual blood is easily noticed. The remedy is to decrease the blood by using enemas and cupping on the abdomen. If the blood is thin, the cause is biliousness, for which the remedy is enemas, thickening of blood, suppositories, and rubbing sandalwood oil on the pubis.

If the cause is phlegm, there will be excessive blood, its character being white and thin. The remedy is decreasing the blood temperament. If the cause is excess of black bile, the remedy is to use a laxative to purge the black bile humor.

If the cause is hemorrhoids or ulcer of the womb, consult the section on those conditions.

At the time of rupture of the hymen, there may be blood flow. This can be remedied by sitting in astringent baths and rubbing the vulva with flower oils.

17.3   Vaginal Secretions

This is perhaps the most common nonspecific female complaint. While there may be bacterial infestation in some cases, the origin of most secretions is in imbalance of the medium of the vagina. It must be corrected according to general dietary regimen, using purgatives, and adjustment of either hot or cold intemperament.

Proper circulation of air is important; nylon underwear, girdles, leotards, and tights can cause or aggravate many minor vaginal irritations. Cotton underwear "breathes" and allows better circulation.

NOTE: A seminallike fluid can come from women too. The corruption and conditions of such emissions are the same as those for men, when related to general organ imbalance. Unusual discharge for female sexual fluids (copious discharge of Bartholin glands and excessive wetness of vagina) may be due to slackness of the mouth of the womb. The remedy is to procure emesis and bathe in astringent waters. The best medicine for slackness of the mouth of the womb is 3 teaspoons fennel seeds, and 2 teaspoons root of lily of the valley, added to ½ teaspoon each pomegranate flower and rose hips. Pound and sift, and give 2 teaspoons with buttermilk or a glass of juiced green grapes.

17.4   Itching of the Vagina

To relieve this irritation, the remedy is made as follows: pound and sift equal parts of pennyroyal leaves, skin of pomegranate, and lentils. Mix with ½ cup of vinegar or water. Spread on a thin piece of sterile cloth, a piece of cotton, or a commercial tampon, adding a few drops of oil of violet and oil of rose. Insert in vagina to relieve vulva itching. *Do not use this remedy if you are pregnant.*

17.5 Contraception

Since the traditional cultures of the East prohibit abortion and generally have a positive desire to have large families, the concentration is more upon finding methods to aid conception than vice versa. There are valid physical and mental reasons for men and women to limit the growth of their families. The traditional midwives (*dais*) recommend that the women eat mung beans (*dahl*) and the seeds and flowers of acacia (acacia is an ingredient in several contraceptive jellies). Also recommended is having the woman jump up and down eight or nine times after intercourse, to cause the seminal fluid to fall down from the mouth of the womb. Rubbing the head of the penis with sesame oil is also recommended prior to intercourse.

17.6 False Pregnancy

All of the signs of pregnancy—swollen and tender breasts, absence of menstrual period, even the psychological feeling of being a mother—may appear even though conception has not occurred. The physical causes of the signs of pregnancy are dropsy, hard swelling of the womb, and ovarian cyst; fertilization of the ovum while in the fallopian tube is also considered a false pregnancy. Consult the sections dealing with these signs, if they are present.

17.7 Inability to Conceive

The first cause is either hot, cold, dry, or moist intemperament of the womb. The sign of heat is that the blood expelled during the menstrual period is thick and tending to a blackish color. The sign of cold is scantiness of the menstrual flow and its coming late. The sign of dryness is lack of normal secretions of the vagina, including suppressed menses. The sign of moisture is vaginal discharge and excessive menstrual flow.

With a humoral intemperament, the woman may become pregnant, but the fetus usually does not survive beyond the third month.

Another cause of inability to conceive is obesity, and the remedy is to engage in a program of weight loss to bring the body to a normal weight range. Extreme thinness can also impair conception, and the woman must develop a more efficient metabolism by diet. The following are other imbalances that can prevent conception, along with the corrective measure for each:

Flatulence of womb The signs of this are flatulence of the pubic area and of the vulva, which is noted by the emission of sounds of flatulence during intercourse; or, when you tap over the pubic bone, there is a hollow sound. The remedy is to remove the flatulence by taking 3 teaspoons castor oil with 1 tablespoon cod liver oil every day, adding fowl to the diet, and applying cupping.

Deviation of mouth of womb The lack of proper alignment of internal female parts can cause the semen to be unable to flow into the womb for fertilization. Altering the positions of intercourse and avoiding any quick motions (such as standing up) directly after intercourse are advised.

Injuries to the womb and other conditions may cause inability to conceive. You should make certain that there are no underlying physical conditions before deciding that it is or is not possible to conceive.

Catnip for conception In Afghanistan, the most frequent recommendation to women who desire to conceive was to drink catnip tea several times per day. Other preparations for pregnancy induction include eating ground almonds and a tea made from 1 teaspoon spearmint, 3 teaspoons cardamom seeds, ½ teaspoon ground ginger, and ½ teaspoon each of ground walnuts and pistachios.

One of the problems of applying the remedies of the East to women in the West is that, according to the *dais*, the time conception is most likely to occur is considered to be the days immediately before, during, and after the menstrual period; this is the opposite of the schedule figured out by Western science.

A lack of conception sometimes is due to the male. Thus, the man should be considered in all aspects of his health to find out if there is any physical basis (infertile sperm, for example) for the inability of the couple to conceive *together*. Just as some fruits are unable to fertilize, some men and women are infertile from birth. The method used by the Hakims as a preliminary determination of whether or not the man is infertile is to place his semen in water. If it floats, it is suspected to be impotent.

17.8   Frequent Miscarriage

The cause may be psychological or physical. The underlying conditions must be determined and removed. A decoction of tea of false unicorn is the best herbal preparation.

17.9   Difficult Birth

The traditional midwives advise women who have difficult births to drink milk, as much as they can comfortably consume and digest, from the eighth month of pregnancy. When the time for birth is near, she should avoid cold water, vinegar, and all cold foods. The attendant at the birth should rub sweet almond oil with oil of linseed, half warmed, on the mouth of the womb to facilitate birth. The specific medicine recommended in the healers' text for delivery is the following: ½ teaspoon each of ground cinnamon, senna leaves, and cassia, cooked with syrup of violet or pea water, in tablespoon doses. The mother should not smell perfumes or incense at the time of childbirth.

There are now many groups of midwives operating in the United States, and their number is growing rapidly. Most of the magazines on natural medicine have articles on natural childbirth, and with a little inquiring, you can find someone to provide you with the names of natural practitioners who will deliver at home under natural conditions. It is perfectly legal for a father to deliver his own child, but you should have an expert medical person available as backup in case there are complications in the delivery. There is no time whatsoever to learn during the delivery itself, and if you are planning to deliver your own child at home, the best course would be to have a general education about the procedures and techniques to be employed. Women with kidney disease, high blood pressure, and other abnormal conditions are high-risk mothers who should probably consider hospital births.

17.10 Imprisonment of the Chorion and Death of Fetus

The chorion is the outermost membrane covering the fetus. The signs that the death of the fetus has occurred are that there is no heartbeat, no movement, and the hands of the mother are cold and the pulse is erratic. Of course, removal of a fetus is a procedure for a medical doctor. If none is available, the medicine advised is to boil 3 teaspoons each of musk, maidenhair herb, and juniper berries; add 2 teaspoons pennyroyal, and drink with several tablespoons of sugar. After consuming this, make the mother sneeze by sniffing black pepper and crushed khalonji. When she is about to sneeze, cover the nose and mouth tightly, to transfer the force of the expulsion inward. If no medicines work, the fetus must be separated from the umbilicus and removed, which requires someone trained to do so.

17.11 Imprisonment of the Afterbirth

The advice is the same as given for suppressed menses. The remedy to relieve the back pains sometimes felt after birth is to make a decoction of linseed and bathe the womb with it (malva flowers are also recommended).

17.12 Insufficiency of Milk

The breast has the capacity to convert blood into milk, just as the testicles convert blood into semen. Insufficiency of milk has three causes:

1. *Insufficiency of blood.* This may be due to blood loss during delivery or the effects of chronic conditions. Give foods to increase blood, such as milk, egg yolk, and protein foods.

2. *Corruption of blood due to bad temperament.* This must be corrected according to the directions in the beginning of the Formulary.

3. *Excess of blood.* This means that the breast cannot "digest" the blood and make milk from it, due to the oversupply of blood itself. Apply cupping to the breasts.

Thinness, yellowness, and sharp smell of milk are due to biliousness. Intense whiteness, thickness, and sourness of milk are due to phlegm. Intense thickness, whiteness, and insufficiency of milk are due to black bile humor imbalance. A salty taste of milk is caused by mixing of phlegm with yellow bile. These must be corrected according to the humor affected.

17.13   Excess of Milk

The causes are the opposite of insufficiency of milk. To attempt to diminish the milk, use the remedies that open the menstrual flow. A half-ounce of cumin cooked in a pint of vinegar and rubbed on the breasts is used. In cases of cold intemperament, make a salve of wild rue (leaves and seeds) and seeds of beet for the breasts. Also useful is cumin or lentils in vinegar as a lotion for the breasts.

17.14   Swelling and Stretching of the Breast

This is due to either hot or cold intemperament of the breasts. For hot intemperament, make a salve of vinegar and cucumber. For cold intemperament, make a salve of pounded celery (or feverfew) and mix with anise water and apply to breasts.

17.15   Cessation of Milk Flow

If there is an excess of heat that makes the milk thick, there will be swelling of the breast. Excess of cold and obstruction of the flow will cause the same problem. The remedy is to remove the cause, consulting the sections on hot or cold intemperament and swellings. If the milk does not come out at first when the baby begins sucking, pour a little warm water over the breast, or "milk" the nipple slowly until the flow begins. It is felt that if a nursing mother is exposed to great fright, her milk flow may stop or become lessened.

If the interruption of flow causes infection, the signs are a change in the milk color, swelling, and foul taste of the milk. The infection must be ripened with a salve of linseed, marshmallow, and chamomile. Mix in equal portions. Pound and sift. Mix with beet juice or water and apply as a salve to the breast two to three times per day. If the infection develops into an abscess, it will have to be treated by a doctor.

17.16   Rawness of the Nipples

Apply cocoa butter to nipples if the baby makes them raw from sucking or chewing.

17.17   Pregnancy Tea

During her pregnancy a woman should eat no foods containing any additives of any kind except for what nature placed in them. She should not smoke or take drugs of any kind. She must not drink alcoholic beverages. For the final month of her pregnancy, she should drink herbal teas that are of benefit during the last stages of pregnancy and delivery. The teas are as follows: Use ½ tea-spoon each of squaw vine, spikenard, and raspberry to make 1½ cups of tea. Consume twice daily during the ninth month. Peppermint is added for taste and to alleviate nausea. At the first sign of labor, at the mildest pains, make up a quart of blue cohosh tea, and consume for the remainder of the labor.

17.18   Ulcers and Wounds of the Womb

The sign is a feeling of pain and excretion of rheum or blood or both. In general, there can be no ulcer without the presence of rheum. The remedy is applied by douching the womb with rose oil, violet oil, and sugar water to cleanse the rheum. Then take a rectal enema with rose oil added (4 drops to 1 pint of pure water, warmed). If the ulcer is in the neck of the womb, there is no need to use a douche; instead, apply to a tampon honey or boiled mother's milk and use as a vaginal suppository. This is very useful to purge the womb. If there is pain in the womb, add a little saffron (one grain) to the tampon mixture.

17.19   Hemorrhoids of the Womb

These are similar to hemorrhoids of the anus, and the remedy is the same as in 12.1 and 12.2.

17.20   Boils of the Womb

If the boils are in the neck of the womb, use an enema. Boils can usually be felt by inserting the finger into the vagina. The remedy is to adjust any intem-perament and apply rose oil.

17.21   Protrusion of the Womb

This causes great pain in the pubis, anus, and groin. Trembling of the body is often present, and the distension of soft tissue can be felt in the vulva. First, purge the stomach and urinary bladder by giving diuretics. Then take 10 drops each of saffron oil and water lily oil with some musk oil, and apply, half warmed, to the womb. Then, on some soft sterile cloth, put an astringent such as false acacia (finely ground) and musk, and while the woman is lying on her back, insert the cloth. Leave the cloth in the womb this way for three days. Also apply astringents on the pubis and vulva area, and apply cupping on the waist close to the navel. The woman should have perfumes to smell constantly. On the fourth day, renew the soaked cloth.

Surgical correction is possible for this condition, and a medical doctor should be consulted in every case.

17.22   Inclination of the Womb to One Side

This can be felt by the inserted fingers. There is pain on intercourse. The condition causes dysentery and constipation. Have the woman sit in a tub of warm water and afterward massage the body with oil of feverfew. If there is excess moisture in the womb, use an enema. If this course fails, a nurse or midwife may be able to correct it with her fingers.

17.23 Swelling of the Womb

If the cause is hot substances or hot intemperament, the signs are fever, elevated pulse, bad digestion, and pain in the pubis and groin. If the swelling occurs on both sides of the womb, the remedy is the same as given for swelling of the urinary bladder in 15.1. The swelling may run rheum and ulcers may form, which must be treated according to 17.18. If the cause is imbalance of the phlegm humor, the pubic area is very painful (remedy in 15.1). If the cause is imbalance of the black bile humor, the signs are hardness of the womb, inclination to one side, and little pain but prevalent heaviness of the womb. Use the black bile purgative, laxatives, and oils for massaging the pubis. Also, bathing twice a day in water of cooked marshmallow and common dill is useful.

17.24 Enlarged Swelling of the Womb

When there is a swelling that has ripened but has not "pierced," it is called enlarged swelling. If it is in the mouth of the womb, the swelling can be pierced mechanically by a physician. If the swelling is deep in the womb, give diuretics. Boil figs and mustard seeds (about one part figs to one-half part seed by volume) in 1 pint water. Strain off the sediment and use the water for a douche. Use the sediment remaining as a pomade to the pubis. After the swelling comes to a head and bursts, use the remedy for cleansing rheum (17.18).

17.25 Cancer of the Womb

Cancer may appear after a warm-natured swelling of the womb. The signs are hardness of the womb, heat, palpitation, and pain. The diaphragm is projected and the back of the feet swollen. In advanced stages, there is bleeding. Most women receive an annual checkup known as the Pap Test, which checks for presence of cancer cell growth. Information on drugless, natural therapies is available from local chapters of the International Association of Cancer Victors and Friends. Many herbs have been used in the treatment of cancer, not only of the womb but other parts of the body. The attitude of natural medicine is that cancer is the final degenerated condition of an organ or bodily system. As such, the establishment of a way of life based upon proper nutrition and harmony of the spirit is the best suggestion for avoiding such a final condition. Among the most prominent nontoxic therapies for cancer are the Gerson therapy, Hoxsey herbs, the Koch therapy, and laetrile. IACVF can supply details of how to discover physicians skilled in administering these therapies. When a bodily condition has degenerated into a full cancerous tumor, the therapy of choice is surgery. No curative claims are made for chemotherapy or radiation, these being palliative procedures designed to slow tumor growth.

While there are some cases of remission of tumors following various herbal and other natural treatments, there is no scientific evidence to support the recommendation of one herb to be used in any particular case. Since the liver has been damaged in all cases of cancer, care of this organ is vital to prevent cancer, as well as during its treatment. Cancer can be prevented, but seldom cured. (See also 20.15). Purging of the black bile humor, cupping, and laxatives are always included in treatment.

17.26 Strangulation of the Womb

This is similar to fainting and epilepsy; there is no foaming at the mouth and little nervous anxiety, but there is frequent fainting. The treatment is the same as for epilepsy and fainting (see 2.12 and 8.2).

The cause is sometimes attributed to pent-up sexual energy, so intercourse is recommended, if possible. Imprisonment of menses is another cause and was discussed in 17.1.

Section 18

The Back, Legs, and Feet

General Considerations

The spine is made up of a series of bones called vertebrae. This vertebral column is the main axis of the body, providing general flexibility, yet also keeping the posture erect for walking. It is also the enclosing protective casing for the spinal cord and roots of the spinal nerves. It is the support by which the ribs, skull, and pelvis are connected to the spine, along with an important plexus of nerves, muscles, and ligaments. The spinal column is composed of four sets of vetebrae, called the cervical (7 vertebrae), thoracic (12), lumbar (5), the sacrum (5 fused vertebrae), and the coccyx (3 to 5 rudimentary vertebrae).

Since the spinal cord and nerves are so closely connected with the spinal column, it is imperative that there be no misalignment of the column. A study done at the Palmer College of Chiropractic revealed that 60 millimeters of pressure (about enough to feel the finger touching the skin) applied to a spinal nerve will impede nearly 40 percent of nerve impulses across that vertebra. Since the nerve connections of the spinal column activate many functions in the body, it is easy to see that any misalignment of the spinal column can itself lead to lowered vitality and function of any organ.

Chiropractic, osteopathy, and naprapathy are branches of natural medicine specializing in the treatment and alignment of the spine. Osteopaths are most like medical doctors, although they avoid the use of drugs; chiropractors usually work only on the spine though some today practice nutritional counseling, hydrotherapy, and other modalities. Naprapathy, a science developed in the early 1900s, involves gentle applications of pressure to the ligamentous tissue surrounding the spinal column to balance muscles that may be in spasm. In addition to these forms of treatment, all of which involve manipulation of the spine, there are many other systems of bodywork that center on the goal of insuring full nerve impulse flow along the spinal column. Shiatsu, kinesiology, Rolfing, acupressure, yoga, and t'ai chi are a few of these, but each has its special terminology and exercise patterns. It would be well to consider one or more of these forms of therapy if you have signs of pain, tension, and restricted movement in any muscles of the body.

18.1 Convexity

Convexity is the natural-medicine term used to describe the movement of one or more of the individual spinal processes out of place. This movement can be either upward, downward, to the right or left, forward or backward.

atlas

2nd-7th cervical vertebrae

1st-12th thoracic vertebrae

1st-5th lumbar vertebrae

sacrum

coccyx

The Spinal Column

Convexity has several causes:

1. Swelling of the vertebra area (pain with fever)
2. Thick flatulency imprisoned under the vertebrae (severe pain without fever)
3. Spinous fluids absorbed by the ligaments in the back of the head (paleness of the face)
4. Convulsion or spasm of the ligament (can be felt, raised tissue)
5. Falls, injuries, or blows to the spine (signs are clear)

The natural remedies to be applied along with any form of massage or corrective manipulation are:

1. Swelling: Laxatives, arnicated oil for pain. Consult Section 20 on swellings.
2. Flatulence: Consult 10.7 and 14.6.
3. Moisture: Remedy same as for 2.
4. Spasm: See sections on swellings (section 20 and 2.24).
5. Injuries, falls: Correct the vertebra. If it has gone downward from its proper position, apply cupping on both sides to the top of the vertebra affected. If it has gone upward, place the cupping below, on both sides. If it is forward or backward in projection, apply astringent salve. It would be best in any case of injury to the spine to have it treated by a specialist

as the muscles are interconnected among three vertebrae, not simply attached to one, and wrong application of a technique can easily aggravate the condition. Use arnicated oil for pain; it works almost immediately.

18.2   Backache

If the cause is bad temperament, the sign of coldness is pain without heaviness, and gas. The remedy is keeping warm, sun baths, and showers directing streams of hot water on the area affected. If the cause is production of phlegm, the sign is pain with heaviness; it often occurs after experiencing severe anger, fatigue, and the like, which stimulate formation of phlegm. The remedy is to purge the phlegm humor and use suppositories for phlegm. If the phlegm (ache) stays in one place, use salves to soothe it (arnicated oil, lobelia, peppermint oil, for instance). Also recommended is back massage with rose oil and saffron, and abstaining from intercourse. If relief doesn't result, resort to purgatives.

Weakness of the kidneys can also cause backache, as was discussed in 14.3.

Excess blood in the veins of the back also causes ache, and the sign is that pain is felt along the entire spinal column, from the first vertebra to the last. The remedy is to apply cupping every five inches along both sides of the spinal column. For backache in women due to suppressed menstrual flow or excess superfluous matter, the remedy is to use diuretics to open the flow (see 17.1), and rub the back with rose oil.

18.3   Pelvis Ache

It sometimes occurs that the femur bone becomes slightly separated from the tissue that holds it in place in the pelvis, which is called a microevulsion of the femur head. It is probably best treated by a qualified practitioner, but you can try this remedy first: Lie down on a hard floor (carpeted is all right), and place a thick telephone book or other large book at an angle so the corner of the book is underneath and supporting the pelvis. This should be applied to one side at a time, and leave the book in place for about ten to twenty minutes. This will allow the tissue to repair itself while the femur head is properly positioned. If this problem recurs, you most likely need to do exercises to strengthen the pelvic muscles that support the femur and keep it positioned properly. Consult a practitoner.

18.4   Joint Ache or Arthritis

This can occur with or without swelling. If it originates in the joints of the hips, it is called ischium; if it continues on down into the feet, it is called sciatica. If it affects the feet or toes, it is called podogra. Many people lump all these pains together and call it arthritis or rheumatism of the joints.

If it comes over many months or even years, gradually worsening, it is caused by intemperament of the body, poor diet, excessive sugar consumption, and the buildup of toxic materials in the body.

If it is caused by bad temperament of the humors, it is recognized by moist swelling in the joints, but no pain. Salves recommended include: marshmallow and violet oil or feverfew seed and melilot. Valerian root, hops, and chamomile are combined as a tea for pain.

If the cause is black bile mixing with the blood humor, the sign is extreme burning pain. Use laxatives to move the bowels, detoxify, and purge the black bile humor. Salves in this case are not of use except to palliate the pain; lobelia and valerian root are recommended. Very sour oxymel is also helpful.

If the imbalance of the phlegm humour is causing joint ache, the remedy is to cleanse the entire system of phlegm with the tincture-of-lobelia emetic. Afterward, use hot-natured diuretics.

If the cause is prevalence of black bile alone, the signs are change of skin color, little pain, need to stretch all the time, excess of hard swelling in the joints. Use the black bile purgatives and apply cupping.

NOTE: Joint ache is caused by different substances in wrong concentrations. The single most useful herb for severe arthritis is meadow saffron. However, it should be taken with cumin and ginger (one part saffron to five parts cumin and ginger), to avoid harming the stomach balance. Use *extreme caution* with meadow saffron. It is an irritant poison and can damage the kidneys and cause severe depression. Excessive use can be fatal.

In addition, rub the joints with oil to which some beeswax has been added. There are several less drastic pain-relieving preparations:

3 teaspoons ground dry coriander with 3 teaspoons gur. Take ½ teaspoon.

or

1 teaspoon each of valerian root and chamomile and ½ teaspoon hops; make 2 cups of tea and drink as desired. Do not repeat this mixture for more than three days.

2 teaspoons marshmallow seeds, 2 teaspoons of sugar of honey. Take ½ teaspoon.

In sciatica, the points to apply massage to relieve pain are about eight fingers' distance above the ankle bone on the side affected, the base of the little finger on the side affected, and the area of the Achilles tendon on the foot.

18.5 Swelling of the Veins of the Leg

The remedy is purging the black bile humor, eating foods that open the bowels, and vomiting to cleanse the stomach. Afterward, apply the white of an egg over the vein to reduce swelling.

18.6 Heel Ache

The cause may be ulcers of the heel, which should be treated with salves of scabious (devil's bit), ammoniac in rosewater, and cupping. If the cause is from a fall or stepping down hard and bruising the heel, add rosewater and apply cupping to the side and just above the heel. If the cause is heat intemperament, rub with rose oil and, in case of coldness, rub with oil of feverfew. An ice pack will also reduce pain and swelling.

18.7   Sole Ache

If pain is in the soles and causes problems in walking, make a salve of lentils cooked in vinegar and apply, lukewarm, to the soles of the feet.

Hair and Nails

General Considerations

The bulb of the hair root consists of many cells massed together, which constantly multiply and grow. Hairs in different parts of the body have different periods of growth, after which they are shed and replaced. In human beings this process goes on continuously. The life of individual scalp hairs is two to five years, of eyebrows and eyelashes three to five months. As children grow, the hairs of eyebrows, lashes, and scalp become progressively larger and coarser than the preceding set. The sex hormones affect the growth of hair in the armpits and pubic area at puberty in both sexes, and on the chest and face of males. Hair grows at an average rate of 1.5 to 3.0 millimeters per week.

19.1 Baldness (Alopecia)

Falling out of hair, with or without loss of adjacent skin, is called baldness. In both cases, there is some corruption of the skin. The cure is to be found in adusting the phlegm humor. If there is no attendant skin eruption, shaving the entire head sometimes helps to promote new vigorous growth of hair. Rubbing the head with myrtle oil and date water is also recommended.

If only the hair on the crown of the head falls out, the remedy is the same as above. If it happens as part of the normal process of aging, there is no cure.

19.2 Split Ends of Hair

The remedy is to drink fresh fruit juices and apply olive oil or other oils to the hair, along with scalp massage twice a day. Purge the phlegm humor.

19.3 Oily Head

The remedy is purging the body. See beginning of Formulary.

19.4 Whiteness of Hair

Hair will turn white as part of the aging process, which is normal. For hair that turns white prematurely, the Hakims recommended this procedure: eat date jam every morning for a month; during the last week of the month, drink water that has been gathered at a holy shrine. Then, allow one month to pass, avoiding all sour foods and sexual intercourse. Finally, take a phlegm purgative and detoxify the system.

19.5 Care of the Hair

Henna treatment is the best conditioner to ensure healthy, luxurious hair.

Here are recommendations for various general applications for the hair on the head and body:

To prevent hair loss: Rub with oil of cistus or oil of myrtle.

To make the hair grow long: Wash the head with myrtle and date water; if available, geranium blossoms can be added.

To stimulate the roots of the hair: Rub with olive oil and cucumber water. Adjust the phlegm humor.

To remove hair: Apply slaked lime and olive oil as a depilatory paste, but do not apply on the armpits, genitals, or other sensitive areas of the body. Ordinarily, shaving or plucking the hairs out as they first appear is the comfortable method.

To stop hair growth at the roots: Rubbing with opium, vinegar, or gallnut is recommended by the Hakims.

To soften the hair: Apply a decoction of lavender flowers several times a day for a week.

To straighten the hair: Mix olive oil with lukewarm water and rub on the hair.

To redden hair: A color between red and yellow is obtained by washing the hair with henna. This is also effective for coloring gray hair.

19.6 Whitening of Nails
The remedy is to pound linseed and milk, mix with honey, and apply to the nails. If this does not work, use a purgative and detoxify the system.

19.7 Nails Turning Yellow
The remedy is to reduce biliousness and apply vinegar to the nails.

19.8 Aching Nails
Pound leaves of myrtle with leaves of cedar and make a salve of the resultant juices; apply to nails.

19.9 Thickening of Nails
This mostly happens at the base, or roots, of the nails. The remedy is to purge the black bile humor.

19.10   Cracking of Nails

This occurs along the vertical axis of the nails; the remedy is to give moistening foods and purge the black bile humor.

19.11   Lack of Nail Growth

If there is no pain in the nail, the remedy is purging the phlegm humor. If it is accompanied by pain, pricking the fingertip of the affected fingers to let a little blood out is suggested. If it is a toenail that is lacking growth, the remedy is to apply syrup of jujube.

19.12   Itching of the Nails

Wash in fresh, flowing stream or river water, and apply a salve of pounded figs. Scrupulous hygiene is important.

19.13   Bruised Nails

The remedy is applying a salve made of pounded pomegranate leaves and myrtle leaves as soon as the injury occurs. After a few hours, apply a poultice of whole wheat flour and olive oil.

19.14   Breaking Nails (and Whiteness)

The remedy is to mix rose preserve and oxymel with almond oil (in equal parts), and apply to nails.

19.15   Blood under the Nail

After a forceful blow to the nail, blood will usually settle and become "dead" under the nail. Mix equal parts of resin and wheat flour and rub the nail in it. Wash the nail frequently in vinegar. The object is to soften the dead nail, so even sucking on the affected finger is helpful. If you want the nail to come off, make a salve of milk and ground apricot kernels; apply and wrap with a clean cloth.

Section 20
Boils, Swellings, Infections, and Aches

General Considerations

When there are toxic matters in the body, including bacteria and other path-
ogens, the body tries to expel them as quickly as possible. However, the normal
systems of elimination, especially the lymphatic channels and ducts, are sometimes already congested. The body then tries to send the toxins out through
other openings, including the pores of the skin. Since the skin is not designed
to eliminate this type of matter, the pores themselves become clogged, and a
boil is formed.

A single bubblelike eruption is called a boil. When this small swelling is
accompanied by heat, pain, and redness, apply a salve of such herbs as sandalwood, false acacia, rose, and common field scabious, gallnut, and chickory.
If the boil has not begun to dry up after one day, apply a second pomade or
poultice made of barley flour, fresh coriander, and marshmallow in equal parts.
The boil may be reduced by being "drained" away internally. If it needs to be
ripened, do so with ground fig seeds and linseed made into a salve or poultice.
If it ripens within a day or two by itself, it will "point" and drain away from
the surface. Do not squeeze or pinch it. If it becomes larger or spreads, it will
probably have to be lanced by a physician.

The above applies to boils and swellings on the body, *except when located behind the ear, under the arms, or on the groin.* For these cases, see 20.9.

20.1 Gangrene

Gangrene is the end result of an unchecked infection and ultimately leads to
the putrefaction of the limb or body part. It is very serious and can lead to
death. The signs of systemic infection are high fever, loss of appetite, diarrhea,
and flushing. When this condition of any infection of the entire system is present, a physician is urgently needed. If medical help is inaccessible, use antibiotics if available, to check the spreading of infection. When the limb has turned
black, however, it must be amputated to prevent infection of other parts of the
body.

20.2 Swelling with Redness

Redness occurring as the sole sign is indicative of bilious swelling. If only the
yellow bile humor is affected, it is called "pure redness": the skin appears shiny
and is a little yellowish in color, and there is a burning sensation. For this,
purge the yellow bile humor and consume cold and moist foods and herbs.

If there is yellow bile mixed with blood humor, there is no burning sensation, but the swollen part is very red. In this case as well, purge the yellow bile humor.

20.3   Skin Cancer

If there is any swelling, reddened area, growth, or wound on the skin that does not heal, a physician should be consulted to test for cancer (see also 20.15). Skin cancer has many forms and names in allopathic medicine. In general, a mild skin cancer is treatable by surgical excision of the affected area, if discovered soon enough. The signs are often that the skin is greatly swollen, there is redness that spreads quickly, and the heat of the swelling may feel as though a fire had been touched to the skin. Some cancers of the skin are painless, however. The herbal application is first to purge the black bile humor and detoxify the system (this all must be carried out under medical supervision). The preparation to put on the cancer is a half-pint of vinegar heated to boiling temperature, mixed with 2 teaspoons of camphor, and, after cooling, applied to the skin.

Another skin cancer salve (also reputed to be effective for removing plantar warts) is made as follows: Take one ounce red clover blossoms and simmer in two pints distilled water for one hour. Strain, add another ounce of red clover blossoms to the liquid, and slowly boil another hour. Strain again, and simmer until the liquid is driven off. When the liquid is nearly all evaporated, you must watch the mixture carefully to avoid scorching it. When it has reached the consistency of tar, remove from the flame and put in a clean, low, wide-mouthed jar. It will harden somewhat as it cools. Apply to the affected part of and cover with a piece of moleskin or soft, sterile cloth.

20.4   Small Boils with White Heads and Red Roots

Purge both the phlegm and yellow bile humors. Soak pomegranate skin in vinegar and rose water, and apply to the boils.

20.5   Moist Boil with Severe Burning and Itching

When it appears, the roots dry soon. Red, featherlike lines are seen before it appears. This may be a prelude to skin cancer. Purge the yellow bile humor and apply a salve of rosewater, gallnut, and vinegar.

20.6   Large Boils

These boils sometimes contain a thin watery discharge or thinned blood. The remedy is to thicken the blood and apply cold salves, such as camphor, cucumber, and the like. The boil may be pierced with a sterile needle if it comes to a head.

20.7   Random Boils

They look red; some are big and some small. The main sign is that they appear very suddenly and itch. They are caused by blood and phlegm humor imbalance. In the case of blood humor imbalance, soften the stomach and apply a salve made with rose leaves. In the case of phlegm, use a phlegm purgative, and stop eating phlegm-producing foods.

20.8   Canker

This is a swelling caused by biliousness and blood humor imbalance. It appears in the head. The entire face becomes very red and swollen. The stomach must be kept soft and the humors corrected. Use laxatives first, and apply cold salves on the throat and chest to keep the swelling from coming down from the face to the chest. Mix 1 teaspoon coriander seed powder with 2 teaspoons oxymel and drink the mixture.

20.9   Boils and Carbuncles of the Armpit, Behind the Ear, and in the Groin

If this condition is caused by an ulcer, consult the appropriate sections for these parts. If it is not due to an ulcer, make a salve of violet leaves, violet oil, and beeswax. Do not use cold pomades. When the substance has been drawn to a ripened point, it can be pierced and drained. These are often signs of a systemic infection and should be seen by a physician.

20.10   Abscesses

Infected swellings need treatment by a physician. The natural treatment is to purge the blood and phlegm humors and drink oxymel. For three days apply a poultice of purslane leaves, sandalwood, and betel nut (in equal parts). On the fourth day, apply ½ ounce of yellow dock with white of egg as binder. When it shrinks and ripens to a point, pierce it with a sterile needle. After it is cleaned of rheum and pus, apply a mixture of pounded figs and resin gum. This can be alternated once a day with dough made of whole wheat flour and water, with a little salt, linseed oil, and honey added.

20.11   Soft, White Swelling without Heat and Pain

Purge the phlegm humor and correct for cold intemperament. Apply a salve of aloe vera, vinegar, and rose water.

20.12   Swelling that is Thick and Hard and Moves under the Skin

When palpated, this kind of swelling is given several names by the Hakims, according to the consistencies: honeylike, fatlike, flourlike, oil-like, and curdlike. The remedy is to purge the phlegm humor.

20.13 Skin Tumors

The difference between a tumor and the condition mentioned in 20.12 is that a skin tumor is a hard growth on the surface of the skin. Any tumor should be diagnosed by a physician. After such diagnosis is made, a decision can be reached whether to pursue an orthodox or nontoxic treatment (see 20.15).

20.14 Scrofula

This condition is characterized by chronic swelling of the glands, especially lymphatics. The imbalance is caused either by phlegm or by phlegm mixed with black bile. In both cases, the phlegm humor must be purged. A definitive diagnosis should be sought whenever there is chronic swelling of the lymph glands.

20.15 Cancer

See also sections 10, General Considerations, 17.25, and 20.3. Cancer—in all of its many forms—has become one of the worst plagues in recorded history. Theories about its origin and methods of treatment abound, but it remains a fact that the cure for cancer has still eluded humankind. Some forms are apparently "cured" by surgical removal, although in many cases the cancer reappears, sometimes many years later. The medical doctors who operate the largest clinic in the Western Hemisphere offering nontoxic treatment of cancer have only approximately a 3.5 percent rate of total remission after five years. The "cure" rate in conventional forms of treatment is approximately the same.

It seems futile to focus treatment on the final stages of a process that takes many years to develop. At the time a cancer is diagnosed, there is always to be found degeneration of primary organs, and the organ most frequently affected is the liver. Environmental toxins and cigarette smoking cause a large percentage of cancers.

According to the view of natural medicine, cancer occurs as the degeneration of the human body or its parts over a period of many years, due to faulty and unbalanced living habits. If you will review the chapters on the origin and progression of illness, you will see that the incomplete digestion of nutrients causes congestion of one or more organs (or humors). Since the body is capable of healing and balancing itself and is astoundingly competent at reducing and correcting the effects of abusive dietary habits, the congestion of an organ may be corrected in whole or part for some time, often for years. But the quality of functioning of those organs also degenerates over time, so the self-healing process weakens. The fact that cancer appears in so many forms and affects so many different organs has its explanation in each person's inherited strengths and weaknesses in his or her own body.

The liver is the seat of manufacture of the blood, and it is simple to see that any chronic or degenerated condition of that organ will lead to impurity and faulty production of the blood, which is the medium for carrying the life force by the breath.

Most cancerous tumors appear as a very hard swelling, with a dark color and rounded shape. The surface is puffy or sunken, and the area may exhibit reddish and greenish veins that resemble a crab (*cancer* is the Latin word for "crab.") The black bile humor must be purged constantly, and the liver must be strengthened. In my opinion, anyone who has received a definitive diagnosis of cancer should investigate all available forms of therapy: surgery, chemotherapy, radiation, and all forms of nontoxic therapies. Some of the better-known unorthodox therapies are Koch glyoxylide therapy, Gerson therapy, laetrile (amygdaline), Iscadore, Tekarina, Crofton vaccine, saline-hydrogen peroxide therapy, parabenzoquinine (PBQ), the Nicolini method, the Baumann Electrolyte Rejuvenation Program, Blass oxygen therapy, Neihans cellular therapy, and the Hoxsey herbs.

Many of these treatments were developed by the person whose name they bear, after these people cured themselves of cancer. There are many other such forms, and to investigate them all would require much labor. As unfortunate as it is, there do exist some perverted people who play upon the suffering of others and offer absurd hopes for high fees in promising a cure for cancer. Remember that for any known treatment, orthodox or unorthodox, the absolute cure rate is abysmally low.

Information about unorthodox cancer therapies is available from the International Association of Cancer Victors and Friends, 7740 West Manchester Avenue, Suite 110, Playa Del Rey, CA 90291. They have chapters in most cities, and usually have a listing in the telephone book.

The clinic of Dr. Hans Nieper at 21 Sedanstrasse, 3000 Hanover, West Germany, has a reputation for being the finest facility for treatment of cancer in the world, offering a combination of both orthodox and nontoxic therapies, which are prescribed by medical doctors on an individual basis. The international phone number for the clinic is 0511-31-11-11. A clinic in the United States that operates along similar lines is the Akbar Clinic, 4000 East 3rd Street, Panama City, Florida, 32404. The telephone number is (904) 763-7689.

Avicenna's View of Cancer

In his *Canon*, Avicenna provides a general review of his views on cancer. It should be noted that any treatment plan should be specific to an individual and administered by a qualified physician.

According to Avicenna, cancer is a tumor arising from "burning" of the black bile humor. By burning it is meant that the increase of heat has become pathological. The cancerous tumor is usually differentiated from benign tumors by the signs of pain, acuteness, and some degree of throbbing and rapid increase in size. Swelling is a manifestation of this black bile substance "boiling" at its junction with the organ. Cancerous tumors also send out crablike "tracks," and there is a trend toward blackness, green, and heat. Avicenna notes that cancer occurs mostly in hollow organs and that is why it is more frequent in women. It also is common in the nerves, muscles, tendons, and lymph.

For Avicenna, the first objective in the treatment of cancer is to keep it as stationary as possible so that it will not increase, and to keep it nonulcerated. A cure is most likely if treatment is begun at the earliest stage. Avicenna notes: "When it [cancer] is advanced [well established] it will not cure."

In the case of occult (hidden) cancers becoming manifest after having existed for some time, both Avicenna and Hippocrates believed the best course is to leave the tumor alone. Avicenna writes: "And if it is left and not treated [removed] the patient may remain alive longer with some safety, especially if the diet is corrected and made to cool and to refresh and produce a bland, safe material like barley water, crushed [mashed] fish, egg yolk half-boiled, and the like."

If there is elevated temperature and fever, Avicenna advises a diet of churned cow's milk, strained vegetables, and squash.

Surgery is recommended by Avicenna for "small" cancers. His influence on contemporary surgical procedure is evident in his description of the technique to employ: "If [the small cancer] can be arrested with anything, it can be so by vigorous excision, the radical one extending beyond [the tumor] to a circle . . . to be excised from the surrounding of the tumor including all the vessels supplying the tumor so that nothing of these will be left and that much blood will flow from the vessels."

But Avicenna's view is much more comprehensive, as he immediately qualifies his recommendation that surgery "be preceded by purifying [clearing] the body of the bad material [black bile] by purgation, cupping, and maintaining that purity by good food quantitatively and qualitatively and strengthening the defense [resistance] of the organ involved."

Even with careful surgery and strict dietary therapy, Avicenna adds this strong caution: "Nevertheless, most of the time, [excision] increases the cancer." Further surgery is often needed, and in this "there may be a great danger if the cancer was in the vicinity of the principal organs and the precious vital organs." This is quite often the case when surgery is performed on one breast, for example, and soon arises in the other.

The formula Avicenna recommends for palliation consists of 4 teaspoons of dodder (*Cuscuta Europea*) in honey, given at three-day intervals. It acts as a brisk purgative. Colocynth (Citrullus colocynthis) has a similar effect.

Local medications for cancer are many. There are four purposes to such treatments: (1) total arrest of the cancer (this is difficult); (2) preventing its progress; (3) preventing ulceration; and (4) treatment of ulceration.

These medications given for total arrest of the tumor or reversing the effects of the corrupted black bile should not be overly powerful, since strong medication increases the risk of spreading the cancer. Also, one should avoid irritant medicines. For these purposes Avicenna recommends zinc oxide mixed with essential oils of rose and other flowers.

Preventing the progress and growth of cancer can be accomplished by controlling the black bile by improving diet and reinforcing the organ involved, and by using salves of substances such as dust from millstone and whetstone, mixed with rose oil and coriander water.

Medications that are needed to prevent ulceration should not be irritants. Many salves can be used for this purpose, but Avicenna specially recommends Armenian bole (a kind of earth), houseleek water, and lettuce juice, or mucilage of fleawort. Also of benefit are zinc oxide preparation with the soft part of fluvial crab.

An ointment recommended for treatment of ulceration is made of kernels of wheat mixed with frankincense and Armenian bole and made into an ointment by adding rose oil. Zinc oxide mixed with rose oil is a simple remedy that is said to be effective.

Cancer will be eliminated only when people return to a more balanced, natural lifestyle, and keep the body, mind, and spirit free from impurities.

20.16   Scabs

These appear often with itching after boils come to a point and drain. Some are dry and moist. If the scab is dry, rub beet juice and pea water on it. Wash with warm water afterward and use a purgative. Massage the area of the scab with rose oil and vinegar. For wet scabs, cup the area around the scab, then give a laxative for the phlegm humor. Do not use hot salves or pomades on scabs.

20.17   Itching

If itching persists without any other sign, boil ¼ ounce linseed in 2 ounces honey, add some powered purslane, and apply as a pomade.

For scabs and itching in children, give a tub bath with rose leaves and violet leaves added, and afterward rub the affected parts with olive oil.

20.18   Severe Itching with Prickling and Small Red Boils

The remedy is to apply the biliousness laxative and a salve of salt, henna, and vinegar. Purge the yellow bile humor.

20.19   Itching with Severe Pain

If the itching has just started, rub the area with balsam, dates, and vinegar salve (in equal parts). If the itching persists and the skin becomes thickened from scratching, use a black bile humor laxative and take warm baths. The recommended salve is made from such things as mustard, alum, and myrrh mixed with a little wheat germ oil and vinegar.

20.20   Pimples

These are white pimples that appear most frequently on the nose and forehead. Purge the phlegm humor and apply a salve of celery water and vinegar.

20.21   Pimples on the Buttocks, Anus, or Vulva

Use a general purgative and detoxify the system.

20.22   Broken Blood Vessels

Rupture of the veins just under the skin is caused either by a blow or may appear spontaneously. The skin is discolored by the accumulation of blood and vaporous substances. When the veins contract, swelling may appear; when veins expand, the swelling goes down. If the swelling is chronic, the skin may take on a purplish color. The suggested treatment is to apply salves of astringent herbs, such as gallnut or chestnut. Avoid blood stimulants.

20.23.   Sebaceous Cysts

These appear in different forms. One is small, white, and hard, with roots; a little rheum comes out from time to time. These can appear anywhere. Another appears mostly on the face, is quite hard, red in color, and often as large as a quarter. A third variety usually appears behind the ear and will emit a puslike substance, sometimes with blood mixed in. These can also appear on the back of the neck, and sometimes are quite painful. The treatment for all types of these sebaceous cysts is to use a purgative and cleanse the system. For the last kind, use a purgative as well, but also drop a little violet oil and mother's milk into the nose and rub the same mixture on the neck and head.

Section 21
Miscellaneous

21.1 Blackheads

These appear mostly on the face, but can appear anywhere there is an accumulation of dirt and lack of skin hygiene. Wash the skin daily and apply
a salve of rhubarb and honey. If blackheads keep appearing, detoxify the body.

21.2 Bloodblisters

These occur from a blow to the skin or from a sharp pinching of the skin.
Apply pounded cabbage leaves and pennyroyal herb made into a salve.

21.3 Freckles

This change in skin pigmentation frequently occurs after exposure to the sun.
It is sometimes hereditary. Apply the remedy for blackheads if you wish to get
rid of them. There is no harm in freckles.

21.4 Frostbite

In its mild form, frostbite appears as a dark redness on the face and hands
after exposure to subzero temperatures. Numbness of the affected part is a sign,
and pain follows. The remedy is to give cooked dates until diarrhea occurs, and
apply a salve of red clover blossoms with a little castile soap added. When the
redness subsides, wash frequently with warm water.

21.5 Blackness of Skin after Exposure to Cold

This needs first-aid treatment at a medical facility. If none is available, rub
olive oil on the hands before any swelling begins and before they turn blue.
When the swelling appears, place hands in a solution of cooked dill and melilot
or a decoction of linseed. Cabbage water also works. When the hands are taken
out of the water (when the swelling is checked), rub with rose oil. A pomade
of pounded boiled lentils applied to the affected part is recommended.

21.6 Swelling and Itching of Fingers during Cold Weather

The remedy is to wash the fingers with salty water and also with the water
from turnips and beets.

21.7 Dandruff

The remedy is to put 1 teaspoon salt in beet water and wash the head with
it. If it is chronic, purge the phlegm and black bile humors.

21.8 Cracks of Hands, Face, and Lips

If the cause is external factors such as cold and wind exposure, use an ointment of sweet almond oil. If due to internal causes, use a purgative and consume more fruits.

21.9 Rough Skin

Use a purgative and massage the body with rose oil and olive oil.

21.10 Scratches

For minor surface scratches, apply almond or rose oil with a pinch of ground golden seal.

21.11 Lice

The first recommendation is to purge the body, wash with salt water, and change the clothes frequently. One kind of louse imbeds itself in the roots of hair and moves about when stimulated by heat. Cayenne pepper in vinegar will dislodge these lice, which can then be washed away.

21.12 Severe Perspiration

Often the cause is that the body is full of phlegm; if so, the phlegm purgative should be employed. This condition can also be caused by overeating and engorging the stomach. The remedy is to refrain from eating for a twenty-four-hour period or longer. If perspiration is caused by general debilitation and weakness, undertake to strengthen the health of the person, and burn dried leaves of myrtle and allow the smoke to reach the person's body. Caloric foods imprison perspiration, a normal avenue of excretion of superfluities. However, people sometimes faint from dehydration as a result of excessive perspiration. The following remedy helps to slow down the elimination of perspiration and in preventing fainting: Pour 2 ounces each of apple juice and rose water into 2 ounces sesame oil; heat gradually to a slow boil, and continue boiling until the water is driven off and only the oil remains. Take a teaspoonful as needed.

NOTE: The prevalence of perspiration that is part of the natural expulsion of toxins associated with a healing crisis should not be stopped.

21.13 Bloody Perspiration

This is excretion of blood with perspiration. The remedy is to use strong laxatives, correct for hot intemperament of the blood, and remove any obstruction of the pores of the skin by using astringents.

21.14 Obesity and Thinness

When carried to extremes, these conditions are an imbalance that affects the overall health. To gain weight, use this preparation: almonds, pine nuts (and any other oil-producing seeds or nuts) in equal parts, pounded together. Mix with butter and turbinado sugar and take a portion morning and evening before meals. Eat moist, energetic foods.

To reduce obesity, reduce food intake. The best diet of all is to eat only when there is true hunger, and then only enough to take the edge off the hunger. Rub the body with oils and common dill ground fine. Make the person sleep on the hard ground. A detoxification program, adhered to strictly, generally causes from five to fifteen pounds of weight loss in a ten-day period. Establishing a day of fasting once a week (or even for half-days at first) will help bring a compulsive eater under the control of self-discipline.

21.15 Bad Odor of the Body

Bathe frequently and rub the body with rose oil after bathing. Use a purgative as well. A little powdered bicarbonate of soda or sandalwood powder dusted under the arms will absorb most of the foul odor of the armpits. Any extended period of corrupted body odor calls for corrective treatment by detoxification and looking into the underlying humoral imbalances.

21.16 Burning by Fire

Two treatments are suggested. The first to put fresh aloe vera on the skin that has been exposed to fire. Anything other than minor burns should be treated by a physician, as burns can become infected easily. The second suggestion is to apply fresh purslane that has been cooled in a freezer or on ice to the area, changing often enough to keep cool. If a blister appears, rub some fireplace soot with egg white on it.

21.17 Burning by Hot Oil

The remedy is the same as for fire; also, you may put on egg white mixed with a little olive oil as a first aid measure.

21.18 Burning by Lightning

Anyone struck by lightning needs medical treatment at once. Emergency measures for burns are the same as mentioned for burns by fire.

21.19 Sunburn

For mild overexposure to the sun, apply fresh aloe vera. Use protective oils before going out into the sun, or cover the exposed skin with appropriate clothing.

21.20 Tongue Burns by Caustics

The people in India chew a leafy substance called *pan* with gallnut and limestone added. While the betel leaf and other ingredients do contain all the vitamins necessary for humans, it also can cause tongue burns if made too strong. Some of the substances chewed in the mouth in America (such as coca leaf with lime) may also cause a slight burn, especially to those who try it for the first time. Recommended is to rub oil of sweet almond and a little finely ground nutmeg on the tongue.

21.21   Wounds

The treatment of most wounds is in the province of the medical physician or surgeon, who has the training and materials to set bones, sew the skin, and perform more complicated procedures to repair internal damage to the body. These forms of treatment lie outside the realm of simple treatment by herbs.

In general, the most dangerous wounds are those to the head and brain, or to the heart. Serious wounds to either place are often fatal. If a penlight held to the eyes of a person struck in the head does not cause contraction of the pupil, it is usually a sign that brain damage has occurred. Obviously, emergency medical aid should be sought as soon as possible in such cases.

The kidney, urinary bladder, and intestine are next in order of importance in wounds. Wounds to the kidney and bladder are known from the urine; wounds to the intestine are diagnosed by the feces. Wounds involving nerves are known by pale color in the face, fainting, and convulsions. Knee wounds easily become chronic and are difficult to cure without surgery. Internal injuries to the abdomen are signaled by vomiting and hiccups. Wounds to the chest produce expulsion of large amounts of air and asthma signs. Apply the best first aid you can, and seek emergency help.

21.22   Falls and Blows from the Fist

If there is no swelling or fever, make a salve of gum ammoniac and egg white. If there is swelling and fever, apply cupping and reinforce the specific area of injury (also see Sections 20, General Considerations, and 20.2). For deep muscle bruises, apply arnicated oil for pain and give marijuana tea as a relaxant.

21.23   Welt from Beating with a Whip

If serious, the tissue under the skin is spread out. If any flesh is torn loose, replace it over the exposed flesh. If no emergency medical aid is available, the procedure recommended by the Hakims is to apply fresh meat. This is said to have effect within twenty-four hours. If blood accumulates under the welts, put a salve of ground radish seeds on the wound.

21.24   Broken Bones

The complete dislocation or fracture of a bone, with or without puncture of the flesh, or bruising of the bone or muscles around it, should be treated by a competent physician or bonesetter. Until one is available, rub olive oil on the part, and also put on pounded leaves of myrtle and marshmallow with egg yolk and cover with a sterile cloth.

21.25   Poisons

If an unknown substance of any quantity is ingested, call the emergency room of any hospital and give them whatever information you can about the bottle it was kept in or what the source of the substance was. They will advise you as to what can be done immediately and arrange for an ambulance, if needed. It is a good idea to get a poison chart and tack it up on the wall.

Poisons can be animal, vegetable, or mineral. When someone has eaten a poison, if it is not known what the source is, vomiting should first be employed to attempt to expel the substance as quickly as possible. There are some exceptions to this rule, such as if the poison is an acid caustic, and it is hard to act with certainty if the identity of the ingested substance is not known at all. Lots of sesame oil or butter added to warm water will usually provoke vomiting. Lobelia tincture should *not* be used, as this will also speed digestion of the substance. If the person cannot vomit much, drinking common dill with salt and oil mixed in water will usually induce vomiting. Give as much fresh milk as possible; this provides mucus to coat the stomach and slows absorption of toxins. If the person becomes drowsy and seems to be falling asleep, try to prevent this by giving strong stimulants such as coffee or spearmint in strong decoction. If the person has an irrepressible urge for a particular food, it is probably what the body needs to counteract the poison.

NOTE: If the person faints, the eyes roll back into the sockets or become red, the pulse is not beating, cold perspiration appears, and the tongue is thrown out from the mouth, there is usually little hope for survival.

21.26   Stings of Poisonous Insects and Snakes

These are treated in the following ways:

1. Give something to increase the natural temperature, to reinforce the intestines and kill the poison, or slow down its absorption into the bloodstream. Opium is said to have this effect. Milk, as a drink and enema, will coat the membranes and help slow down absorption.

2. Purge the body of moisture by inducing vomiting or diarrhea.

3. Give antitoxin or antidote if known and available.

4. Give a medicine to stir up the phlegm and repulse the nature of the poison (4 drops of tincture of iodine will accomplish this).

5. Do something to stop the spread of the poison, such as opening the vein and sucking out the toxic blood. A small incision can be made over the point of the bite, and a tourniquet can be applied about five to ten inches above the wound. Cupping can be done over the cut, or the poison can be sucked out with the mouth, although care should be taken not to ingest any of the blood by lubricating the mouth with olive or flower oil before sucking.

Eating three palmfuls of fresh coriander is said to be good for the sting of wasps, bees, and ants. If you have any sulfur-tipped kitchen matches handy, wet the tip of one with saliva and rub on the area of the sting; if done within thirty seconds or so of the sting, there is little swelling or pain.

Despite their reputation, the bites or stings of tarantulas, scorpions, and black widow spiders are not often fatal to adults (they *may* be to children); there is often more danger from the shock experienced after any insect or animal bite than from the wound or poison itself.

21.27 Wound by Bite of Rabid Animal

There are rabies antitoxins, which must be administered by a physician. The people in remote areas without access to medical treatment (such as Afghanistan) take some blood from the dog or animal that bit the person and mix it with water and drink it as an emergency antitoxin. At other times, the animal is killed and its liver fried and eaten. If treated in this way, the wounds usually do not heal for a long time.

Rabies vaccine is effective, even if given some days after the bite—usually within ten days. Skunks and bats are prime carriers of rabies, and cats and dogs have plagues of rabies among their population from time to time, especially in the Western states. Rabies is almost invariably fatal if not treated with an antitoxin.

III
Materia Medica

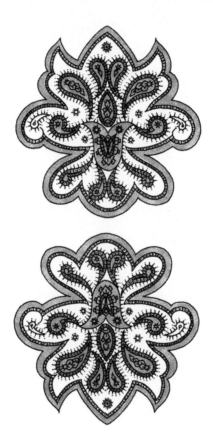

Unani Tibb Botanicals

The following are the herbs referred to in the Formulary. The botanical, common English, and Tibb names are given for each herb, along with information about its native home, properties, and uses. For specific instructions as to use, consult various ailments and sections in the Formulary.

The information about these herbs was gathered from the following sources, which are recommended for more detailed information about the properties and uses of the Unani Tibb herbs.

David M. R. Culbreth. *A Manual of Materia Medica and Pharmacology.* Philadelphia: Lea & Faber, 1927.

J. F. Dastur. *Medicinal Plants of India and Pakistan.* Bombay: D. B. Taraporevala Sons & Co., 1962.

M. Grieve. *A Modern Herbal,* 2 vols. New York: Dover Publications, 1971.

Kamal, Dr. Hassan. *Encyclopedia of Islamic Medicine.* Cairo: General Egyptian Book Organization, 1975.

Al-Samarqandi. *Materia Medica of Al-Samarqandi.* Sidney, New York: Chishti Institute, 1986.

This list is by no means exhaustive. Hakim Ibn Sina includes 273 herbs in his *Canon,* and there exist Tibb herbals giving data on several hundred more. A survey of Tibb medicinal drugs by the Hamdard Institute of India lists some 655 drugs that are used in common by the Tibb and Ayurvedic medicine systems in India. Nonetheless the data provides an overview of some of the most important and useful botanicals. Most of them are available in the United States from various sources. Even most of those indigenous to India or Pakistan can be obtained through Indian stores in major cities such as New York or Chicago, or through the American Institute of Unani Medicine.

For some of the herbs, more than one species is used, as is the case with rose and cumin, for example. You should try to obtain the highest-quality unadulterated herbal substances, grown in your locale, if possible—although sometimes only an imported herb fulfills these criteria, as with ginger.

I have supplied the Tibb name for each herb, although this presents some problems in terminology. The source books used were in Arabic, Persian, and Urdu, all of which have local names for various herbs, sometimes the same but often different. When requesting an herb from a supplier, always use the standard Latin botanical name, as well as any common or foreign names.

A final point to remember is that the great Hakims are known for their mastery of and ability to use a few herbs skillfully on a wide variety of ailments, rather than attempting to use a vast number of herbs on a few ailments.

For your interest, following the list of Tibb Botanicals are given the 21 most-used herbs, as reported by the ten leading Dawakhanas, or Tibb herbal clinics, in Pakistan. It should be of interest that more than half are common nutrient botanicals.

*Indicates medicinal botanicals that require caution in use, as even small amounts may cause adverse reactions. Consult a physician or herbal expert before using.

Acacia, False *(Acacia senegal)*
Ajowan (Ajwain) *(Ptychotis ajowan)*
Aloeswood *(Aquilaria agallocha)*
Aloe Vera *(Aloe vera)*
Ammoniacum
    (Dorema ammoniacum)
Aniseed *(Pimpinella anisum)*
Arabic Gum *(Acacia arabica)*
    (See Acacia, false)
* Asafoetida *(Ferula foetida)*

Balsam Fir *(Abies species)*
Barberry *(Berberis vulgaris)*
Basil *(Ocimum balsilicum)*
Bayberry Bark *(Myrica cerifera)*
Beleric Myrobalen
    (Terminalia belerica)
*Betel Nut *(Areca catechu)*
Black Pepper *(Piper negrum)*
Borage *(Borago officinalis)*

* Camphor *(Cinnamomum camphoru)*
Capers *(See* Sebestan)
Capparis *(See* Hyssop)
* Capsicum *(Capsicum frutescens)*
Caraway (Seed) *(Carum carui)*
Cardamom *(Elettaria cardamomum)*
*Cassia, Purging *(See* Senna)
Catnip *(Nepeta cataria)*
* Celandine *(Chelidonium majus)*
Chamomile *(Anthemis nobilis)*
Chestnut *(Castanea vesca [dentata])*
Chickory *(Chichorium intybus)*

*Chrysanthemum
    (Chrysanthemum roseum)
Cinnamon *(Cinnamomum Loureirii)*
Cistus *(Cistus Ladaniferous)*
Clove *(Caryophyllus aromaticus)*
Cocoa Butter *(Theobromatis cacao)*
Coriander *(Coriandum sativum)*
* Cottonseed *(Gossypium herbaceum)*
Cucumber *(Cucumis sativus)*
Cumin *(Cuminum cyminum)*

Date *(Phoenix dactylifera)*
Dill *(Anethum graveolens)*
*Dodder *(Cuscuta Europea)*
Dragon's Blood *(Daemonorprops draco)*

Embelia *(Embelia ribes)*
Emblic Myrobalen *(Emblica officinalis)*
Eyebright *(Euphrasis officinalis)*

Fennel *(Foeniculum vulgare)*
Fenugreek *(Trigonella foenum-graecum)*
Feverfew
    (Chrysanthemum parthenium)
Fig *(Ficus carica)*
Frankincense *(Boswellia carterii)*

Garlic *(Allium sativum)*
Gentian *(Gentiana lutea)*
Ginger *(Zingiber officinalis)*
*Goldenseal *(Hydrastis canadensis)*
*Gourd, wild *(Citrullus colocynth)*
Grape *(Vitis vinifera)*
Gum Ammoniac *(See* Ammoniacum)

Henna (*Lawsonia inermis*)
Hops (*Humulus lupulus*)
Horehound (*Marrubium vulgare*)
Hyssop (*Hyssop officinalis*)

Jasmine (*Jasminum officinale*)
Jujube (*Zizyphus vulgare*)
Juniper (*Juniperus communis*)

Khalonji (*Nigella sativa*)

Lavender (*Lavandula vera*)
Lemon (*Citrus limonum*)
Licorice (*Glycyrrhiza glaba*)
*Lily of the Valley (*Convallaria majalis*)
Linseed (*Linum usitatissimum*)
*Lobelia (*Lobelia inflata*)

Malabar Nut Tree (*Adhatoda vasica*)
Malva (*Malva sylvestris*)
Mango (*Mangifera indica*)
*Marijuana (Cannabis)
   (*Cannabis sativa*)
Marjoram (*Origanum marjorana*)
Marshmallow (*Althea officinalis*)
Masterwort (*Heracleum lanatum*)
Mastic (*Pistacia lentiscris*)
*Meadow Saffron
   (*Colchicum autumnale*)
Melilot (*Melilotus officinalis*)
*Mugwort (*Artemisis vulgaris*)
*Mustard (*Brassica nigra [juncea]*)
Myrrh (*Commiphora myrrh*)
Myrtle (*Myrtus communis*)

Nutmeg (*Myristica fragrans*)

Olive (*Olea europea*)

*Pellitory (Root) (*Anacyclus Pyrethrum*)
*Pennyroyal (*Hedeoma pulegioides*)
Peppermint (*Mentha piperita*)
Pistachio (*Pistacia vera*)

Plantain (*Plantago major*)
Pomegranate (*Punica granatum*)
Poppy (Seed) (*Papaver somniferum*)
Prickly Ash
   (*Xanthoxylum americanum*)
Pumpkin (*Curcurbita pepo*)
Purslane (*Portulacea Oleracea*)

Quince (*Cydonia vulgaris*)

Radish (*Raphanus sativus*)
Raspberry (*Rubus strigosus*)
Red (Wild) Clover (*Trifolium pratense*)
Rhubarb (*Rheum officinale*)
Rose (*Rosa damascens*) (species)

Safflower (*Carhamus tinctorius*)
*Saffron (*Crocus sativus*)
Sandalwood (*Santalum album*)
Sarsaparilla (*Smilax officinalis*)
Scabious (*Scabiosa succisa*)
Sebestan (Capers) (*Capparis sativa*)
*Senna (*See* Cassia, purgative)
Sesame (*Sesamum orientale*)
Skunk Cabbage
   (*Symplocarpus foetidus*)
Spikenard (*Aralia racemosa*)
Squaw Vine (*Mitchella repens*)
Sumac (*Rhus aromatica*)

Tamarind (*Tamarindus indica*)
Tamarisk (*Tamarix articulata*)
Turmeric (*Curcurma longa*)

*Valerian (*Valeriana officinalis*)

Walnut (*Juglans regia*)
*Water Lily (*Nymphaea lotus [odorata]*)
Watermelon (*Citrullus vulgaris*)
Wild Rue (*Peganum harmala*)
*Wormwood (*Artemisia absinthium*)

Yerba Santa (*Eriodictyon californicum*)

MOST POPULAR BOTANICALS

The twenty-one most-used botanicals as reported by the ten leading Unani herbal clinics of Pakistan

Please note that while several hundred herbal substances are used in healing, these are the *most used*, and at that, they are all but four primarily thought of as food spices, not exotic medicines.

Botanical Name	Common Name	Total Quantity (kg.) Bulk Herb Used by 10 Clinics in One Year
1. *Adhatoda vasica*	Malabar nut	11,500
2. *Althea officinalis*	Marshmallow	4,050
3. *Cassia angustifolia*	Senna	23,610
4. *Cinnamomum zeylanicum*	Cinnamon	19,395
5. *Coriandum sativum*	Coriander	18,155
6. *Cuminum* species	Cumin seed	7,435
7. *Elettaria cardamomum*	Cardamom seed	5,220
8. *Emblica species*	Myrobalen	24,900
9. *Foeniculum vulgare*	Fennel	20,400
10. *Glycyrrhiza glabra*	Licorice root	17,040
11. *Malva sylvestris*	Mallow Leaves	11,240
12. *Mentha* species	Peppermint	15,990
13. *Nymphaea lotus*	Water lily	9,590
14. *Piper negrum*	Black pepper	18,670
15. *Ptychotis ajowan*	Ajowan	24,200
16. *Rheum emodi*	Rhubarb	7,210
17. *Rosa damascena*	Red rose	13,325
18. *Sesamum indicum*	Sesame seed	19,290
19. *Terminalia* species	Beleric myrobalen	35,305
20. *Viola odorata*	Violet	13,790
21. *Zingiber officinale*	Ginger root	12,420

Herbs marked with an asterisk (*) may produce adverse reactions. Consult a physician or herbal expert before using.

Acacia, False *(Acacia senegal)*

Common Names: Gum arabic, gum senegal, Egyptian thorn, Indian gum tree, Gum acacia.

Tibb Name: Aqaquiya, اقاقيا

Habitat: East and West Africa, Senegal, Egypt, Abyssinia, India, Nubia, Upper Nile.

Properties: Demulcent, emollient, protective, nutritive. By its viscidity sheaths inflammed surfaces; as a dilutant, lessens acridity of irritating medicines.

Uses: Coughs, laryngitis, gastritis, typhoid fever, dysentery, diarrhea.

Quality: Hot and dry in second degree.

Ajowan [Ajwain] *(Ptychotis ajowan)*
Common Name: Ajwain.

Tibb Name: Ajwain, ajowan, اجوان

Habitat: India, Pakistan.

Properties: Of main ingredient (thymol): stimulant, antiseptic, deodorant, disinfectant, parasiticide, antipyretic, local anesthetic, anthelmintic, tonic, emmenagogue, antispasmodic.

Uses: Gastritis, hookworm, stomatitis, diphtheria, bronchitis, coryza, rhinitis, ozena, conjunctivitis, otorrhea, gonorrhea, uterine lochia, cancer, leukorrhea, warts, skin diseases (psoriasis, eczema, etc.), diarrhea, dysentery, typhoid fever, diabetes, rheumatism, neuraligia; externally for sores, ulcers, gangrene.

Quality: Hot and dry in second degree.

Aloeswood *(Aquilaria aqallocha)*
Common Names: 'Ud, aloes, aloeswood.

Tibb Name: 'Oud, sabr, lowah, عـود

Habitat: A genus of liliaceous plants growing only in India and Arabia.

Properties: Stimulant, stomachic, laxative (purgative in large amounts), aphrodisiac.

Uses: Its chief effect is on the colon. Prescribed in anemia, amenorrhea, atonic dyspepsia, obstructive jaundice, and painful piles, and as an anthelmentic. Externally the powder is dusted over wounds to expedite healing.

Quality: Hot and dry in second degree.

Aloe Vera (*Aloe vera*)
Common names: Aloe, Barbados aloe, Curaçao aloe.

Tibb Name: Sabir, صبر

Habitat: East Africa, Socotra (West Indies), Italy, South Africa, southwestern United States.

Properties: Cathartic, drastic, emmenagogue, vermifuge, stomachic. The action on colon and large intestine causes irritation to uterus and inflamed hemorrhoids, stimulates liver functions, and intestinal secretions generally, increases flow of bile; acts in about 15 hours.

Uses: Costiveness, atonic dyspepsia, jaundice, nonactive hemorrhoids, amenorrhelaster, ascardies (for last two may be given by enema); externally, raw juice applied to burns.

Quality: Cold and moist in second degree.

Ammoniacum (*Dorema ammoniacum*)
Common Name: Gum ammoniac.

Tibb Name: Ushaq, اشق

Habitat: Middle and Near East, India, Persia.

Properties: Expectorant, diuretic, antispasmodic, stimulant, diaphoretic, emmenagogue.

Uses: For fistulas, abscesses, eye problems, tumors, insanity, as a poultice.

Note: Ammoniac has been used since antiquity and was mentioned by Hippocrates.

Quality: Cold and moist in second degree.

Aniseed *(Pimpinella anisum)*
Common Names: Anise, anise seed, sweet cumin.

Tibb Name: Anisun, انيسون

Habitat: Egypt, Crete, Cyprus, Near East.

Properties: Aromatic stimulant and carminative, stomachic, galactagogue, emmenagogue.

Uses: Digestive aid, cough mixtures, flavoring agent.

Quality: Hot and dry in second degree.

Arabic Gum *(Acacia arabica): See* Acacia, false

* Asafoetida *(Ferula foetida)*
Common Names: Gum asafoetida, devil's dung, food of the gods.

Tibb Name: Hing, Hiltit, حلتيت حنك

Habitat: Persia, Afghanistan, Turkey; mountain slopes; barren, desolate wastes; deserts.

Properties: Stimulant, antispasmodic, expectorant, laxative, emmenagogue, anthelmentic, condiment.

Uses: Hysteria, hypochondriasis, convulsions, spasms, whooping cough, measles, asthma, coughs, catarrhs, flatulent constipation, chorea, nervous apoplexy, consumption. Used in India and Near East as a condiment for flavoring, like garlic and onions; acts here as a stimulant to the bowels and digestion. Tolerance of odor and taste is acquired, as on first contact may seem nauseating.

Quality: Hot and dry in third degree.

Balsam Fir (*Abies* species)
Common Name: Balm of Gilead.

Tibb Name: Tanub, تنوب

Habitat: U.S.A., Canada, Europe, worldwide in mountainous elevations.

Properties: Similiar to oil of turpentine; stimulant, irritant.

Uses: Hysteria, whooping cough, intestinal irritation, amenorrhea, rheumatism, liniments, plasters.

Quality: Hot and moist in second degree.

Barberry (*Berberis vulgaris*)
Common Names: Barberry bark, jaundice berry, pepperidge, sowberry.

Tibb Name: Amir Baris, امیرباریس

Habitat: Deciduous shrub that grows in northeastern states and rich soils of western states of U.S.A.

Properties: Anthelmintic, tenifuge, astringent.

Uses: Vermifuge, astringent. Root: hepatic, laxative. Berries: laxative, refrigerant. Lowers blood pressure, purgative. Juice of fresh fruit used to strengthen gums and relieve pyorrhea.

Quality: Cold in second degree.

Basil (*Ocimun basilicum*)
Common Names: Common basil, St. Josephwort, sweet basil.

Tibb Name: Shahfaram. شاهفرم

Habitat: Annual plant growing in Sri Lanka, Indochina, Persia, Java, and tropical and subtropical regions of the world.

Properties: Cordial, cephalic, diuretic, nervine.

Uses: Flatulence, bad eyesight, melancholy, rheumatism, influenza.

Quality: Hot and dry in first degree.

Bayberry Bark *(Myrica cerifera)*
Common Name: Wax myrtle.

Habitat: Southern U.S.A.; dry woods, fields.

Properties: Alterative, cholagogue, diuretic, sialagogue, astringent, tonic.

Uses: Diarrhea, scrofula, jaundice.

Beleric Myrobalen *(Terminalia belerica)*
Common Name: Beleric Myrobalen.

Tibb Name: Bahera, بحرا

Habitat: India and Pakistan.

Properties: Astringent, tonic, laxative, purgative.

Uses: Piles, diarrhea, fever, dropsy, cough, hoarseness, dyspepsia, catarrh.

Quality: Hot and dry in second degree.

* Betel Nut *(Areca catechu)*
Common Names: Areca nut, paan, siparu.

Tibb Name: Faufal, paan, بان فوفل

Habitat: India; cultivated.

Properties: Astringent; nervine; midly narcotic.

Uses: Condiment after meals; astringent, tenifuge.

Quality: Cold in third degree.

Black Pepper *(Piper negrum)*
Tibb Name: Murch siah, مورج سیا

Habitat: South Asia; cultivated worldwide.

Properties: Stimulant, tonic, antiperiodic, carminative, rubefacient.

Uses: Intermittent fevers, colic, indigestion, flatulence; gargle for throat; gums, plaster for rheumatism; universal condiment.

Quality: Hot and dry in third degree.

Borage *(Borago officinalis)*
Common Names: Bugloss, borage.

Tibb Name: Lasan al-Thur, لسان الثور

Habitat: Annual plant that grows wild in Mediterranean countries and is cultivated throughout the world.

Properties: Aperient, diaphoretic, febrifuge, galactagogue, pectoral, tonic.

Uses: Reduces fever, antidote for poisons, nervine, pleurisy, peritonitis, increases flow of milk. Fresh leaves may cause dermatitis.

Quality: Cold and moist in second degree.

* Camphor *(Cinnamomun camphoru)*
Common Names: Camphor laurel, gum camphor tree.

Tibb Name: Kafur, كافور

Habitat: China, Japan, Taiwan, Borneo; cultivated in Italy, California, Florida, wherever frosts are light.

Properties: Antispasmodic, stimulant, carminative, stomachic, (an)aphrodisiac, antipyretic, nervine, sedative, diaphoretic, rebefacient, resolvent, antiseptic. Has great healing powers; dilates vessels, increases flow of gastric juice and peristalsis.

Uses: Refrigerant, anaphrodisiac, hysteria, dysmenorrhea, nervousness, diarrhea, colic, flatulence, rheumatism, gout, tenesmus, asthma, cough, coryza, toothache, headache, spasms, chorea, epilepsy, nausea, typhoid condition, mania. Externally: as a wash, liniment, ointment for ulcers, gangrene, scabies, sprains, bruises, rheumatic pains, convulsions.

Note: Ibn Masawaih considers camphor one of the five most important aromas. Al-Razi employed camphor for headache, but said it causes insomnia. Ibn Sina prescribed camphor for abscesses, kidney calculi, and bladder stones.

Quality: Cold and moist in third degree.

* Capsicum *(Capsicum frutescens)*

Common Names: Cayenne pepper, African cayenne, chili pepper, red pepper.

Tibb Name: Filfil ah, فلفل اح

Habitat: South and Central America, East India, Java, Africa; cultivated in U.S.A. and in tropics.

Properties: Stimulant, stomachic, rubefacient, condiment, diaphoretic; stimulates flow from salivary, gastric, and intestinal glands, also the stomach walls and heart. Long, continuous use may produce chronic gastritis, abdominal pain. Large quantity may produce acute gastritis, renal inflammation, strangury.

Uses: Indigestion, dyspepsia, atonic gout, alcoholism, delirium tremens, inter-mittents; flatulent colic, low fevers, cholera, menorrhagia, seasickness, tonsillitis, scarlet fever, diphtheria, hemorrhoids. Externally: lumbago, rheumatism, neuralgia, relaxed uvula.

Note: Capsicum has been used medicinally since the origins of recorded history.

Quality: Hot and dry in fourth degree.

Caraway (Seed) *(Carum carui)*

Common Names: Caraway seed, carvies.

Tibb Name: Karawyah, كراوية

Habitat: Central and West Asia, Himalayas. Caucasus, Europe, Siberia; cultivated in England, Norway, Russia, Germany, Holland, Morocco, U.S.A.

Properties: Carminative, stimulant, diuretic, stomachic.

Uses: Flatulent colic, especially of infants, corrective to nauseous purgatives, flavoring, toothache, as a cooking spice. Mainly the distilled oil is used.

Quality: Hot and dry in second degree.

Cardamom *(Elettaria cardamomun)*
Tibb Name: Qaqullah, قاقله

Habitat: Malabar, cultivated; India, Sri Lanka, Annam, Thailand.

Properties: Stomachic, carminative, anticolic, heart stimulant, aphrodisiac, emmenagogue, relaxant, tonic, purgative, condiment, aromatic, digestive.

Uses: Corrective to tonics, purgatives, flavoring agent in cakes, tea, puddings, etc.

Quality: Hot and dry in second degree.

* Cassia, Purging: *See* Senna

Catnip *(Nepeta hindostana [Cataria])*
Common Names: Catmint, catrup, catswort, field balm.

Habitat: Asia, Europe, naturalized in U.S.A.

Properties: Carminative, stimulant, tonic, diaphoretic, emmenagogue, antispasmodic, aphrodisiac (cats).

Uses: Hysteria, chlorosis, colic, amenorrhea, toothache.

Quality: Hot and dry in second degree.

* Celandine *(Chelidonium majus)*
Common Names: Chelidonium, garden celandine, great celandine, tetterwort.

Tibb Name: Mamiran Kabir, ما ميران كبير

Habitat: Biennial or perennial plant that grows widely in damp, rich soil in northeastern U.S.A., along fences, roads, and hedges; also in wastelands in Europe.

Properties: Cathartic, diuretic, diaphoretic, expectorant, rubefacient, purgative, cholagogue.

Uses: Jaundice, dropsy, intermittent fever, scrofula, skin diseases. Externally: warts, corns, eczema, urticaria, itching eruptions. Fresh herb in amenorrhea, as a vulnerary. In Russia it is used against cancer.

Quality: Hot and dry in fourth degree.

Chamomile *(Anthemis nobilis)*
Common Names: Roman chamomile, chamomile, matricaria, ground apple, whig plant.

Tibb Name: Babunag, بابونج

Habitat: Roman chamomile is a low European perennial found in dry fields and around gardens and cultivated fields. Widely cultivated.

Properties: Bitter, stomachic, carminative, anti-epileptic, antipyretic, nervine, emmenagogue. In large quantities, emetic, cathartic.

Uses: Intermittent fevers, torpid liver, delirium tremens, dyspepsia. Externally: colic, toothache, earache, rheumatism, ulcers, sprains. Oil used for rheumatism, flatulent colic.

Quality: Hot and dry in first degree.

Chestnut *(Castanea vesca [dentata])*
Common Names: Chestnut.

Tibb Name: Qastal, قسطل

Habitat: A huge tree of beautiful appearance growing in North America, western Asia, southern Europe.

Properties: Tonic, mild sedative, astringent; skin—antipyretic.

Uses: Leaves used in whooping cough, controlling paroxysms, dysentery; nuts a delicacy, thoroughly edible.

Quality: Cold and moist in second degree.

Chickory *(Chichorium intybus)*
Common Names: Succory, wild chickory.

Tibb Name: Hindbah, هندبا

Habitat: A perennial plant, grows wild in the U.S.A. and Europe, and is also cultivated.

Properties: Stomachic, tonic, digestive, diuretic, cholagogue.

Uses: Roasted chickory root is one of the most effective herbs to tone the liver and is often prescribed in jaundice. Gastritis, gallstones, digestive problems. Roasted chickory is a common adulterant in coffee, due to its quality of off-setting the bitter principle of coffee.

Quality: Hot and dry in second degree.

* Chrysanthemum *(Chrysanthimum roseum)*
Common Names: Persian pellitory, Persian insect powder.

Habitat: Western Asia, Persia; cultivated.

Properties: Cardiac depressant.

Uses: Due to toxicity, often used as a insecticide; cardiac conditions.

Quality: Use with caution, only under medical supervision.

Cinnamon *(Cinnamomum Loureirii)*
Common Names: God's cinnamon, Annam.

Tibb Name: Dar Chini, درصينى

Habitat: Cochin China (South Vietnam).

Properties: Carminative, stomachic, stimulant, astringent, hemostatic, aromatic, antispasmodic, germicide.

Uses: As a spice; diarrhea, flatulence, nausea, vomiting, menorrhagia, parturient, to correct griping medicines; for flavoring preparations.

Quality: Hot and dry in third degree.

Cistus *(Cistus Landaniferous)*
Common Names: Landanum cistus, rock rose.

Tibb Name: Ladan, لادن

Habitat: Grecian Islands.

Properties: Stimulant, expectorant, emmenagogue.

Uses: Adhesive, in plasters, catarrh, dysentery.

Quality: Cold and moist in first degree.

Clove *(Caryophyllus aromaticus)*
Common Names: Cloves, mother cloves.

Tibb Name: Qaranful, kabbash (fruits), قرنفل

Habitat: Molucca Islands, cultivated in Indian Ocean Islands, Sumatra, Malacca, Penang, South America (Brazil), Guyana, Africa, Zanzibar.

Properties: Stimulant, stomachic, carminative, anti-emetic, aromatic, anti-spasmodic, rubefacient, germicide, antiseptic. Increases temperature, circulation, digestion, nutrition. Excreted by kidneys, skin, liver, bronchi—stimulating and disinfecting each.

Uses: Nausea, vomiting, flatulence, colic, indigestion, condiment, corrective. Externally: in rheumatism, neuralgia, toothache; in liniments; as a poultice over nape of neck for infantile convulsions.

Quality: Hot and dry in third degree.

Cocoa Butter *(Theobromatis cacao)*
Common Name: Cacao butter.

Habitat: South America (Brazil), Central America, Mexico, West Indies; cultivated in the tropics.

Properties: Nutrient, demulcent, emollient.

Uses: Seldom used internally; usually used in suppositories, as a carrier for other medicines; externally in cosmetic ointments, pill coatings, for abraded or sunburned skin.

Quality: Cold and moist in second degree.

Comfrey *(Symphytum officinale)*
Common Names: Blackwort, bruisewort, gum plant, healing herb, slippery root.

Tibb Name: 'Irq Injbar, عرق انجبار

Habitat: A perennial plant common in moist areas of the U.S.A. and Europe.

Properties: Anodyne, astringent, demulcent, emollient, expectorant, hemostatic, refrigerant, vulnary.

Uses: Diarrhea, simple hemorrhages, gargle, mouthwash, digestive problems, leukorrhea, dysentery. Externally: as a poultice for sprains, bruises, sores, and insect bites.

Quality: Cold in second degree.

Coriander *(Coriandum sativum)*
Common Name: Coriander seed.

Tibb Name: Kuzbarah, كزبرة

Habitat: The fruit of an umbelliferous plant in Europe and Asia; cultivated in the U.S.A.

Properties: Aromatic, carminative, stimulant, stomachic, aromatic.

Uses: Indigestion, flatulence, corrective to griping medicines, flavoring in cooking, rheumatism, neuralgia. The tender leaves and shoots are used to flavor salads and soups. Enters prominently into Middle and Near Eastern and Indian cooking.

Note: Hakim Ibn Sina held this plant in particularly high regard, due to the dictum of the Prophet Muhammad (s.a.s.) to the effect that seed of coriander was the cure of every disease; this remark is also attributed about the herb known as khalonji.

Quality: Hot and dry in second degree.

* Cottonseed *(Gossypium herbaceum)*
Common Names: Absorbent cotton, cotton, cotton wool.

Tibb Name: Cotn, قطن

Habitat: Central Asia, India, China, Arabia, Northeast Africa, Egypt; cultivated in the U.S.A., West Indies, North Africa, Spain, Australia, Central and South America.

Properties: Hairs: protective. Oil: Demulcent, nutrient.

Uses: Hairs: dressings on burns, scalds, erysipelas, blisters, surgical wounds; prevents entrance of germs that cause infection and septic disease. Oil: similar to olive and almond oils; used for liniments, salves, etc. Seed: mucilaginous, as a remedy for coughs.

Note: Most of the commercially grown cotton crop in the U.S.A. is sprayed with highly toxic chemicals and is unsuitable for medicinal use.

Quality: Hot and dry in third degree.

Cucumber *(Cucumis sativus)*
Tibb Name: Khiyar, خيار

Habitat: A fleshy, creeping, or climbing vine that grows worldwide in hot and tropical climates.

Properties: Aperient, diuretic, sedative, cooling, antipyretic.

Uses: Excellent to remove water for those with kidney and heart problems; helps dissolve uric acid accumulations such as kidney and bladder stones. An ointment made from fleshy part is used for beautifying the skin and for fissures of the nipple.

Quality: Cold and moist in second degree.

Cumin *(Cuminum cyminum)*
Tibb Name: Kammun, كمّون

Habitat: Near, Middle, and Far East, and Mediterranean countries; cultivated worldwide.

Properties: Seeds aromatic, carminative, digestive.

Uses: Digestive aid; powdered seeds used for deafness; mixed with honey and pepper as aphrodisiac.

Note: Cumin enters into virtually all of the compound formulas of the ancient Hakims. It is believed that cumin is one of the only herbs that pass through the stomach unaffected by digestion and release their action only at the site of the liver.

Quality: Hot and dry in third degree.

Date *(Phoenix dactylifera)*
Common Name: Date palm.

Tibb Name: Nakhil; when dried, called Tamr, نخيل

Habitat: One of the oldest trees known to man. Native to Middle and Near East. Cultivated in southwestern U.S.A.

Properties: Nutrient, demulcent, emollient.

Uses: Primarily as a nutrient.

Quality: Hot and dry in first degree.

Dill *(Anethum graveolens)*
Common Name: Dill seed.

Tibb Name: Shabat, شبت

Habitat: Southern Europe, Asia, cultivated in the U.S.A.

Properties: Carminative, cardiac tonic, soporific, stomachic, stimulant, condiment, flavoring.

Uses: Flatulent colic, hiccup, indigestion; cardiac ailments. Ancient physicians used decoction as an eyewash, said to innoculate against diseases of cornea.

Quality: Hot and dry in second degree.

* Dodder *(Cuscuta Europaea [reflexa])*
Common Names: Beggarweed, Scaldweed.

Tibb Name: Kasoos, طحم كسوس

Habitat: Grows parasitically on clover, thyme, heath, milk vetch, and other small plants; Great Britain, Persia, India.

Properties: Tonic for liver, carminative, abortifacient, purgative, attenuant, antiobstructive.

Uses: Jaundice, sciatica, scrofulous tumors.

Quality: Hot and dry in third degree.

Dragon's Blood *(Daemonorprops draco)*
Tibb Name: Dam Al-Ak, دم الك

Habitat: Borneo, Sumatra.

Properties: Mild stimulant, astringent.

Uses: In tooth powders, plasters, etc.

Quality: Hot and dry in second degree.

Embelia *(Embelia ribes)*
Tibb Name: Abranajah, ابرنجة

Habitat: Throughout India and Pakistan.

Properties: Anthelmintic, carminative, stomachic, alterative, tonic.

Uses: Berries are specific for tapeworm; skin diseases, dyspepsia, flatulence, ringworm, headache.

Quality: Hot and dry in second degree.

Emblic Myrobalen *(Emblica officinalis)*
Common Names: Emblic myrobalen, Indian gooseberry.

Tibb Name: Amlaj, املج

Habitat: India and Pakistan.

Properties: Refrigerant, tonic, antiscorbutic, diuretic, laxative, anthelmintic.

Uses: One of the richest sources of vitamin C; fevers, hiccups, vomiting, indigestion, habitual constipation, to expel worms, blood purifier, diarrhea, dysentery, hemorrhage, gonorrhea, ophthalmia, scabies.

Quality: Cold and dry in third degree.

Eyebright *(Euphrasia officinalis)*

Common Names: Red eyebright, euphrasy, eye-bright.

Habitat: Annual herb common in grassy areas, meadows of Europe and western Asia; naturalized in U.S.A.

Properties: Astringent, tonic.

Uses: As name suggests, used to soothe eyes, usually prepared as a decoction and used as eyewash; for hayfever.

Quality: Cold and moist in first degree.

Fennel *(Foeniculum vulgare)*

Common Name: Fennel seed.

Tibb Name: Shamar, شمر

Habitat: Southern Europe, western Asia; cultivated worldwide.

Properties: Carminative, stimulant, diaphoretic, aromatic, stomachic, galactagogue, emmenagogue, aphrodisiac, lactagogue.

Uses: Nausea, colic, amenorrhea, infantile flatulency; increases secretion of milk, perspiration, urine, mucus; as a corrective to griping medicines such as senna, and rhubarb. Much used in veterinary medicine, especially for cattle.

Quality: Hot and dry in second degree.

Fenugreek *(Trigonella foenum-graecum)*

Tibb Name: Hulba, farigah, فريقة حلبة

Habitat: India, Europe; cultivated in France, Germany, etc.

Properties: Sedative, stomachic, anthelmintic, expectorant, restorative, aphrodisiac.

Uses: Coughs, tuberculosis, bronchitis, fevers, sore throat, neuralgia, sciatica, swollen glands, skin eruptions, wounds, tumors, sores, furuncles, asthma, emphysema.

Note: Fenugreek is one of the oldest herbs in use, common since the time of Hippocrates. Avicenna valued it highly, due to the dictum of the Prophet Muhammad (s.a.s.): "If you knew the value of fenugreek, you would pay its weight in gold."

Quality: Hot and dry in third degree.

Fig *(Ficus carica)*
Tibb Name: Tin, تـــين

Habitat: Indigenous to Persia, Asia Minor, and Syria. Now grows wild in most Mediterranean countries. Cultivated in temperate zones of Europe and U.S.A.

Properties: Laxative, demulcent, nutritive.

Uses: Habitual constipation. Split open and applied as poultice.

Quality: Hot and dry in second degree.

Frankincense *(Boswellia carterii)*
Common Names: Frankincense, olibanum. لبان الكنك

Tibb Name: Loban; resin is called loban or Al-Kunnuk

Habitat: East Africa, Arabia.

Properties: Stimulant, expectorant, emmenagogue, sudorific.

Uses: Bronchial and laryngeal infections; locally for chilblains; prevents hemoptysis; deadens toothache; fumigant.

Quality: Hot and dry in second degree.

Garlic *(Allium sativum)*
Common Name: Clove garlic.

Tibb Name: Thum, ثـــوم

Habitat: Central Asia, southern Europe; widely cultivated.

Properties: Stimulant, anthelmintic, antispasmodic, carminative, condiment, diuretic, expectorant, rubefacient, stomachic, antipyretic, febrifuge, intestinal antiseptic, emmenagogue, aphrodisiac.

Uses: Bronchitis, indigestion, chronic cough, stomach and intestinal catarrh, dysentery, cholera, typhoid; beneficial action on circulation and heart action; urinary stones.

Quality: Hot and dry in third degree.

Gentian *(Gentiana lutea)*
Tibb Name: Jantiana, جنطيانا

Habitat: Mountains.

Properties: Roots are stimulant, bitter stomachic, antipyretic, appetizer, digestive.

Uses: Anemia, dyspepsia, pregnancy, and convalescence.

Quality: Cold in second degree.

Ginger *(Zingiber officinalis)*
Common Names: Ginger, Jamaican ginger.

Tibb Name: Zanjabil, زنجبيل

Habitat: India; cultivated in West Indies, Africa.

Properties: Aromatic, carminative, stimulant, sternutatory, rubefacient, anodyne, sialagogue, cardiac tonic, aphrodisiac.

Uses: Atonic dyspepsia, flatulent colic, atonic gout, diarrhea, cholera, chronic bronchitis, alcoholic gastritis, corrective to nauseous medicines, condiment.

Quality: Hot and dry in third degree.

* Goldenseal *(Hydrastis canadensis)*
Common Names: Goldenseal, yellow root.

Habitat: North America; rich woodlands, mountains.

Properties: Upon the digestive, circulatory, respiratory, and nervous system, similar to but much weaker than strychnine; bitter tonic, increases appetite, digestion, gastric secretions, and flow of bile; antiperiodic, protoplasmic poison, alterative to mucous membranes, antiseptic, cholagogue, diuretic.

Uses: Chronic dyspepsia and cystitis, catarrhs of the stomach, duodenum, gall ducts, bladder, vagina; constipation, bronchitis, malaria, intermittent fever, jaundice; locally in gonorrhea, leukorrhea, otorrhea, gleet, chronic nasal catarrh and pharyngitis, syphilitic sores, chronic ulcers and sores, cancers, fistulas, hemorrhoids, fissured nipples, conjunctivitis, tonsillitis, hemorrhage.

Note: Large doses, while nontoxic, produce warmth in the stomach and ringing in the ears.

Quality: Hot and dry in third degree.

* Gourd, Wild *(Citrullus colocynth)*

Common Names: Colocynth, bitter apple.

Tibb Name: Hanzal, حنظل

Habitat: South and West Asia, North and South Africa, in deserts of Arabia, Syria, Egypt, Morocco, Greece, Spain, Japan, Pakistan; cultivated.

Properties: Drastic hydragogue cathartic, hepatic stimulant, diuretic, abortifacient; small doses bitter, stomachic; large doses emetic, irritant poison, causing violent griping, dangerous bowel inflammations.

Uses: Evacuant, dropsy, melancholia, coma, apoplexy, paralysis, antisyphilitic, to promote bile secretions, cancer, arthritis.

Quality: Hot and dry in fourth degree.

Note: Never to be used in pregnancy, nor where gastric or intestinal inflammation exists. It is very harsh and seldom used alone. In event of poisoning, evacuate stomach, give demulcents, stimulants, etc.

Grape *(Vitis vinifera)*

Common Name: Grape vine.

Habitat: West Asia; cultivated universally.

Properties: Stimulant, depressant, astringent, tonic, diaphoretic, laxative.

Uses: Bronchitis, fevers, general debility, irritable stomach, ulceration, gangrene, tetanus, old age.

Quality: Hot and moist in second degree.

Henna *(Lawsonia inermis)*
Tibb Name: Henna, حناء

Habitat: India, Arabia.

Properties: Dye, sedative.

Uses: Mainly to dye hair and hands reddish color. When leaves are cooked and eaten, henna is said to purify the blood; when infused with vinegar, it is a sedative. The flowers are fragrant and used to make perfume. The ancient Egyptians used henna in mummification.

Quality: Cold and moist in second degree.

Hops *(Humulus lupulus)*
Tibb Name: Hashishah al-dinar, حشيشة الدينار

Habitat: Northern temperate zone; North America, Central Asia; cultivated.

Properties: Anodyne, nervine, tonic, stimulant, nervous sedative, hypnotic, diuretic.

Uses: Nervous insomnia, dyspepsia, delirium tremens, hysteria, irritable bladder, rheumatism, abscesses (poultice).
Note: Large doses can be harmful.

Quality: Cold in third degree.

Horehound *(Marrubium vulgare)*
Common Names: Hoarhound, marrubium, white horehound.

Tibb Name: Farasiun, فراسيون

Habitat: Europe, Central Asia, North America; cultivated in waste places, gardens, etc.

Properties: Stimulant, tonic, bitter stomachic, expectorant, resolvent, anthelmintic, heart tonic; large doses: diuretic, diaphoretic, laxative.

Uses: Dyspepsia, bronchitis, chronic hepatitis, jaundice, amenorrhea, phthisis, cachexia, catarrh, chronic rheumatism, typhoid fever, to calm heart action.

Quality: Hot and dry in third degree.

Hyssop *(Hyssop officinalis)*
Tibb Name: Zufa, زوفــا

Habitat: Southern Europe; cultivated in temperate U.S.A.

Properties: Cathartic, carminative, stimulant, sudorific, emmenagogue, expectorant, tonic, stomachic.

Uses: Dyspepsia, amenorrhea, rheumatism, bruises, bronchitis, sore throat, chronic catarrhs, flatulence, scrofula, dropsy; as a wash for burns, bruises, and skin irritations.

Quality: Cold and moist in second degree.

Jasmine *(Jasminum officinale)*
Tibb Name: Yasmin, ياسمين

Habitat: Warm parts of Eastern Hemisphere; India, the Middle East; now cultivated in gardens in southern U.S.A.

Properties: Calmative.

Uses: To calm the nerves, aphrodisiac, rheumatism, gout.

Note: When used as a natural perfume (without alcohol), jasmine is said to be unparalleled in its ability to lessen depression.

Quality: Cold and dry in first degree. Attar of jasmine is hot and dry in second degree.

Jujube *(Zizyphus vulgare)*
Tibb Name: 'Onnab, عنّاب

Habitat: Native to China, but now cultivated in several Mediterranean countries.

Properties: Pectoral, astringent.

Uses: In Tibb, used as a flavoring for lozenges known as jujubes. Infusion of leaves is used for relaxation, diuresis, and purgation.

Quality: Cold and dry in first degree.

Juniper *(Juniperus communis)*
Common Name: Juniper berry.

Tibb Name: 'Ar'Ar, عرعر

Habitat: North America, Asia, Europe, North Africa; dry hills, woods.

Properties: Stimulant, diuretic, anodyne, emmenagogue, carminative, stomachic, antiseptic, sudorific, laxative.

Uses: Renal dropsy, vesical catarrh, rheumatic pains, swellings, analgesic, urinary conditions, female reproductive diseases, digestive problems.

Note: Usually taken as a tea made from the berries. In large doses can damage kidneys; not recommended for pregnant women.

Quality: Cold and dry in third degree.

Khalonji *(Nigella sativa)*
Common Names: Khalonji, black seeds.

Tibb Name: Khalonji, thuniz, حبة السوداء

Habitat: Arabia, Egypt, India, Pakistan, Afghanistan.

Properties: Diuretic, emmenagogue, galactagogue, abortifacient, anthelmintic, carminative, stimulant.

Uses: Lung and bronchial complaints, coughs, jaundice, tertian fever, paralysis, piles; decoction of seeds is given to promote contraction of uterus after birth and also to secrete milk; given in amenorrhea and dysmenorrhea, eruptive skin diseases.

Note: A remark is attributed to the Prophet Muhammad (s.a.w.s.) to the effect that the seeds of khalonji are the cure of every disease except the decline of old age (death).

Quality: Hot and dry in second degree.

Lavender *(Lavandula vera)*
Common Name: True lavender.

Tibb Name: Ustokhudus, اسطوخودوس

Habitat: Southern Europe (France, Italy, Spain), Northwest Africa; sunny hills and mountains; cultivated.

Properties: Stimulant, carminative, nervine, errhine, antispasmodic, diuretic, sedative, stomachic, tonic.

Uses: Nausea, flatulence, nervous headache, fainting, dizziness, perfumery, hair rinse. Usually in form of the expressed oil.

Quality: Hot and dry in third degree.

Lemon *(Citrus limonum)*
Tibb Name: Laimun, ليمون

Habitat: Known throughout the world; highest quality grown in Florida and California.

Properties: Astringent, refrigerant, stomachic, tonic. Seeds: antipyretic and anthelementic. Juice: acid, astringent.

Uses: Soothing in inflammations, dental caries, vomiting, rheumatism, headache, colds, coughs, sore throat; hair rinse, facial astringent. Externally: sunburn, warts, corns.

Qualities: Juice is cold and dry in first degree. Pith is cold and moist in first degree. Seeds, peel, and blossom are hot and dry in first degree.

Licorice *(Glycyrrhiza glaba)*
Common Names: Licorice root, sweet licorice.

Tibb Name: Meluthi, ملوثى

Habitat: Southern Europe, western Asia, Syria, Persia, North Africa; cultivated in Russia, Spain, England, France, Germany, U.S.A., China; rich lowlands, river valleys.

Properties: Demulcent, expectorant, laxative, diuretic.

Uses: Primarily for bronchial problems; bowel and urinary infections; in pharmacy to mask unpleasant taste of bitter medicines.

Quality: Hot and dry in second degree.

* Lily of the Valley *(Convallaria majalis)*
Tibb Name: Mad'af, Zanbaq al-wadi, زنبق الوادى مضعف

Habitat: U.S.A.; cultivated.

Properties: Heart tonic, diuretic, emetic, purgative.

Uses: Greatly slows heart; arrhythmia; similar in action to digitalis.

Quality: Hot and dry in third degree.

Linseed *(Linum usitatissimum)*
Common Names: Flaxseed, linseed, lint-bells.

Tibb Name: Kittan, كتّان

Habitat: Central Asia, Egypt, southern Europe; spontaneous in most temperate climates; cultivated in Russia, Egypt, India, U.S.A., southern Europe, England, Holland.

Properties: Demulcent, emollient diluent, diuretic.

Uses: Infusion for inflammation of the mucous membranes of respiratory, digestive, and urinary organs; renal and vesical irritation, catarrh, dysentery, calculi, strangury; poultice of ground residue applied to enlarged glands, swellings, boils, pneumonia, welts, etc. Coat skin with olive oil, glycerin, or other oil before applying. Linseed oil is excellent in piles; also added to purgative enemas and to cover irritated skin surfaces.

Quality: Cold and moist in second degree.

* Lobelia *(Lobelia inflata)*
Common Names: Indian tobacco, emetic herb, lobelia.

Habitat: North America; in fields and open places.

Properties: Expectorant, emetic, nervine, purgative, narcotic, diuretic, diaphoretic. Similar to epicac, but causes more intense nausea and prostration. Larges doses emetic, causing severe vomiting.

Uses: Spasmodic asthma, catarrh, croup, bronchial spasms, whooping cough, strangulated hernia, constipation (when feces are hard and dry); externally for poison ivy (and oak), eczema.

Note: Do not give to children under age five; under twelve only with supervision of physician. A very effective, though potent herb. Use with caution.

Quality: Hot and dry in third degree.

Malabar Nut Tree *(Adhatoda vasica)*
Tibb Name: Arusa, اروسا

Habitat: Pakistan, India.

Properties: Expectorant, antispasmodic, febrifuge, tonic.

Uses: Chest diseases, bronchitis, asthma, diarrhea, dysentery, malarial fevers.

Quality: Cold and moist in second degree.

Malva *(Malva sylvestris)*
Common Names: Malva flowers, mallow leaves.

Tibb Name: Kubbazi, خبازی

Habitat: Europe, Asia, cultivated in U.S.A.

Properties: Demulcent, emollient.

Uses: Dysentery, catarrh, kidney troubles. Leaves are soothing to skin. Enters into poultices and dressings; via rectal enema for acute enteritis.

Quality: Cold and moist in first degree.

Mango *(Mangifera indica)*
Common Names: Mango tree, mango fruit.

Tibb Name: Manju, مانجو

Habitat: India, Mexico.

Properties: Bark: astringent. Flowers: nervine, tonic.

Uses: Diarrhea, diabetes, hiccup, ash of leaves for burns and scalds, mouth-wash, toothache, menorrhagia, leukorrhea, purulent discharges from uterus and bowels, dysentery, bleeding piles, skin diseases, diphtheria, flatulent colic, fevers, dyspepsia. Mixture of ½ ounce juice of the bark and 180 grams of lime water is given for seven days as a specific for gonorrhea.

Quality: Cold and moist in second degree.

* Marijuana *(Cannabis sativa)*

Common Names: Indian hemp, marijuana, bhang, ganja.

Tibb Name: Qanab, قنّب

Habitat: Asia, Persia, hills of North India; cultivated in India, Europe, Central and South Russia, Brazil, western and southern U.S.A.; cultivated worldwide.

Properties: Anodyne, nervine, sudorific, narcotic, aphrodisiac, increases appetite. Perverts perception, condition, and relation of objects. Large habitual doses bloat face, infect eyes, makes limbs tremulous, cause weakness, mental confusion, loss of short-term memory.

Uses: Neuralgia, distressing cough, quiets tickling in throat, gout, delirium tremens, tetanus convulsions, chorea, hysteria, mental depression, epilepsy, morphine habit, nervous vomiting.

Quality: Cold and dry in third degree.

Marjoram *(Origanum marjorana)*

Common Name: Wild marjoram.

Tibb Name: Bardaqush, بردقوش

Habitat: Asia, Europe, North Africa, naturalized in U.S.A.

Properties: Carminative, stimulant, emmenagogue, diaphoretic, tonic, fomentation, stomachic, anti-inflammatory.

Uses: Dyspepsia, indigestion, nausea, colic, rheumatism, neuralgia, sneezing, cough, respiratory ailments, menstrual cramps.

Quality: Hot and dry in second degree.

Marshmallow *(Althea officinalis)*
Common Names: Marsh mallow, white mallow, mortification root, sweet weed.

Tibb Name: Khatmiyah, خطمية

Habitat: Europe, western and northern Asia; naturalized in salt marshes, New England, New York, Australia; cultivated in Europe.

Properties: Emollient, sedative, protective.

Uses: Inflammations of pulmonary, digestive, urinary organs, mucous membranes; skin eruptions, gingivitis, ear bath in otitis, herpes, psoriasis, enema for vaginal and rectal irritation. In pharmacy, powdered root used to harden pills.

Quality: Hot in first degree.

Masterwort *(Heracleum lanatum)*
Common Names: Cow parsnip, hogweed, madnep, youthwort, masterwort.

Habitat: North America.

Properties: Stimulant, carminative, antispasmodic.

Uses: Epilepsy, dyspepsia, warts, escharotic, colds, asthma.

Note: The fresh leaves can produce dermatitis; cattle have reportedly been killed from eating masterwort.

Quality: Hot and dry in third degree.

Mastic *(Pistacia lentiscris)*
Tibb Name: Mustaki, مصطكى

Habitat: Mediterranean Basin, Island of Scio, Grecian Archipelago, etc.

Properties: Stimulant, diuretic, protective (solution).

Uses: Bronchial and vesical catarrhs, leukorrhea, gastric debility, chronic diarrhea, toothache, fumigation; saturated etheral solution allowed to harden in teeth as temporary filling; with alcohol or oil of turpentine as a varnish; fumigation; seldom used internally.

Quality: Cold and dry in second degree.

* Meadow Saffron *(Colchicum autumnale)*
Common Names: Colchicum root, upstart.

Tibb Name: Lilah, حلاح

Habitat: Central and southern Europe, North Africa; moist and high meadows.

Properties: Alternative, cathartic, emetic, sedative, diuretic, diaphoretic, gastrointestinal irritant. Small doses increase secretions. Normal doses produce pains and loose bowels.

Uses: Gout, rheumatism, increases urea and uric acid elimination from blood, urticaria, asthma.

Signs of Poisoning: Nausea, vomiting, thirst, pain in throat, suppressed urine, dilated pupils, cold extremities, weak pulse, spasm, stupor, death. Evacuate stomach, give morphine, demulcent drinks, stimulants, heat to extremities.

Quality: Hot and dry in fourth degree.

Melilot *(Melilotus officinalis)*
Common Names: Yellow melilot, yellow sweet clover, sweet trifoil.

Tibb Name: Iklil al-malik, handuq, حندوق أكليل الملك

Habitat: Europe, U.S.A.

Properties: Astringent, stimulant, resolvent.

Uses: To allay pain in abdomen, joints, diarrhea, dysmenorrhea, rheumatism.

Quality: Cold and moist in second degree.

* Mugwort *(Artemisis vulgaris)*
Common Names: Common mugwort, felon herb, sailor's tobacco.

Tibb Name: Swaila, سويلا

Habitat: Europe, Aisa, North and South America.

Properties: Appetizer, digestive, cholagogue, purgative, bitter, fragrant, emmena-gogue, antihysteric, anti-epileptic.

Uses: Hysteria, epilespy, catarrh, digestive aid, regulates menstruation, gout, rheumatism. Large doses may produce symptoms of poisoning.

Quality: Hot and dry in third degree.

* Mustard *(Brassica nigra [juncea])*
Common Names: Mustard seed, brown mustard.

Tibb Name: Saljam, سلجم

Habitat: Asia, southern Europe, Africa; cultivated in gardens; wild in the U.S.A.

Properties: Stimulant, emetic, tonic, diuretic, laxative, rubefacient, irritant, epispastic, carminative, condiment, vesicant; dilates the vessels, causing redness, warmth, and irritates sensory nerves, giving burning pain.

Uses: Atonic dyspepsia with constipation, delirium tremens, atonic dropsy, hiccup, narcotic poisoning. Externally: for rheumatism, gout, atrophy, neuralgia, colic, gastralgia, inflammation of throat or lungs, toothache, earache, headache, vomiting, diarrhea, dysentery, amenorrhea, dysmenorrhea; stimulant to heart, vascular system, and respiratory system.

Note: Large doses of black mustard either internally or externally can cause severe inflammation and burns. Never let undiluted mustard oil touch the skin, mucous membranes, or eyes.

Quality: Hot and dry in fourth degree.

Myrrh *(Commiphora [Balsamodendron] myrrha)*
Common Names: Myrrh, gum myrrh, Somali myrrh.

Tibb Name: Murr, مُرّ

Habitat: East Africa, southwestern Arabia, Somalia.

Properties: Antiseptic, astringent, carminative, stomachic, stimulant, tonic, expectorant, emmenagogue, vulnerary: increases circulation and the number of white corpuscles; it is eliminated by the genito-urinary and bronchial mucous membranes, augmenting and disinfecting their secretions. Large doses purge, cause vomiting. Externally: stimulant, disinfectant, and antiseptic to mucous membranes, ulcerated surfaces.

Uses: Atonic dyspepsia, amenorrhea, anemia, bronchial catarrh, cystitis, pharyngitis, chronic uterine and vaginal leukorrhea. Externally: ulcerated and spongy gums, relaxed throat, ptyalism, indolent ulcers. Myrrh powder applied to ulcers and wounds as disinfectant.

Quality: Cold and dry in second degree.

Myrtle *(Myrtus communis)*
Tibb Name: As, marsin, مرسين آس

Habitat: Egypt, India; temperate climates, tropics.

Properties: Astringent, carminative, emetic, diuretic, anthelmintic, antiseptic.

Uses: Chronic bronchitis, gonorrhea, uterine inflammation and discharge, rheumatism; as an incense to purify air; when cooked, used as hair dye.

Quality: Cold and dry in second degree.

Remarks: May substitute huckleberry.

Nutmeg *(Myristica fragrans)*
Tibb Name: Juz al-tibb; *Seeds:* Bisbasah, بسباسة جوز الطبّ

Habitat: Molucca Islands; cultivated in tropics, India, Philippine Islands, New Guinea, East and West Indies, South America, Sri Lanka, Sumatra.

Properties: Aromatic, stimulant, stomachic, narcotic, flavoring, condiment, increases gastric juice, digestion, appetite. Large doses, like camphor, act on cerebrum, causing stupor, delirium.

Uses: Rheumatism, hair tonic, flatulence, gastric debility, diarrhea, dysentery, vomiting, colic, dyspepsia, flavoring, condiments.

Quality: Hot and dry in third degree.

Olive *(Olea europea)*
Tibb Name: Zaitun, زیتون

Habitat: Asia, Egypt, Middle East, southern Europe, Algeria; cultivated in southern U.S.A., South America.

Properties: Antipyretic, nutritious, demulcent, emollient, laxative, protection of mucous membranes. Increases secretion of bile and peristalsis, and dissolves cholesterin, the chief constituent of gallstones.

Uses: Gallstones, cantharides, and other poisonings; infantile constipation in enema. Externally: burns, skin inflammations, insect bites, stings, bruises, wounds, engorged mammaries. As a lubricant; to make liniments, plasters, ointments, etc.

Quality: Older oil is hot and moist in second degree. Fresh oil is cold and dry in first degree.

* Pellitory (Root) *(Anacyclus pyrethrum)*
Tibb Name: 'Aquir Qarha, عاقیر قرحا

Habitat: North Africa, Algeria; highlands, cultivated in gardens.

Properties: Irritant, rubefacient, sialagogue, sternutatory (poisonous).

Uses: Headache, rheumatism, neuralgia, toothache, paralysis of tongue or throat, relaxed uvula, chronic catarrh.

Quality: Hot and dry in fourth degree.

* Pennyroyal *(Hedeoma pulegioides)*
Common Names: American pennyroyal, squaw balm, mosquito plant.

Habitat: North America, sandy fields, hills, open woods.

Properties: Stimulant, carminative, emmenagogue, aromatic.

Uses: Flatulent colic, nausea, indigestion, corrective to purgatives; hot infusion: diarrhea, bronchitis, rheumatism, amenorrhea. Odor repels mosquitoes, etc. Large doses induce abortion.

Note: Within the last decade, a woman in the United States died while attempting to use essential oil of pennyroyal to induce abortion.

Quality: Hot and dry in third degree.

Peppermint *(Mentha piperita)*
Common Names: Mint, peppermint, lamb mint.

Tibb Name: Na'na', نعناع

Habitat: Asia, Europe, North America; cultivated worldwide.

Properties: Carminative, stimulant, nervine, antispasmodic.

Uses: As tea or essential oil: Spasmodic stomach and bowel pains, flatulency, nausea, cholera, morbus, diarrhea, dysentery, colic, dysmenorrhea, nervous headache, hiccup, heart palpitations, vomiting. As a flavoring agent. Externally (oil): rheumatism, neuralgia, toothache, antibacterial.

Quality: Hot and dry in second degree.

Pistachio *(Pistacia vera)*
Common Name: Pistachio nuts.

Tibb Name: Fastaq, فستق

Habitat: Temperate countries.

Properties: Main constituent is albuminoids.

Uses: Mainly used in cooking; skins of nuts for diarrhea, especially in children.

Quality: Hot and dry in second degree.

Plantain *(Plantago major)*
Common Names: Plantain, ribwort, buckhorn, soldier's herb.

Tibb Name: Lisan, al-hamal, لسان الحمل

Habitat: Meadows, roadsides, argricultural lands in U.S.A., Canada, Asia, Europe.

Properties: Astringent, demulcent, expectorant. Root and leaves: hemostatic, refrigerant, diuretic.

Uses: Cough, irritated throat, gastritis, respiratory problems; to eliminate mucus, catarrh. Externally: fresh leaves are crushed and applied for cuts, wounds, sores, bruises, insect bites, hemorrhoids.

Quality: Cold and dry in second degree.

Pomegranate *(Punica granatum)*
Tibb Name: Raman, رمان

Habitat: Southwest Asia, India, Persia, Arabia, China, Japan, East and West Indies; naturalized in subtropics, southern U.S.A.

Properties: Astringent, anthelmintic, tenifuge. Leaves and flowers: styptic, tonic.

Uses: To expel worms, tenia, externally and internally astringent; large doses cause vomiting, purging, cramps, numbness in legs, giddiness, dim vision, increased urine. Rind is also astringent in diarrhea, leukorrhea, hemorrhage, cancerous and other ulcers of uterus and rectum; intermittent fever. For tapeworm a tea is made from the bark, taken at one-hour intervals on an empty stomach. Also used for tanning, dying. Fruit is used as a cooling article of food.

Quality: Cold and dry in second degree.

Poppy (Seed) *(Papaver somniferum)*
Common Names: Poppy, opium poppy, marble flower.

Tibb Name: Khashkhas, خشنماش

Habitat: Western Asia, Persia, China, Africa, India, Italy, Greece, England, U.S.A.; cultivated.

Properties: Narcotic, anesthetic, soporific, sedative, anodyne, antispasmodic, hypnotic, diaphoretic, chiefly due to morphine.

Uses: Relieves pain, except in acute inflammation of the brain; induces sleep in insomnia of low fevers; relieves irritation; checks secretions—diarrhea, dysentery, diabetes; supports metabolism in low fevers; peritonitis, cerebrospinal meningitis, delirium tremens, mania spasms, melancholia, sciatica, neuralgia, cancer, renal and hepatic colic from calculi, cough without secretion; locks bowels when required by inflammation, hemorrhages, angina pectoris, cerebral anemia. Externally: applied in poultices for gout, rheumatism, ophthalmia, periodontitis, inflamed gums.

Note: Opium is illegal in the U.S.A. Children are very susceptible to its effects, and it should never be given to them without medical supervision. Also, women are affected more easily than men. Some persons cannot tolerate even the smallest dose.

Quality: Cold and dry in fourth degree.

Prickly Ash *(Zanthoxylum americanum)*
Common Name: Prickly ash bark.

Habitat: North America: Canada to Virginia to Florida.

Properties: Alterative, stimulant, sialagogue, diaphoretic, diuretic. Causes salivation, tingling in tongue, increased cardiac action and arterial tension, also secretion from stomach, intestines, liver, pancreas.

Uses: Chronic rheumatism, myalgia, lumbago, dropsy, chronic dyspepsia, diarrhea, syphilis. Externally: counterirritant in female pelvic diseases.

Quality: Hot and dry in fourth degree.

Pumpkin *(Curcurbita pepo)*
Common Name: Pumpkin seed.

Tibb Name: Qar', قرع

Habitat: Widely cultivated in warm and temperate climates.

Properties: Anthelmintic.

Uses: Large amounts of pumpkin seeds are used to expel worms in children and adults. Oil of pumpkin seed is used externally for burns and scalds.

Quality: Cold and moist in second degree.

Purslane *(Portulacea Oleracea)*
Tibb Name: Rijla, رجلة

Habitat: Cultivated in warm, moist climates.

Properties: Laxative, diuretic, sedative, anthelmintic.

Uses: Constipation, nervous indigestion, to expel worms. Flowers made into a tea are sedative. Leaves are applied as a poultice to cure carbuncles.

Quality: Cold and moist in second degree.

Quince *(Cydonia vulgaris)*
Tibb Name: Safarjal, سفرجل

Habitat: Western Asia.

Properties: Demulcent, protective. Fruit is astringent.

Uses: Chronic diarrhea, hemoptysis. Seeds are soaked in water, and the resulting mucilage is administerd to children for cough and also to stop the falling of hair.

Quality: Cold and dry in third degree.

Radish *(Raphanus sativus)*
Common Names: Radish seed, wild radish, garden radish.

Tibb Name: Fujl, فجـل

Habitat: Mild climates worldwide.

Properties: Diuretic, galactagogue, antispasmodic, astringent, cholagogue.

Uses: Coughs, rheumatism, gallbladder problems, flatulence, diarrhea, headache, insomnia. Not to be used when stomach or bowels are inflamed. Prevents dental caries. Juice used to dissolve biliary calculi.

Quality: Hot and dry in second degree.

Raspberry *(Rubus stringosus)*
Tibb Name: 'Aliq asuo, عليق اسود

Habitat: Europe, North Asia, North America.

Properties: Anti-emetic, astringent, laxative.

Uses: Edible fruit, for preparing syrup, diarrhea, nausea, vomiting, constipation.

Quality: Cold and moist in first degree.

Red (Wild) Clover *(Trifolium pratense)*
Common Name: Red clover blossoms.

Tibb Name: Barsim, برسيم

Habitat: Hejaz, Yemen, Turkey, Europe; naturalized in North America.

Properties: Alterative, deobstruent, sedative, diuretic, expectorant.

Uses: Whooping cough, liver problems, constipation, sluggish appetite, spasmodic cough. Externally: rheumatic or gouty pains; syrupy extract as a treatment for persistent sores and tumors.

Quality: Hot and dry in second degree.

Rhubarb *(Rheum officinale)*
Tibb Name: Rawand, رواند

Habitat: China, Tibet; mountains; cultivated in light, loose, sandy, and rich black soil.

Properties: Aperient, purgative, astringent, stomachic, tonic.

Uses: Diarrhea, hemorrhoids, infant cholera, chronic dysentery, dyspepsia, thread worm.

Quality: Hot and dry in first degree. Some species cold.

Rose *(Rosa damascens)* (species)
Common Name: Red rose.

Tibb Name: Ward, Gulab, كول آب ورد

Habitat: Western Asia, southern Europe; cultivated worldwide.

Properties: Tonic, mild astringent, carminative, aperient, stomachic.

Uses: Gargles, enemas, uterine and other hemorrhages, ulcers of the mouth, ears, anus, inflamed eyes, chapped hands and lips, burns, flavoring vehicle, perfumery; ointment: abrasions, ulcers, frostbite.

Note: More than 100 species of rose are used in medicine.

Quality: Cold and dry in second degree.

Remarks: When using rose petals as a remedy, which is called for in a number of formulas, it is very important that they be organically grown and not from a commercial greenhouse operation which uses many chemicals and pesticides. You may find roses growing wild in most areas of the country, or a neighbor may be able to supply some. Almost all of the herb suppliers sell rose petals, but they are sprayed with toxic chemicals and are intended only for use in potpourri and not for internal consumption.

Safflower *(Carthamus tinctorius)*
Common Names: Safflower; bay saffron.

Tibb Name: Qurtum, قرطم

Habitat: India; cultivated in U.S.A., Europe, etc.

Properties: Diaphoretic, tonic, laxative, purgative, emmenagogue, diuretic.

Uses: Colds, mixed with honey for skin diseases, measles, catarrh, rheumatism.

Quality: Hot and dry in second degree.

* Saffron *(Crocus sativus)*
Common Names: Crocus, saffron.

Tibb Name: Za'faran, زعفران

Habitat: Western Asia, Spain, France.

Properties: Stomachic, emmenagogue, diaphoretic, sedative, aphrodisiac, anodyne, carminative.

Uses: Coughs, whooping cough, stomach gas, colic, insomnia, measles, conjunctivitis.

Quality: Hot and dry in third degree.

Sandalwood *(Santalum album)*
Common Name: White sandalwood.

Tibb Name: Sandal, ﻨﺪﻝ

Habitat: Southern India, East Indian Islands, Malabar, Macassar, Australia; cultivated.

Properties: Astringent, stimulant, diuretic, disinfectant, expectorant, sudorific, heart tonic.

Uses: Heart disease, bronchitis, gonorrhea, chronic and subacute inflammations of mucous membranes, cystitis, chronic diarrhea, perfumery.

Quality: Cold and dry in second degree.

Sarsaparilla *(Smilax officinalis)*
Tibb Name: Oshbah, Sabarina, سبارينا عشبة

Habitat: Tropical Americas, Mexico to Brazil; Andes and Chinqui Mountains; indigenous to U.S.A.; cultivated.

Properties: Alterative, diuretic, diaphoretic, tonic.

Uses: As a blood purifier in scrofula, cutaneous diseases, abscesses, ulcers, gout, rheumatism, venereal diseases.

Quality: Hot and dry in second degree.

Scabious *(Scabiosa succisa)*
Common Name: Devil's bit.

Habitat: Grows wild in open meadows and cornfields of Europe.

Properties: Diaphoretic, demulcent, febrifuge.

Uses: Coughs, fevers, internal inflammations, poisonings, plagues.

Quality: Cold and dry in second degree.

Sebestan *(Capparis sativa; C. spinosa)*
Common Name: Caper plant.

Tibb Name: Qabber, قبّار

Habitat: Deciduous shrub found on the Mediterranean shores.

Properties: Roots: diuretic. Fruit: carminative, sedative.

Uses: Flower buds gathered and preserved in salt and vinegar for use in sauces and salad dressings. Berries and roots in rheumatism and for toothache.

Quality: Hot and dry in second degree.

Senna: *(Cassia angustifolia)*
Tibb Name: Sana makkak

Habitat: East and Central Africa, India.

Properties: Cathartic and cholagogue: the active principle is cathartic acid, an unstable glucoside. Acts on nearly the entire intestinal tract (especially the colon), increasing peristalsis and intestinal secretions, except bile; produces copious yellow stools in four to six hours, with griping and flatulence; does not cause hypercatharsis or constipation. Large doses cause vomiting, but never poison. Even the odor acts as cathartic on susceptible persons.

Uses: To promote menstruation, for skin afflictions, habitual constipation, detoxification, hemorrhoids, anal fissures, fevers. Griping and flatulent qualities are lessened by addition of coriander, peppermint, tamarind, fennel, or Epsom salt.

Quality: Hot and dry in third degree.

Sesame *(Sesamum orientale)*
Tibb Name: Sem sem, سمسم

Habitat: India, Egypt, Africa, cultivated in U.S.A.

Properties: Laxative, demulcent, emollient, nutritious; similar to olive oil, but less agreeable and digestible.

Uses: Hair preparations, liniments; as a cooking oil; in poultice and as oil to allay pain.

Quality: Cold and moist in first degree.

Skunk Cabbage *(Symplocarpus foetidus)*
Common Names: Collard, meadow cabbage, polecat weed.

Habitat: Native American perennial plant found in the swamps of eastern North America.

Properties: Emetic, diuretic, antispasmodic, stimulant, narcotic.

Uses: Asthma, chronic catarrh, rheumatism, chorea, hysteria, dropsy, bronchitis, respiratory ailments.

Quality: Hot and dry in third degree.

Spikenard *(Aralia racemosa)*
Common Names: American spikenard, Indian root, nard.

Habitat: U.S.A.: Georgia to Canada, west to Rocky Mountains.

Properties: Stimulant, diaphoretic, alterative, expectorant.

Uses: Syphilis, chronic rheumatism and cutaneous affections, asthma, coughs, before labor to make childbirth easier; externally in poultice for bruises, sprains, swellings, inflammations.

Quality: Hot and dry in third degree.

Squaw Vine *(Mitchella repens)*
Common Names: Checkerberry, deerberry, squawberry, winter clover.

Habitat: North America.

Properties: Tonic, astringent, diuretic.

Uses: Mainly recommended in a combination of herbs to be taken the last few weeks of pregnancy to make childbirth easier.

Quality: Hot and dry in second degree.

Sumac *(Rhus aromatica)*
Common Names: Dwarf sumac, mountain sumac.

Tibb Name: Sumaq, سُماق

Habitat: Indigenous to North America.

Properties: Astringent, diuretic, emmenagogue, febrifuge, refrigerant, tonic.

Uses: Sore throat, diarrhea, leukorrhea, urinary problems, inflammation of the bladder, gonorrhea. Externally: leaves applied as poultice to relieve symptoms of poison ivy.

Quality: Cold and dry in second degree.

Tamarind *(Tamarindus indica)*
Tibb Name: Tamr-hindi, تمرهندى

Habitat: Evergreen tree growing in tropical regions.

Properties: Anthelmintic, laxative, refrigerant, antipyretic.

Uses: Flowers have beneficial effect in liver diseases. Commonly used in cooking and made into cooling beverage.

Quality: Hot and dry in second degree.

Tamarisk *(Tamarix articulata)*
Tibb Name: Tarfa, طرفاء

Habitat: There are now more than sixty species of Tamarisk trees, an evergreen that grows in extensive woods.

Properties: The gallnut, the nut of the Tamarisk tree, is abrasive; astringent, tonic.

Uses: To check secretions, as a tooth powder to polish teeth, to treat bad breath.

Quality: Cold and dry in third degree.

Turmeric *(Curcurma longa)*
Common Names: Tumeric, turmeric.

Tibb Name: Korkum, كركم

Habitat: South Asia, India, Indian Ocean Islands.

Properties: Stimulant, stomachic, diuretic, salivant, appetizer.

Uses: As a condiment, for jaundice, to prevent tooth caries.

Quality: Hot and dry in third degree.

* Valerian *(Valeriana officinalis)*
Common Names: Valerian root, all-heal, cat's valerian.

Tibb Name: Waleriana, Hashish al-har, والريانا حشيشة اهر

Habitat: Europe, North Asia, in moist and dry localities: naturalized in New England and New York; cultivated.

Properties: Stimulant, anodyne, nervine, antispasmodic, vermifuge; increases heart action and temperature, causing exhilaration, stimulates circulation, secretion and peristalsis of stomach and intestines; it is eliminated by kidneys, bronchial and genito-urinary mucous membranes; if used continuously may produce melancholia, hysteria. Large doses cause nausea, diarrhea, urination, delirium. Oil paralyzes the brain and spine, slows pulse, lowers blood pressure.

Uses: Hysteria, hypochondriasis, hemicrania, nervous cough, whooping cough, diabetes, delirium tremens, typhoid fever, dysmennorrhea, vertigo, epilepsy, convulsions, flatulence, reflex neuralgia, fevers.

Note: Although catnip is ordinarily thought to excite cats, valerian is actually much preferred by felines.

Quality: Hot and dry in third degree.

Violet *(Viola odorata)*
Common Name: Violet flowers.

Tibb Name: Banafsa, بنفسج

Habitat: Europe, North America; cultivated.

Properties: Alterative, expectorant, large doses emetic, cathartic, laxative, sudorific.

Uses: Flowers: bronchial problems, headache, perfumery; root produces emesis; skin diseases, scrofula, syphilis, nephritis.

Quality: Cold and moist in first degree. Some varieties with dark flowers may be hot.

Walnut *(Juglans regia)*
Common Names: Butternut, oil nut, white walnut.

Tibb Name: Juz, جـوز

Habitat: Persia, Himalayas, China; cultivated in Europe.

Properties: Astringent, anthelmintic, cathartic, tonic.

Uses: Decoction of leaves in leukorrhea, meningitis; decoction of leaves, rind, or bark in checking mammary secretions, ulcers, diarrhea, sore mouth, tonsils, uterine hemorrhages, carbuncles, scrofula.

Quality: Hot and dry in second degree.

* Water Lily *(Nymphaea lotus [odorata])*
Common Names: White pond lily, cow cabbage, nenufar, water lily, water cabbage.

Tibb Name: Bashnin, بشنين

Habitat: Aquatic perennial plant commonly found in ponds or slow streams in North America.

Properties: Sedative, soporific, antiaphrodisiac (said to cause sterility), antiseptic, astringent, demulcent.

Uses: Gargle for inflammation of mouth and throat, eyewash, antiseptic vaginal douche; as lotion or poultice, to soothe skin, as relief for skin irritations, wounds, bruises, cuts, etc.

Quality: Cold and moist in second degree.

Watermelon *(Citrullus vulgaris)*
Tibb Name: Tarbuz, تربوز

Habitat: South Asia; cultivated worldwide.

Properties: Seeds are diuretic, tenifuge, anthelmintic.

Uses: Mainly as a cooling food in summertime; seeds used to expel worms.

Quality: Cold and moist in second degree.

Wild Rue *(Peganum harmala)*
Common Name: Rue.

Tibb Name: Harmal, حرمل

Habitat: Persia, Arabia, Syria, North Africa, southern Europe.

Properties: Seeds are antispasmodic, narcotic, hypnotic, anodyne, emetic, emmenagogue, stimulant, alterative, aphrodisiac, lactagogue, and anthelmintic.

Uses: Insanity, epilepsy, ointment for baldness, hemorrhoids, intermittent fevers, colic, retention of urine, hiccup, hysteria, rheumatism, calculi of ureter, gallstones, jaundice, dysmenorrhea, neuralgia, lumbago. Powdered seeds are a particularly powerful expeller of tapeworms. Seeds are burned immediately after childbirth, as the smoke is believed to dispel malevolent and distressing psychic forces.

Quality: Cold and dry in second degree.

* Wormwood *(Artemisia absinthium)*
Tibb Name: Shih, شیح

Habitat: Europe, North Asia, North Africa.

Properties: Tonic, stomachic, stimulant, febrifuge, anthelmintic, emmenagogue.

Uses: Atonic dyspepsia, worms, stimulant in cerebral exhaustion, locally as anesthetic for rheumatism, neuralgia.

Quality: Cold and dry in third degree.

Yerba Santa *(Eriodictyon californicum)*

Common Names: Eriodityon, yerba santa, bear's weed, mountain balm.

Habitat: California, northern Mexico; dry hills, mountains.

Properties: Stimulant, expectorant, bitter tonic, antispasmodic, febrifuge.

Uses: Colds, chronic laryngitis, bronchitis, lung problems, asthma. Externally: poultice for bruises, sprains, wounds and insect bites. Leaves are smoked or chewed as cure for asthma.

Quality: Cold and moist in second degree.

TABLE OF WEIGHTS AND MEASURES

In the Formulary, any measures given in drams can be measured approximately as one level teaspoon of dried herb. The liquid measure of one dram is $\frac{1}{8}$ ounce.

U.S.

1 tablespoon = 3 teaspoons
1 ounce = 2 tablespoons
1 cup = 8 fluid ounces
1 pint = 2 cups
1 quart = 2 pints
1 gallon = 4 quarts

Metric

1 centiliter = 0.34 fluid ounces
1 deciliter = 3.38 fluid ounces
1 liter = 1.06 quarts
10 liters = 2.64 gallons

Apothecary

1 minim = 0.06 mililiters
1 fluid dram = 60 minims
 (approximately 1 teaspoon)
1 fluid dram = $\frac{1}{8}$ fluid ounce

Avoirdupois

1 grain = 0.06 grams
1 dram = 1.77 grams
1 ounce = 16 drams
1 pound = 12 ounces

Household Measures

Less than 1 teaspoon = a few grains
1 teaspoon = 1 dram
1 dessert spoon = 2 drams
1 tablespoon = 4 drams
1 cup = 7 ounces
1 fruit jar = 1 pint

APPENDIX II
THERAPEUTIC ACTION
OF BOTANICALS

The actions of various herbs are given under the heading of "Properties" in the Materia Medica section. The following list defines and explains the pharmacological terms used.

Property	Therapeutic Action
Abortifacient	Causes abortion
Alkali	Stimulates alkali acid and checks alkaline secretions
Alterative	Alters morbid conditions; furthers metabolism
Anaphrodisiac	Lessens sexual appetite
Anesthetic	Causes loss of sense of touch or feeling
Anodyne	Relieves pain
Anthelmintic	Kills or expels intestinal worms
Antiemetic	Lessens nausea and vomiting
Antihydrotic	Checks perspiration
Antilithic	Prevents formation of urinary stones
Antiperiodic	Prevents or modifies fevers
Antiphlogistic	Reduces inflammation of membranes
Antiscorbutic	Corrects scurvy
Antiseptic	Prevents decay or putrefaction
Antispasmodic	See stimulant
Antizymotic	Arrests fermentation
Aperient	Acts as gentle purgative
Aphrodisiac	Stimulates sexual appetite
Aromatic	See carminative
Astringent	Contracts muscular fiber by irritation; arrests discharges
Bitter	Increases tone of gastrointestinal tissue
Cardiac Depressant	Lessens force and frequency of heart action
Cardiac Stimulant	Slows and strengthens contractions of heart
Carminative	Expels gases from stomach and intestines
Cathartic	Hastens intestinal evacuations
Caustic	See escharotic
Cephalic	Acts on head
Cerebral Depressant	See sedative
Cerebral Excitant	See stimulant
Cholagogue	Promotes discharge of bile

Ciliary Excitant	Promotes bronchial mucus elimination
Cordial	Acts as strong aromatic
Demulcent	Soothes skin and membranes
Dental Anodyne	Stems pain of caries
Deobstruent	Removes obstructions
Diaphoretic	Increases perspiration
Disinfectant	Destroys infection
Diuretic	Increases kidney secretions
Drastic	Acts as violent purgative
Ecbolic	Causes abortion
Emetic	Causes vomiting
Emmenagogue	Restores menstrual function
Emollient	Softens and relaxes skin
Epispastic	See vesicant
Errhine	Increases nasal secretion
Escharotic	Destroys tissue, skin
Expectorant	Promotes mucus membrane secretions
Febrifuge	See antiperiodics
Galactagogue	Increases flow of breast milk
Germicide	See parasiticide
Hemostatic	See styptic
Hypnotic	Causes sleep
Irritant	Causes activity on skin surface
Lactagogue	See galactagogue
Laxative	See aperient
Lithotropic	Dissolves urinary stones
Motor Depressant	Lowers activity of motor functions and ultimately paralyzes
Motor Excitant	Increases motor activities and reflex excitability
Mydriatic	Dilates pupil
Myotic	Contracts pupil
Narcotic	Produces stupor or unconsciousness
Nervine	Reduces nervous excitement
Oxytocic	See ecbolic
Parasiticide	Kills parasites
Pectoral	Is good for diseases of chest
Protective	Protects injured parts
Pulmonary Sedative	Lessens irritability of respiratory nerves
Purgative	Activates peristalsis
Pustulant	Causes pustules
Refrigerant	Allays thirst; cools
Resolvent	Promotes resolution of disease
Respiratory Depressant	Lowers function of respiratory center

Respiratory Stumulant	Increases function of respiratory center
Restorative	Restores strength and vitality
Rubefacient	Causes temporary skin redness
Sedative	Lessens higher brain functions but initially excites
Sialagogue	Promotes secretion of saliva
Soporific	Produces deep sleep
Spinant	See motor excitant
Sternutatory	Causes sneezing
Stimulant	Increases functional activity of brain
Stomachic	Acts as gastric stimulant
Styptic	Arrests hemorrhage
Sudorific	Causes profuse perspiration
Tenifuge	Expels tapeworms
Tonic	Produces and restores normal tissue tone
Vermifuge	Expels intestinal worms
Vesicant	Causes inflammation of skin, blisters
Vulnerary	Promotes healing of wounds

DIGESTION TIME OF FOODS*

1 ¼ Hours
parsley

1 ½ Hours
lemon
Irish moss

1 ¾ Hours
avocado
grapes
mango
olive, ripe
raspberry

2 Hours
blueberry
sweet cherry
grapefruit
orange
raisin
coconut milk
artichoke
beet greens
garlic
potato
tomato
brown rice

2 ¼ Hours
fig, fresh
pear, fresh
pineapple
strawberry
asparagus
carrot
cauliflower
lettuce: cos, loose leaf,
   iceberg

2 ½ Hours
blackberry
date
fig, dried
gooseberry
peach, fresh
almond
dandelion greens
leek
mushroom
okra
lima bean
white rice
basmati rice

2 ¾ Hours
apple, fresh
apricot, fresh
currant
peach, dried
plum
watermelon
chestnut
coconut meat, fresh
pecan
pignolia
beet
summer squash
wheat bran

3 Hours
lime
prune, dried
filbert nut
walnut
broccoli
cabbage
Swiss chard
sweet corn
endive (escarole)
kohlrabi
rhubarb
spinach
winter squash
white bean
lentil
soybean
wheat germ

*Source: Ford Heritage, *Composition and Facts about Foods* (Mokelumne Hill, Calif.: Health Research, 1971).

3 ¼ Hours
cranberry
cantaloupe
casaba melon
honeydew melon
olive oil
pomegranate
cashew nut
coconut meat, dried
celery
cucumber
onion
sweet green pepper
pumpkin
radish
rutabaga
sweet potato
turnip greens
watercress
snap bean
peas, fresh
peanut
millet

3 ½ Hours
safflower oil
sesame seed oil
eggplant
mustard greens
peas, dried
soybean oil
rye

3 ¾ Hours
persimmon
quince
red cabbage
barley
wheat

4 Hours
Brussels sprouts
horseradish
turnip

SOURCES OF UNANI TIBB HERBS

Local health food and herbs stores may have some of the herbs and spices mentioned in this book. If you have difficulty locating what you want, the Unani spices and herbs may be obtained by mail order from the following sources. You should be as specific as possible when ordering. Be prepared to send prepayment or make cash payment for COD orders.

The Chishti Order's Institute of Unani Medicine, founded in 1975 to promote Unani traditional healing, specializes in books, booklets, audio and video cassettes, and tools for the Unani healer. They also offer various workshops and seminars, and a correspondence course for training as a Unani practitioner. Write to:

The Institute of Unani Medicine
P.O. Box 820
Oxford, NY 13830
(607) 843-6011

Attar Bazaar carries an extensive line of the best quality East Indian natural attar perfume oils. They offer a correspondence course in Spiritual Aromatherapy, plus practitioner kits and tools.

Attar Bazaar
P.O. Box 7249
Endicott, NY 13761
(800) 344-7172

Spice and Sweet Mahal is an excellent source for Unani cooking supplies such as chapati flour, basmati rice, garam masala, chili peppers, and bulk spices, as well as frying pans and other utensils.

Spice and Sweet Mahal
135 Lexington Avenue
New York, NY 10016
(212) 683-0900

Meadowsweet Herbal Apothecary carries one of the most complete lines of medicinal botanicals in the U.S. They strive to carry as many of the Unani herbs mentioned in this book as possible.

Meadowsweet Herbal Apothecary
77 East 4th Street
New York, NY 10003
(212) 254-2870

The following sources also carry extensive lines of herbs and spices.

Aphrodisia	Frontier Cooperative	Penn Herb
282 Bleeker Street	Box 299	603 North Second
Brooklyn, NY 10014	Norway, IA 52318	Philadelphia, PA 19123
(212) 989-6440	(319) 227-7991	(215) 925-3336

Bibliography

Children and Natural Childbirth

Benson, Ralph C. *Handbook of Obstetrics and Gynecology*. Los Altos, Calif.: Lange Medical Publications, 1974.

Eiger, Marvin, and Sally Olds, *The Complete Book of Breastfeeding*. New York: Bantam Books, 1972.

Elolesser, Leo; Edith Galt; and Isabel Hemingway. *Pregnancy, Childbirth and the Newborn: A Manual for Rural Midwives*. Ninos Heroes, Mexico: Inter-American Indian Institute, 1973.

Khan, Hazrat Inayat. *The Sufi Message of Hazrat Inayat Khan*, Vol. III. London: Barrie & Jenkins, 1971.

Myles, Margaret. *Textbook for Midwives*. New York: Longmans, *1974*.

Ostrander, Sheila, and Lynn Schroeder. *Natural Birth Control*. New York: Bantam Books, 1973.

Sousa, Marion. *Childbirth at Home*. New York: Bantam Books, 1976.

Diets and Fasting

Al-Ghazzali. *The Mysteries of Fasting*. Lahore: Ashraf Press, 1968.

Bragg, Paul. *The Miracle of Fasting*. Santa Ana, Calif.: Health Science, n.d.

Ehret, Arnold, *Mucusless Diet Healing System*. Beaumont, Calif.: Ehret Publishing Company, 1922.

Howell, Edward, M.D. *Enzyme Nutrition: The Food Enzyme Concept*. Wayne, N.J.: Avery, 1985.

McKellar, Doris. *Afghan Cookery*. Kabul: Afghan Books, 1972.

New Age Vegetarian Cookbook, 4th ed. Oceanside, Calif.: Rosicrucian Fellowship, 1973.

Newman, Laura. *Make Your Juicer Your Drug Store*. New York: Benedict Lust Publications, 1972.

Robertson, Laurel; Carol Flinders; and Bronwen Godfrey. *Laurel's Kitchen: A Handbook for Vegetarian Cookery and Nutrition*. Berkeley: Nilgiri Press, 1977.

Torre, Teofilo de la, N.D., O.D. (ed.). *Edena* v 5-8, nos. 17-32. Santa Ana, Costa Rica: 1955-1958.

Walker, N. W. *Raw Vegetable Juices*. New York: Pyramid Books, 1970.

Yacoubi, Ahmed. *Alchemist's Cookbook: Moroccan Scientific Cuisine*. Tucson: Omen Press, 1972.

Esoteric Healing

Bailey, Alice A. *Esoteric Healing,* vol. IV. New York: Lucis Publishing Company, 1953.

Dehellvi, Hazrat Maulana Ahmad Saeed. *Prophetic Medical Sciences (The Savior).* Delhi: Arshad Saeed, 1977.

Dickinson, Martin (ed.). *The Sufi Messenger Quarterly.* Geneva: International Headquarters of the Sufi Movement, July 1970.

Gaines, Thomas. *Vitalic Breathing: The Miracle Air Discovery.* Hollywood, Calif.: Concord Press, 1947.

Heindel, Max. *Occult Principles of Health and Healing.* Oceanside, Calif.: Rosicrucian Fellowship, 1938.

Khan, Hazrat Inayat. *The Sufi Message of Hazrat Inayat Khan,* vol. IV. London: Barrie & Jenkins, 1961.

Healing in Afghanistan

Al-Faruqi, Ismail R., Ph.D. "Moral Values in Medicine and Science." *Journal of the IMA* 8, nos. 1-2. Pittsburgh, March-Sept. 1977.

Abdullah, Mawlawi, and Maulawi Ala'addin (eds.). *Mizan-ul-Tebb* (in Persian). Bombay: Haidari Press, n.d.

Akhgar, Najiba. "Popular Medical Treatments" (in Persian). *Folklore Magazine* 3, no. 1 (June-July 1975). Kabul: Ministry of Information and Culture.

Ali, Mohammed. *The Afghans.* Kabul: Prof. Mohammed Ali, 1969.

Amin, Hamidullah. *Agricultural Geography of Afghanistan* (in Persian). Kabul: Faculty of Letters and Humanities, 1974.

Blumhagen, Rex V., M.D., and Jeanne Blumhagen, M.D. *Family Health Care: A Rural Health Care Delivery Scheme.* Wheaton, Ill.: Medical Assistance Programs, 1974.

Colvin, Diana. "Folk Medicine in Afghanistan." *Folklore Magazine* 1, nos. 2, 3 (Aug-Nov. 1973). Kabul: Ministry of Information and Culture.

Dupree, Louis. *Afghanistan.* Princeton: Princeton University Press, 1974.

Dupree, Nancy Hatch. *An Historical Guide to Afghanistan.* Kabal: Afghan Tourist Organization, 1971.

el-Salakawy, Ahmad A. *Spotlights on Medical Terminology: The Human Body Systems* (in Arabic). 1972.

_____ .*Fundamentals of Medical Terminology* (in Arabic). Dar Al Maaref, Cairo, Egypt, 1968.

Elgood, Cyril (trans.). *Tibb-ul-Nabbi or Medicine of the Prophet, Being a Translation of Two Works of the Same Name.* Vol. I: *The Tibb-Ul-Nabbi of Al-Suyuti.* Vol. II: *The Tibb-Ul-Nabbi of Mahmud Bin Mohamed Al-Chaghhayni, Together with Introduction, Notes & Glossary.* N.A.

Eltorai, I., M.D. "Avicenna's View on Cancer from His Canon." *American Journal of Chinese Medicine* 7 no. 3, pp. 276-284. Institute for Advanced Research in Asian Science and Medicine, 1979.

Elkadi, Ahmad, M.D. "Professional Ethics: Ethics in the Medical Profession." *Journal of IMA* 7, no. 2. Pittsburgh, Sept. 1976.

Faculty of Medicine and Pharmacy. *Medical Education in Afghanistan.* Kabul: University of Kabul, 1965.

Gobar, Dr. A. H. "Narcotic Drugs Abuse Problem in Afghanistan" (in Persian). *Afghan Medical Journal* 19, no. 1-2 (March 1975). Kabul.

Gruner, O. Cameron, M.D. *A Treatise on The Canon of Medicine of Avicenna, Incorporating a Translation of the First Book.* New York: Augustus M. Kelley, 1970.

Hunte, Pam; Mahbouba Safi; Anne Macey; and Graham Kerr. *Indigenous Fertility Regulation Methods in Afghanistan.* Kabul: Ministry of Public Health, 1975.

Ibn Sina. *Qamus al-qanun fi'l tibb.* New Delhi: Idarah ta'rikh al-tibb wa'l-tahqiq al-tibbi, 1967.

Kerr, Graham, B.; Anne Macey; Pam Hunte; Hassan Kamiab; and Mahbouba Safi. *Afghan Family Guidance Clients and Their Husbands Compared with Non-Client Neighbors and Their Husbands.* Kabul: Ministry of Public Health, 1975.

Kahn, Sayed Mohammad Husain. *Qarabadin-e Kabir* (in Persian). Bombay: Munshi Nool, publisher, n.d.

Kumorek, Martin. *Afghanistan: A Cross Cultural View.* Kabul: Peace Corps, 1976.

Levey, Martin, and Al-Khaledy. *The Medical Formulary of Al-Samarqandi and the Relation of Early Arabic Simples to Those Found in the Indigenous Medicine of the Near East and India.* Philadelphia: University of Pennsylvania Press, 1967.

Macey, Anne; Pam Hunte; and Mahbouba Safi. *The Dai: A Traditional Birth Attendant in Afghanistan.* Kabul: Ministry of Public Health, 1975.

Macey, Anne; Pam Hunte; and Hassan Kamiab. *Indigenous Health Practitioners In Afghanistan.* Kabul: Ministry of Public Health, 1975.

Mohebi, Farokhsha. "Folk Medicine" (in Persian). *Folklore Magazine* 3, no. 1 (June-July 1975). Kabul: Ministry of Information and Culture.

Patcha, Lal. "Zadrans' Popular Medicine" (in Persian). *Folklore Magazine* 5, no. 1 (June-July 1977). Kabul: Ministry of Information and Culture.

Rashid, Abdul; Mohammad Azam; Ahmad Jan; and Mohammad Ebrahim. *Rahat-ul-Atfal* (in Persian). Kabul: Government Printing House, Reign of Habibullah.
Kabul: Ministry of Information and Culture.

Sameii, Dr. B. A. "Hemp and Alcohol" (in Persian). *Afghan Medical Journal* 19, no. 1-2 (March 1975). Kabul.

Sekandar, Dr. Nasar Mohammad. *A Field Survey of Health Needs, Practices and Resources in Rural Afghanistan.* Cambridge, Mass.: Management Sciences for Health, 1975.

Stone, Russell A.; Saxon Graham; and Graham B. Kerr. *Afghan Pharmacists: Their Knowledge of and Attitude toward Family Guidance.* Kabul: Ministry of Public Health, 1973.

Tabibi, Dr. Abdul H. *Sir-i Tassawf-i Afghanistan* (in Persian). Kabul: Ministry of Information and Culture, 1977.

Herbalogy

Abdul Wahid, Hakim, and Dr. H. H. Siddiqui. *A Survey of Drugs, with Particular Reference to the Arab (Unani) Medicine and Ayurveda,* 2nd. ed. Delhi: Institute of the History of Medicine and Medical Research, 1961.

Bach, Edward, *The Twelve Healers and Other Remedies.* London: C. W. Daniel, 1975.

Christopher, Dr. John Raymond. *School of Natural Healing,* Vols. 1 and II. Provo, Utah: Christopher Distributing, 1975.

Committe of Manufacturers of Tibbi Medicine. *Medicinal Plants.* Karachi: Hamdard Foundation Press, 1983.

Culpeper, Nicholas. *Culpeper's Complete Herbal.* London: W. Foulsham & Co., Ltd, 1651

Dastur, J. F. *Medicinal Plants of India and Pakistan.* Bombay: D. B. Taraporevala Sons, n.d.

Edinger, Philip (ed.). *How to Grow Herbs: A Sunset Book.* Menlo Park, Calif.: Lane Books, 1974.

Fazal, Dr. Hakima Ummul, and Hakim M. A. Razzack. *A Hand Book of Common Remedies in Unani System of Medicine.* New Delhi: Central Council for Research in Indian Medicine and Homeopathy, 1976.

Gonzales, Dr. Pedro Alvarez. *Yerbas Medicinales: Como Curarse con Plantas.* University of Mexico, Mexico City, Mexico, n.d.

Grieve, M. *A Modern Herbal,* Vols. I and II. New York: Dover Publications, 1971.

Harper-Shove, Lt.-Col. F. *Prescriber and Clinical Repertory of Medicinal Herbs.* Bradford, England: Health Science Press, 1952.

Heffern, Richard. *The Herb Buyer's Guide.* New York: Pyramid Books, 1975.

Herb Society of America. *The Herbalist.* Boston: 1974.

Hutchens, Alma R. *Indian Herbalogy of North America.* Ontario: Merco, 1974.

Kirk, Donald R. *Wild Edible Plants of the Western United States.* Healdsburg, Calif.: Naturegraph Publishers, 1975.

Kloss, Jethro. *Back to Eden.* New York: Lancer Books, 1971.

Meyer, Joseph E., and Clarence Meyer. *The Herbalist.,* n.d.

Nature's Herb Company. *Herbs and Spices for Home Use.* San Francisco, n.d.

Pelt, J.M., and Younos, J. C., "Plantes medicinales et drogues de L'Afghanistan." Extract from *Bulletin de la Societe de Pharmacie de Nancy*, no. 66 (September 1965).

Powell, Eric F. *The Modern Botanic Prescriber*. London: L. N. Fowler & Co., 1971.

Royal, Penny C. *Herbally Yours*. Provo, Utah: Bi-World Publishers, 1976.

Sherman, Ingrid, Ph.D., Pss.D., N.D., D.O. (GB). *Natural Remedies for Better Health*. Healdsburg, Calif.: Naturegraph Publishers, 1970.

Shook, Dr. Edward E., N.D., D.C. *Advanced Treatise on Herbology*. Mokelumne Hill, Calif.: Health Research, 1974.

Sweet, Muriel. *Common Edible and Useful Plants of the West*. Healdsburg, Calif.: Naturegraph Company, 1962.

Thomson, Samuel, *Guide to Health; or Botanic Family Physician*. Boston: J. Q. Adams, 1835.

History and Philosophy of Natural Medicine

Al-Ghazzali. *The Mysteries of Purity*. Lahore: Ashraf Press, 1970.

Bach, Edward. *Heal Thyself: An Explanation of the Real Cause and Cure of Disease*. London: C. W. Daniel, 1974.

Brock, J. Arthur (trans.). *Greek Medicine, Being Extracts Illustrative of Medical Writers from Hippocrates to Galen*. New York: E. P. Dutton, 1972.

Browne, E. G. *Arabian Medicine*. Cambridge: Cambridge University Press, 1962.

Haggard, Howard W., M.D. *Mystery, Magic and Medicine*. New York: Doubleday, Doran, 1933.

Hall, Manly P. *Healing: The Divine Art*. Los Angeles: Philosophical Research Society, 1971.

Khaldun, Ibn. *The Muquaddimah: An Introduction to History*. Trans. Franz Rosenthal. Princeton: Princeton University Press, 1970.

Khusrau, Amir. *Differentiation in the Fundamental and the Subsidiary Principles of Music*. Hyderabad Sind, Pakistan: Sind University Press, 1975.

Leslie, Charles. *Asian Medical Systems*. Berkeley: University of California Press, 1976.

Lindlahr, Henry, M.D. *Philosophy of Natural Therapeutics*, Vol. I. Chicago: Lindlahr Publishing Co., 1922.

Mysticism

Ali, Sufi Abu Anees Muhammad Barkat. *Maksboofat-e-manazal-e-ehsan*, vols. 1 & 2. Trans. Muhammad Iqbal. Dar-ul-Ehsan, Faisalabad, Pakistan: Dar-ul-Ehsan Publications, 1978.

Begg, W. D. *The Big Five of India in Sufism*. Ajmer, India: W. D. Begg, 1972.

———. *The Holy Biography of Hazrat Khwaja Muinuddin Chishti*. Tucson: Chishti Sufi Mission of America, 1977.

Chisti, H. Moinuddin. *The Book of Sufi Healing.* New York: Inner Traditions International, 1985.

de Jong-Keesing, Elisabeth. *Inayat Answers.* London: Fine Books Oriental, 1977.

Karim, Alhaj Maulana Fazlul. *Gazzqali's Ihya ulum-id-din, or The Revival of Religious Sciences, The Book of Constructive Virtues,* Part I. Dacca: F. K. Islam Mission Trust, 1971.

Nicholson, R. A. (trans.). *Kashf Al-Mahjub of Al-Hujwiri.* London: Luzac & Co., 1970.

Schimmel, Annemarie. *Mystical Dimensions of Islam.* Chapel Hill: University of North Carolina Press, 1976.

Smith, Margaret. *Rabi'a, The Mystic, A.D. 717-801, and Her Fellow Saints in Islam.* San Francisco: The Rainbow Bridge, 1977.

Sprenger, Aloys, M.D. *Abdu-R-Razzaq's Dictionary of the Technical Terms of the Sufis.* Lahore: Zulfiqar Ahmad, 1974.

Suhrawardi, Shaikh Shahab-Ud-Din 'Umar B. Muhammad. *The 'Awarif-ul-Ma'arif.* Lahore: Ashraf Press, 1973.

Valiuddin, Dr. Mir. *Contemplative Disciplines in Sufism.* London: East-West Publications, 1980.

Naturopathy, Naprapathy, Homeopathy, and Chiropractic

Airola, Paavo O. *Health Secrets from Europe.* New York: Arco Publishing Co., 1970.

_____. *How to Get Well.* Phoenix: Health Plus, 1976.

Biron, W. A.; B. F. Wells; and R. H. Houser. *Chiropractic Principles and Technic.* Chicago: National College of Chiropractic, 1939.

Garten, M. O. *The Health Secrets of a Naturopathic Doctor.* New York: Lancer Books, 1967.

Jensen, Bernard. *The Joy of Living and How to Attain It.* Solana Beach, Calif.: Bernard Jensen Products, 1970.

_____. *The Science and Practice of Iridology.* Escondido, Calif.: Bernard Jensen, 1974.

Naprapathic Principles. Chicago: Chicago College of Naprapathy, 1942.

Pawlikowski, Timothy (ed.). *The Digest of Naprapathy/Journal of the A.T.X. Naprapathic Fraternity.* Chicago: June 1977.

Perry, Edward L., M.D. *Luyties Homeopathic Practice.* St. Louis: Formur, 1976.

Smith, Oakley. *Naprapathic Technique.* Chicago: Chicago College of Naprapathy, 1933.

Thomson, Robert, N. D. *Natural Medicine.* New York: McGraw-Hill Book Co., 1978.

_____. *The Grosset Encyclopedia of Natural Medicine.* New York: Grosset & Dunlap, 1980.

_____ . *A Handbook of Common Herbal Remedies.* Orem, Utah: BiWorld Publishers, 1981.

_____ . "Application of Tibb-ul-Nabbi to Modern Medical Practice." *Journal of the Islamic Medical Association* 2, nos. 1 & 2 (April 1980).

_____ . "Medicines for The Soul." Unpublished manuscript.

Thomson, William. "Rice, The Superstar of Grains," *East West Journal* 14, no. 4 (April 1984).

Walther, David S. *Applied Kinesiology.* Pueblo: Systems DC, 1976.

Washington State Naturopathic Association. "The Reader's Health Digest," n.d.

Wendel, Paul. *Diseases of the Stomach and Intestines Naturopathic.* Brooklyn: Dr. Paul Wendel, n.d.

_____ . *Standardized Naturopathy.* Brooklyn: Dr. Paul Wendel, 1951.

Nutrition

Beiler, Henry G., M.D. *Food Is Your Best Medicine.* London: Neville Spearman, 1968.

Borsook, Henry, M.D. *Vitamins: What They Are and How They Can Benefit You.* New York: Pyramid Books, 1971.

Deal, Sheldon C. *New Life through Nutrition.* Tucson: New Life Publishing, 1974.

Heritage, Ford. *Composition and Facts about Foods and Their Relationship to the Human Body.* Mokelumne Hill, Calif.: Health Research, 1971.

Lee Foundation for Nutritional Research. *Portfolio of Reprints for the Doctor.* Milwaukee: Lee Foundation for Nutritional Research, 1974.

Snyder, Arthur W. *Foods That Preserve the Alkaline Reserve.* Los Angeles: Hansen's, n.d.

Stebbing, Lionel (ed.). *Honey as Healer.* Sussex, England: Emerson Press, 1975.

Pharmacology

History of Pharmacy. New York: Parke, Davis & Company, n.d.

Huff, Barbara (ed.). *Physician's Desk Reference,* 30th ed. Oradell, N.J.: Medical Economics Company, 1976.

"Instructions to Laboratory Users," N.R. Laboratory. Chicago: Uro-Biochemical Research, 1976.

Weil, Andrew, M.D. *The Natural Mind.* Boston: Houghton Mifflin, 1972.

Wright, Harold N., and Mildred Montag. *A Textbook of Materia Medica Pharmacology and Therapeutics.* Philadelphia: W. B. Saunders, 1945.

Reference Works

Beaurecueil, S. de Laugier, O.P. *Manuscrits d'Afghanistan.* Le Caire, France: Imprimerie de L'Institut Francais d'Archeologie Orientale, 1964.

Chen, Philip S. *Chemistry: Inorganic, Organic, and Biological.* New York: Barnes & Noble, 1968.

Compact Edition of the Oxford English Dictionary, Vols. I & II. Oxford: Oxford University Press, 1971.

DeGowin, Richard L., and Elmer L. DeGowin. *Bedside Diagnostic Examination.* New York: Macmillan, 1969.

Dunmire, John R. (ed.). *Sunset Western Garden Book.* Menlo Park, Calif.: Lane Magazine and Book Company, 1973.

Elias, Elias A. *Elias' Pocket Dictionary: English-Arabic.* Cairo: Elias' Modern Press, n.d.

Frohse, Franz, Max Brodel, and Leon Schlossberg. *Atlas of Human Anatomy.* New York: Barnes & Noble, 1970.

Gray, Henry, F.R.S. *Anatomy, Descriptive and Surgical.* Philadelphia: Running Press, 1974.

Healing Canadian Whole Earth Almanac 2, no. 3. (Fall). Toronto, Canadian Whole Earth Research Foundation, 1971.

Kamal, Dr. Hassan. *Encyclopedia of Islamic Medicine.* Cairo: General Egyptian Book Organization, 1975.

Khan, Dr. Muhammad Muhsin Khan (trans.). *Sahih al-bukhari,* vols. 1-12. Al-Medina Al-Munaurwara, Saudi Arabia: Islamic University, 1974, 1976 (revised).

Law, Donald. *A Guide to Alternative Medicine.* New York: Doubleday, 1976.

The Merck Manual of Diagnosis and Therapy, 14th ed. Rahway, N.J.: Merck Sharp & Dohme Research Laboratories, 1982.

Park Seed Flowers and Vegetables, 1977. Greenwood, N.C.: 1977.

Popenoe, Cris. *Wellness.* Washington, D.C.: Yes! Inc., 1977.

Rodale, Robert (ed.). *The Encyclopedia of Organic Gardening.* Emmaus, Pa.: Rodale Books, 1971.

Steen, Edwin B., and Ashley Montagu. *Anatomy and Physiology,* Vols. I and II. New York: Barnes & Noble, 1959.

Steingass, F. *Persian-English Dictionary.* London: Routledge & Kegan Paul, 1963.

Wilson, John L. *Handbook of Surgery,* 4th ed. Los Altos, Calif.: Lange Medical Publications, 1969.

Windholz, Martha (ed.). *The Merck Index: An Encyclopedia of Chemicals and Drugs,* 9th ed. Rahway, N.J.: Merck & Co., 1976.

Religious and Divine Healing

Ali, A. Yusuf. *The Meaning of the Illustrious Qur'an.* Lahore: Ashraf Press, 1967.

Fox, Emmet. *The Golden Key* (pamphlet).

Gibbings, Cecil. *Divine Healing.* The Hague: East-West Publications, 1976.

Holy Bible. Cambridge: Cambridge University Press, n.d.

The Medical Group, Theosophical Research Center, London. *The Mystery of Healing.* Wheaton, Ill.: The Theosophical Publishing House, 1968.

Osborn, T. L. *Healing the Sick.* Tulsa: OSFO Publications, 1959.

Szekely, Edmond Bordeaux. *The Essene Science of Life: According to the Essene Gospel of Peace.* San Diego: Academy Books, 1975.

Zikria, Faiz A. (ed.). *Spiritual Dimension: Islam Ideas and Philosophy*, Vol. I. Squirrel Hill, Pa.: Zikria Bros., 1976.

Traditional Eastern Medicine

Abdul Hameed, Hakim. *Avicenna's Tract on Cardiac Drugs and Essays on Arab Cardiotherapy.* Karachi: Hamdard Foundation Press, 1983.

Al-Ghazzali. *The Alchemy of Happiness.* Lahore: Ashraf Press, 1964.

A Barefoot Doctor's Manual (The American Translation of the Official Chinese Paramedical Manual). Philadelphia: Running Press, 1977.

Garde, R. K., M.D. *Ayurveda for Health and Long Life.* Bombay: D. B. Taraporevala Sons & Co., 1975.

Gohlman, William E. *The Life of Ibn Sina.* New York: State University of New York Press, 1974.

Ibn Ishaq, Hunayn. *Questions on Medicine for Scholars.* Cairo: Al-Ahram Center for Scientific Translations, 1980.

Khan, Hazrat Inayat. *Healing.* Tuscon: Ikhwan Press, 1975.

Moss, Louis, M.D. *Acupuncture and You.* New York: Dell, 1972.

Muramoto, Naboru. *Healing Ourselves.* New York: Swan House, 1973.

Quinn, Joseph R. (ed.). *Medicine and Public Health in the People's Republic of China.* Bethesda, Md.: Geographic Health Studies, NIH, U.S. Dept. of HEW, 1973.

Said, Hakim Mohammad. *Personalities Noble, Glimpses of Renowned Scientists and Thinkers of the Muslim Era.* Karachi: Hamdard Foundation Pakistan, 1983.

_____ . *Traditional Greco-Arabic and Modern Western Medicine: Conflict or Symbiosis.* Karachi: Hamdard Academy, n.d.

_____ . *Greco-Arab Concepts on Cardiovascular Diseases.* Karachi: Hamdard Foundation Press, 1983.

Veith, Ilza. *The Yellow Emperor's Classic of Internal Medicine.* Berkeley: University of California Press, 1973.

Unorthodox Therapies

Benjamin, Harry. *Better Sight without Glasses.* London: Health for All Publishing Company, 1929.

Brown, Arlin J. *March of Truth on Cancer,* 7th ed. Fort Belvoir, Va.: Arlin J. Brown Information Center, 1971.

Gerson, Max, M.D. *A Cancer Therapy: Results of Fifty Cases.* Del Mar, Calif.: Totality Books, 1975.

Griffin, Edward G. *World without Cancer, Parts I and II.* Westlake Village, Calif.: American Media, 1974.

Heline, Corinne. *Healing and Regeneration through Music.* Oceanside, Calif.: New Age Press, 1965.

_____ . *Healing and Regeneration through Color.* Oceanside, Calif.: New Age Press, 1967.

Hendren, Julie S. (publisher). *Newsreal Series,* no. 4, August 1977.

Kelley, William Donald. *One Answer to Cancer: An Ecological Approach to the Successful Treatment of Malignancy.* Grapevine, Calif.: Kelley Research Foundation, 1969.

Richardson, John, M.D., and Patricia Griffin, R.N. *Laetrile Case Histories: The Richardson Cancer Clinic Experience.* Westlake Village, Calif.: American Media, 1977.

Western Medicine

Goetz, John T. (ed). *Advanced First Aid and Emergency Care* (The American National Red Cross). New York: Doubleday, 1973.

Gould, George M., and Walter L. Pyle. *Anomalies and Curiosities of Medicine.* New York: Sydenham, 1937.

_____ . *Pocket Cyclopedia of Medicine and Surgery.* Philadelphia: Blakiston, 1926.

Vogel, Virgil J. *American Indian Medicine.* New York: Ballantine, 1973.

Index